HERBS, VITAMINS, & SUPPLEMENTS for WELLNESS & BEAUTY

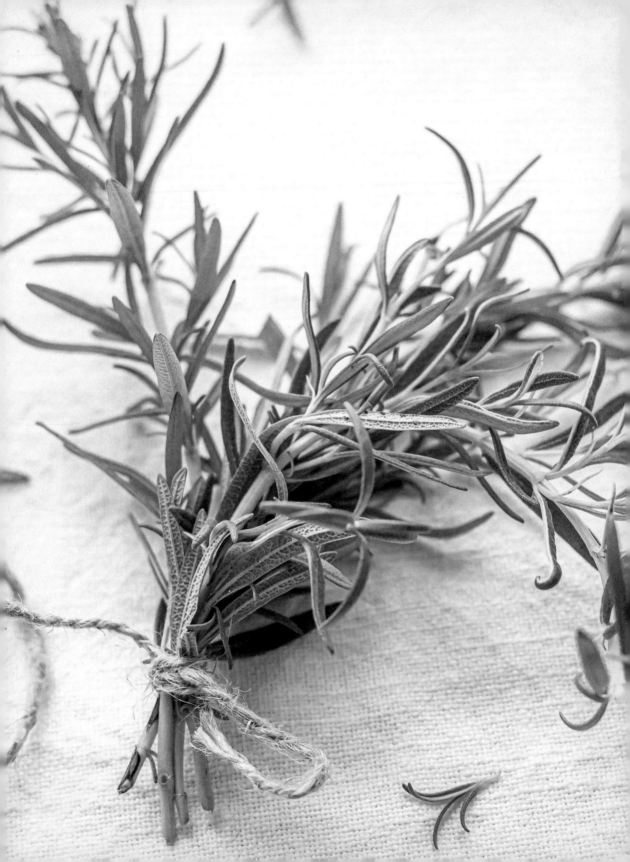

HERBS, VITAMINS, & SUPPLEMENTS for WELLNESS & BEAUTY

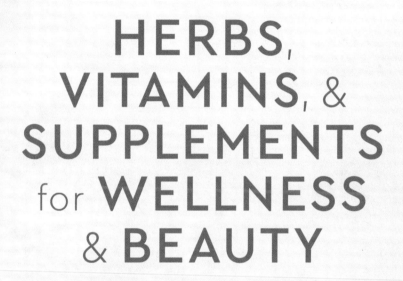

The Ultimate Guide

JANET WEINER
ROCKSTAR ENERGY DRINK CFO & COO

MICHAEL WEINER, PhD
NURITION & EPIDEMIOLOGY
AKA MICHAEL SAVAGE

Post Hill PRESS

A POST HILL PRESS BOOK
ISBN: 979-8-88845-835-8

Herbs, Vitamins, & Supplements for Wellness & Beauty: The Ultimate Guide
© 2024 by Janet Weiner and Michael Weiner, PhD
Based on *Herbs That Heal* © 1994, 1999 by Janet Weiner and Michael A. Weiner
All Rights Reserved

Cover and interior book design by Timothy Shaner, NightandDayDesign.biz

Library of Congress Cataloging in Publication Data
Card Number 93-086281

Post Hill Press
New York • Nashville
posthillpress.com

Published in the United States of America

1 2 3 4 5 6 7 8 9 10

Printed in Canada

For Russ

To the Moon and Stars

Always our Champion

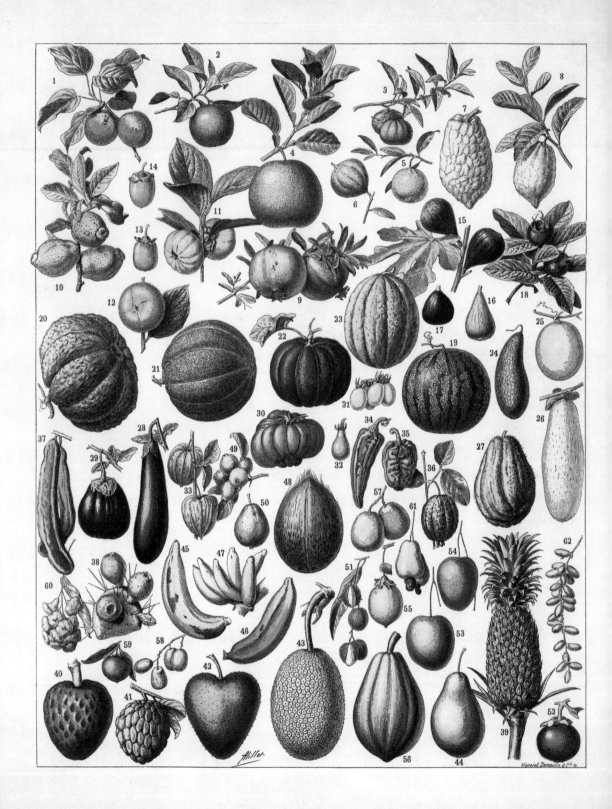

CONTENTS

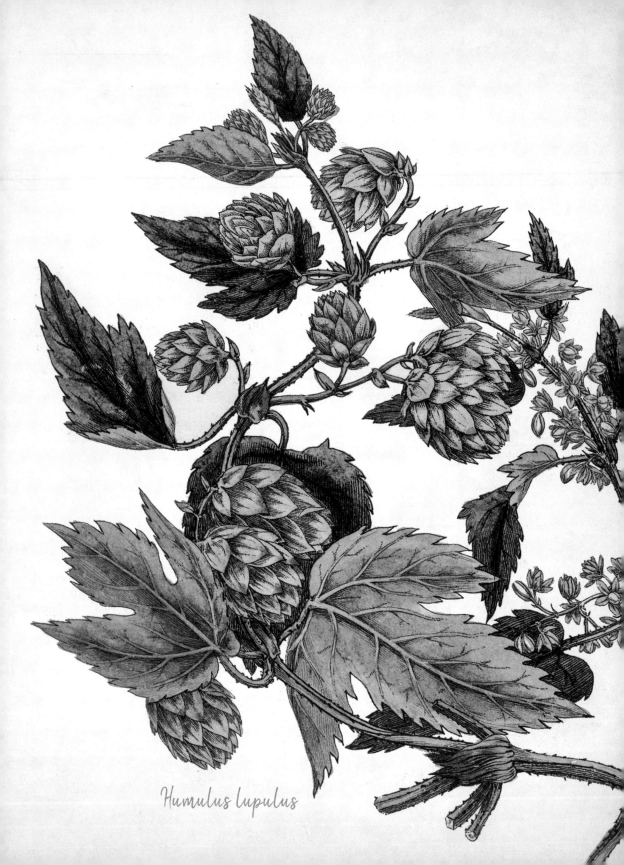

Humulus Lupulus

A History of Herbal Medicine

Welcome to the 2024 fully revised and updated "Herbs That Heal" with latest scientific herbal updates and now including for the first time a fully current, scientifically validated, state of the art supplement section! This volume encompasses every herb, vitamin, and supplement about which you need to have full information. This is your comprehensive and complete guide.

Long before the beginning of society, before the dawn of history, herbal medicine was man's first line of defense against the many ills and accidents that plagued us. Ancient humans learned from instinct, from the observation of animals, from birds, and by using leaves, earth, mud, and water.

These were the first soothing applications. Through trial and error, early humans learned what served them best. Eventually this knowledge was applied to helping others. Though the early methods were basic and crude, several of today's medicines still spring from sources as simple as those that were within reach of ancient man.

In the earliest times, the application of herbs and other healing substances, such as minerals, animal products, and extracts, were often accompanied by magical rites. While such spiritual rites still accompany the application of herbal medicine in the few primitive societies that remain, herbal medicine is today the only medicine available to treat their many ills. In the technological world in which we dwell, many of our most useful drugs are still connected to the early medical folklore of plants. Examples of these are reserpine from *Rauwolfia serpentina* (Indian snakeroot), digitoxin

> *All that man needs for health and healing has been provided by God in nature, the challenge of science is to find it.* —PARACELSUS

from *Digitalis purpurea* (foxglove), quinine from *Cinchona* species (Peruvian bark), morphine from *Papaver somniferum* (opium poppy), cocaine from *Erythroxylum coca* (coca leaves), atropine from *Atropa belladonna* (deadly nightshade), and d-tubocurarine from *Strychnos* and other species (arrow poisons). These are but some of the drugs of today that have their roots in folk medicine, and new experimental drugs, such as Taxol from the Pacific yew (*Taxus brevifolia*), are showing enormous promise against certain forms of cancer. Others, of course, exist. And even in an age of synthetic pharmaceuticals approximately 25 percent of all prescription drugs sold in the United States are derived from a plant.

MESOPOTAMIA, CHINA, AND EGYPT

Ancient Mesopotamia, often called the cradle of civilization, provides us with the earliest known record of the practice of the art of medicine as we know it today. In those days, medicine was largely herbal medicine. In this era, about 2600 B.C., the Babylonians already had a primitive form of medicine. The practitioners of healing in this era were priests, physicians, and pharmacists all in one. Clay tablets describe early medical treatments and the first symptomology for illnesses, as well as the prescription and the directions for compounding various remedies. This early medicine in ancient Babylonia is thought to have spread to the neighboring countries along the caravan routes to and from India, Arabia, and Egypt.

In China during this same period, people of the Hsia and Shang dynasties employed similar methods to combat various diseases. The records we have from this early time show 36 names of diseases but mention only prayers for healing with no reference to herbal treatments. While many other medical classics were thought to have been written in China, only the *Shan Hai Ching* survived. It dates from about 250 B.C. Another document is the *Hai Ching,* dating from 120 B.C. These records describe approximately 250 plants and animals, 68 of which are used medicinally. Of these, 21 are from plants and 47 from animals. Included in these early descriptions of herbal remedies are cinnamon, angelica, gambier, peony, juju, dragon bone, and talc. Tracing the development of herbal medicine in China through contemporary times, we note a dictionary of Chinese herb drugs, which covers 5,767 various kinds of medicinal substances, that was recently published by the People's Republic of China. In clinical practice, however, approximately 200 herbs, including ginseng, are most commonly used. In Japan, about 250 herbs are commonly used. Chinese herbology is a part of Chinese medicine and is a comprehensive system of health that teaches that health and disease are due to the balance and imbalance of living forces acting on man and animals alike. Consequently, Chinese herbs are rarely utilized individually but are always compounded in a carefully balanced mixture, aiming always to reestablish the inner harmony of the human organism.

Egyptian medicine dates from the royal courts of King Zoser in about 2900 B.C., but truly accurate records of medical practices have not been uncovered that date earlier than 1900 B.C. The best known and most important record of early drug making is the *Papyrus Ebers,* a sort of formulary or collection of various prescriptions, which contains about 800 different prescriptions and mentions 700 drugs of vegetable, mineral, and animal origin. In addition to formulas for inhalations, suppositories, gargles, snuffs, enemas, poultices, decoctions, infusions, pills, lotions, ointments, plasters and fumigations, we find that beer, milk, wine, and honey were common vehicles for most of the drugs that were mixed together. The Egyptian herbologist was very aware of beauty as well, for we find approximately 74 prescriptions pertaining to hair washes, dyes, oils, and depilatories. In ancient Egypt, there were several echelons in the preparation of drugs. They were the gatherers and preparers of drugs and "chiefs of fabrication," or the equivalent of chief herbalists. They are thought to have worked in the "house of life."

ANCIENT GREECE AND ROME

Moving to ancient Europe, we focus on Theophrastus of Eresos, an early Greek philosopher and natural scientist who is known as the father of botany. Theophrastus is still recognized today for his intensely accurate observations on all types of subjects, including botanical subjects. He is credited as being one of the earliest scientific observers. It is in his ninth book, *The History of Plants,* that we find him dealing with the medical qualities and peculiarities of herbs. Not only does he accurately describe herbs, but he also very aptly describes the preparation and uses of drugs obtained from plants.

In the first century A.D., Dioscorides was born in Anazarbos, which was in a part of Asia Minor that was then a part of the Roman Empire. In order to study the herbs then known, he accompanied Roman armies throughout Asia Minor and traveled in Spain, Greece, Italy, and Gaul. Recording what he observed as he observed it, he wrote a book based on his travels that made him famous. Galen, a Roman scientist who lived a century later, stated, "In his book, Dioscorides has written in a useful way on the entire materia medica because he not only deals with the herbs but includes the trees, fruits, seeds, the natural and artificial juices and, furthermore, the metals and animal substances. In my opinion, he is the one among the various authors who has presented the most perfect discussion of the drugs." For 15 centuries, Galen's words maintained the supremacy of Dioscorides in the world of plant drugs, his texts considered basic science in the field as late as the 16th century. Mentioned previously, Galen, who lived between A.D. 130 and 200, was not only a historian of sorts, but practiced and taught medicine and early pharmacy in Rome. He created principles for the preparation and compounding of medicines that were maintained for over 1,500 years. Galen went beyond his predecessors by attempting to find a scientific basis for the dispensing of drugs and in his introduction of cautious dosage. He developed many methods for mixing, extracting, refining, and combining plants and other drugs.

THE MIDDLE AGES

During the Middle Ages, known also as the Dark Ages, much of the cultural and scientific knowledge of earlier civilizations in the Western world was destroyed. Fortunately, however, the more ancient knowledge of herbalism and medicine was preserved and utilized mainly in the monasteries. During this period, it was the monks who did much to take care of the evolving science. Thus, for example, Latin writings on medicine were preserved in the libraries of monasteries. The early knowledge of herbal medicine was taught in the cloisters as early as the seventh century.

Manuscripts from many ancient writers and many ancient lands were translated and copied for monastic libraries. Gathering herbs in the field, the monks planted them in their own herb gardens. They prepared and used these for the benefit of the sick and injured amongst themselves and the surrounding areas. In many countries today, herb gardens may still be found in monasteries.

Before turning to the modern era, or post-Medieval times, we should make note of several scientists who were writing in Arabic. The findings of al-Razi, also known as Rhazes, who worked in about the year 923, was of scientific importance in the history of herbalism. Another important figure from this part of the world is the Spanish-born Ibn al-Baitar, who lived between 1197 until 1248. He compiled a methodical and critical compendium of more than 2,000 herbal drugs. Yet when discussing the Arabian era

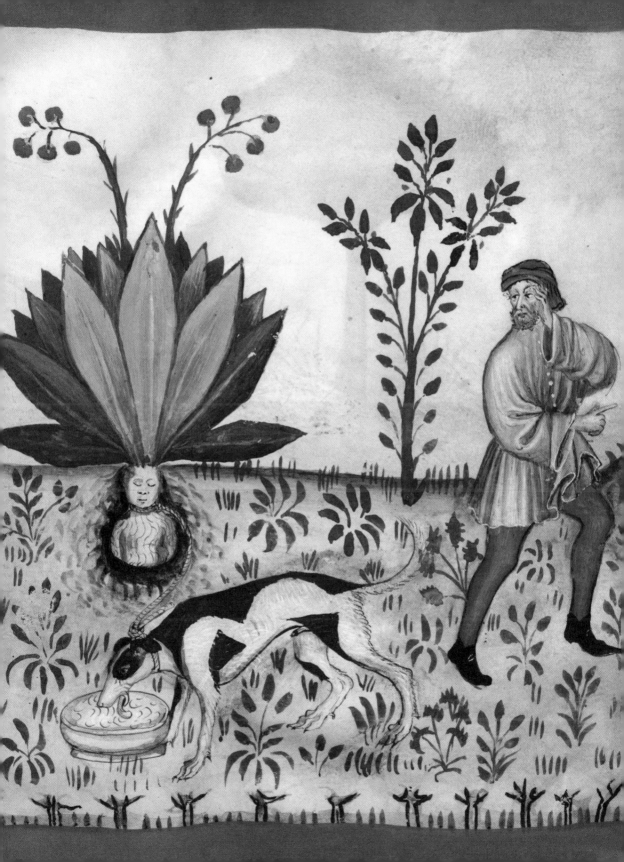

in the history of herbal medicine, one genius stands above all the others, the Persian Ibn Sina, also known as Avicenna in the English language. Sometimes known as the "Persian Galen," Avicenna lived from about 980 until 1037. He has been called an intellectual giant who was an herbalist, physician, poet, philosopher, and diplomat. His works were accepted as authoritative in the Western world until as late as the 17th century, and they are still considered influential in parts of the Orient. So, here we have an early herbal scientist whose work dominated through the long Middle Ages and even into the Renaissance. It should be noted that Avicenna first adopted and then elaborated on Galen's ideas.

At this point in the history of herbal medicine, we see the development of the first official pharmacopoeia. (A pharmacopoeia is a book of standards used by pharmacists in preparing and dispensing medicines as dictated by physicians.) In 1498, the *Nuovo Receptario* was published and was based almost solely on the Greek and Arabic drug therapy that preceded it. This pharmacopoeia, the first of its kind, was written in Italian and was translated into Latin in 1518 and soon became available throughout the Western world. Soon thereafter, official pharmacopoeias began to appear in other regions of Europe.

HERBAL MEDICINE IN THE NEW WORLD

In the beginning of the 1600s, early settlements began to appear in North America. This period marks the beginning of the first new age in herbalism because it was the interaction between the Europeans and the Native Americans that brought forth a pollination in the science of herbs. Many Europeans brought with them their knowledge of healing plants. They cultivated their own herb gardens upon arriving in the New World. These early American herbalists often learned about new drug plants from Native Americans. The earliest records demonstrate that many Native American plants were soon adopted by the European settlers. These included boneset, mullein, goldenseal, and jack-in-the-pulpit.

We now enter the first truly modern period of herbal medicine. The German chemist Friedrich Serturner began experimenting with opium in 1803 and soon delineated opium's chief narcotic principle, morphine. He also recognized and proved the critical importance of an entire new class of organic substances, the alkaloids. This was based upon the fact that morphine, which was then a new substance, was alkaline in nature, and he saw it as the first of a new class of organic bases that formed salts with organic as well as with inorganic acids. It's interesting to note that this young man was only 23 years of age at the time of his discovery.

Late in the 18th century, there was reported in Europe the value of "Peruvian barks," which were used to alleviate the symptoms of malaria and other strong intermittent fevers. Many scientists then tried to isolate the secret of cinchona bark. It was two young French chemists, Pierre-Joseph Pelletier and Joseph-Bienaimé Caventou, who first discovered quinine and cinchonine in cinchona bark. Soon after this discovery, the large-scale manufacture of quinine was begun, but Pelletier, because of his love for humanity, refused to patent or create a monopoly for the manufacture of this important fever-lowering drug.

Earlier we described herb gardens in monasteries. The concept of obtaining God's healing powers from the earth achieved a renaissance among the Shakers, the Protestant sectarians who settled in North American colonies. While they began their first cultivation and study of medicinal herbs in the early 1700s, their most important community was in New Lebanon, New York. The Shakers gathered and cultivated approximately 200 varieties of medicinal herbs. They dried and ground them and then pressed them into solid bricks that were then sold to pharmacists and physicians around the world. They later made solid and fluid extracts. By 1850, the herb gardens of New Lebanon, then known as "physics gardens," occupied about 50 acres and were largely cultivated with hyoscyamus, belladonna, taraxacum, aconite, poppy, lettuce, sage, summer savory, marjoram, dock, burdock, valerian, and horehound. There were approximately another 50 minor plants raised by these people.

THE 18TH AND 19TH CENTURIES

Focusing on the English-speaking world, the 18th and 19th centuries saw the proliferation of numerous healers whose repertoire consisted largely of herbal remedies. Then as now, there were many healers but few who documented their techniques and remedies in any recognizable or lasting form. Therefore, we can best summarize the history of herbal medicine in these centuries by listing some of the chief books of medicinal plants that survive from this period. These include the beautifully illustrated volumes by Stephenson and Churchill, *Medical Botany* (1836), and by Bentley and Trimen, *Medicinal Plants* (1880). Both sets were published in England. The United States saw the publication of Charles F. Millspaugh's *Medicinal Plants* (1892), which covered 1,000 species. There were several other books published, but none of equal quality.

THE AGE OF TECHNOLOGY

We now enter the age where technological progress permits the manufacture of highly reliable preparations of herbal medicines. Before glancing at some of the processing methods, it may be useful to look at the various ways in which herbs are still prepared in China and compare these with the dominant forms in the United States. Traditional Chinese drugs are often found in the following forms: slices, powder, pills, plasters, medicated liquors, herb distillates, pellets, and medicinal teas. New dosage forms also appear in the Orient. These include tablets, capsules, tinctures, fluid extracts, ointments, instant granules, and others that are the same as those found in Western medicine, including syrups, suppositories, aerosols, injections, and ampules. In today's bustling industrial world, people are too busy to prepare their own herbal remedies and generally do not like the traditional preparations because they are usually odorous, bitter, pungent, and difficult to consume. So even in Asia, scientifically prepared herbal preparations have become very popular and have gained a fine reputation and wide acceptance.

WHY HERBS ARE PROCESSED

In addition to saving time in their preparation, that is, for convenience, there are other goals of drug processing. These include the reduction of toxicity and adverse effects. For example, in their raw states, certain herbs may cause irritation of the throat, which is true for pinellia, a Chinese herb. Processing will reduce or eliminate this side effect. Another example is the Chinese herb genkwa, which generally causes abdominal aching in the raw state, but after fermentation it does not cause this reaction. In addition, herbs may be processed to promote their therapeutic effects. The alkaloids of certain herbs are hardly soluble in water, but after vinegar processing, they are readily soluble, and this enhances their potency. By processing licorice with honey, the effects are increased. Crude drugs are also processed to remove contaminants and unpleasant odors. In the raw state, the contaminants may include mold, rot of other forms, and animal waste. Processing renders the herbal product perfectly safe for human consumption. After processing, herbs may be screened, cut, and extracted. These processes have been developed over thousands of years. Currently in America, we have certified potency herbal products as well as magnified dosages of various components of specific herbs that give them a more powerful therapeutic effect.

THE QUESTION OF "STANDARDIZED HERBS"

There's a potency war brewing. The bottom line, however, may prove that the 1970s aphorism "small is beautiful" or "less is more" is the answer. Simply upping the percentage content of an active constituent in an herbal preparation may yet prove harmful.

For now, the answer is to welcome standardization and to proceed with caution—making standardized herbal extracts *only* from plants that have been subjected to safety

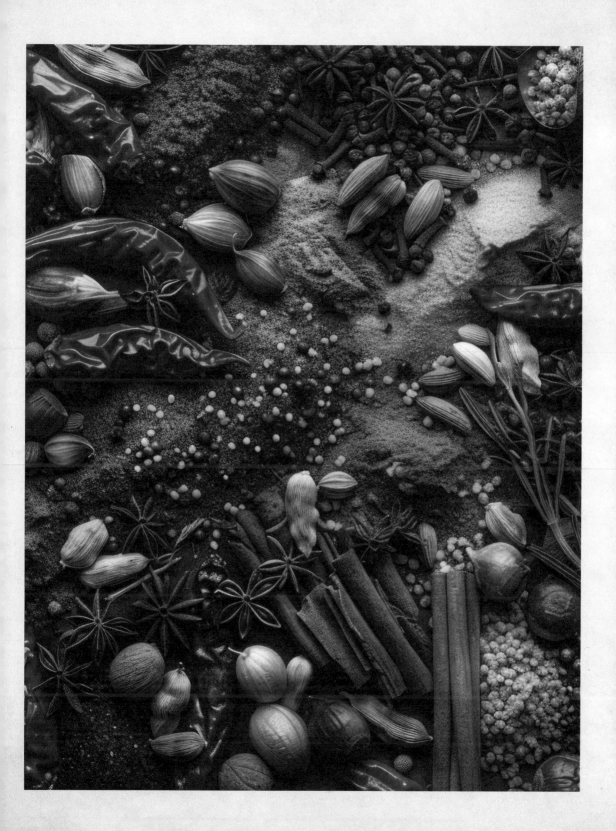

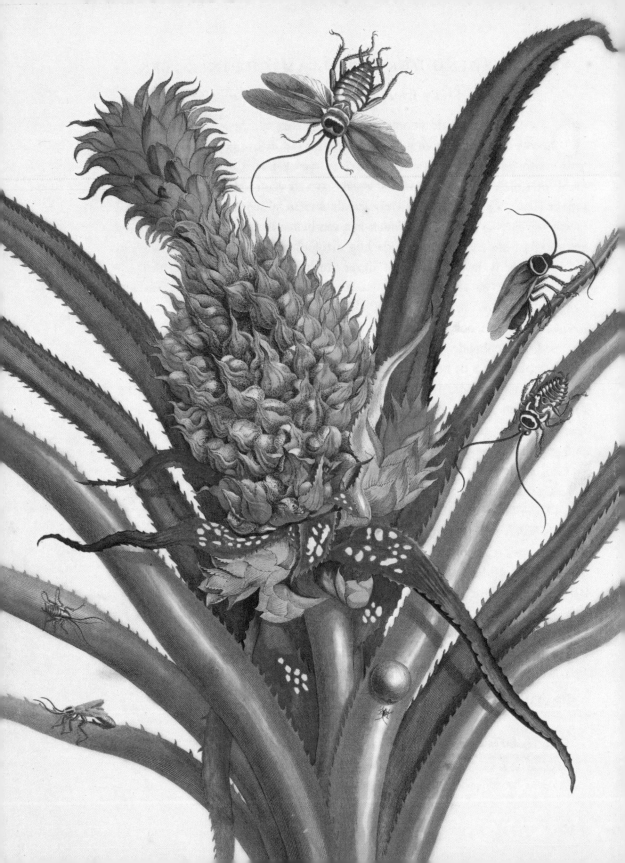

and efficacy studies. Examples include herbs such as ginseng, ginkgo, ginger, milk thistle, echinacea, turmeric, essential oil or orange (d-limonene), valerian, St. John's wort, horsetail, bilberry, and others with good efficacy and safety data.

Standardization was introduced to counter the negative effects of poor quality control, which plagued the herb industry in the 1970s. With standardized herbs, we can reliably count on receiving the same quantity of one or more active constituents per unit taken. Thus, a one-gram capsule of milk thistle said to contain 80% silymarin, the chief active component, can be reliably assumed to contain this consistent quantity.

In nature, herbs vary in their content of active constituents. Soils, climates, harvesting methods, processing, packaging, and storage all affect the relative potency of a finished herbal product. When an active principle in the finished product is so identified on the label, the miscellaneous subjective effects can be objectively controlled, and the consumer can rely upon receiving a stated quantity and balance of activity.

A reasonable course of action, at this stage of knowledge, would be to proceed cautiously, as stated previously, standardizing active constituents of herbs with well-established safety and efficacy. By also including the whole plant in the final product, some measure of the inherent natural "checks and balances" or synergism will be retained. With this method, we see an *enhancement* of natural medicinal activity rather than an imbalanced drug effect.

Increased control of active ingredients and a general increase in sophistication throughout the industry, coupled with greatly rising demand for herbal products at the consumer level, leads me to conclude that being bullish on herbs is a very safe course indeed.

BULLISH ON HERBS

The future of herbal medicine in America is very bright. People have rediscovered plant remedies and are once again looking to nature for solutions to various ills and conditions.

This is a natural progression when we consider that the ethno-medical folklore of preindustrial (so-called "primitive") cultures consists of prescriptions for treating most physical ailments. Taken together with the fact that the main active ingredient of approximately 25% of all prescription drugs sold in the U.S. was derived from plants, we can see why folklore has given life to the new scientific interest in herbs.

Ever since two principle anticancer drugs, vincristine and vinblastine, were isolated from the Madagascar periwinkle (*Catharanthus roseus*) in the 1950s and '60s, we have seen interest in the promise of herbal medicine. These powerful plant-derived drugs arrest cell division so dramatically that one of them, vincristine, is used for the treatment of acute leukemia, especially in children. With other drugs, these plant-derived compounds are used to treat other cancers, including Hodgkin's disease. Currently, Taxol, derived from the Pacific yew tree, is being used to treat "incurable" cancers.

These great success stories stimulated a worldwide investigation of centuries of folk medicine and the consumer usage of herbal preparations, mainly teas, in the United States.

In the late 1970s, the interest in herbs seemed to have waned. A new decade was beginning, one that would lead mankind into the new century, a century of high technology, and herbs were assigned an archaic aura. The new president ushered in a glittering decade. Hippies were dead. "Natural" was passé and all that glittered was thought to be golden.

As the 1980s matured, and the romance with surface realities was reevaluated, people once again wondered if nature, that most unfickle phenomenon, might yet hold some answers for mankind's infirmities.

In the '90s, we saw a new and wonderful outcry to preserve our natural environment. There was a realization that the rainforests were repositories of hundreds if not thousands of potential medicines. Herbal preparations were tried, for the first time by some, again by many.

HERBS IN THE 21ST CENTURY

While estimates of the percent of new prescriptions in the U.S. that contain an active ingredient originating in nature run between 25 and 40%, these compounds represent a very short list with very wide usage. Very few *new* compounds derived from nature have entered the American pharmaceutical marketplace in the past 20 years. The same few developed years ago reappear in new permutations and combinations.

The lack of patent protection, not the lack of efficacy, keeps the pharmaceutical giants in the U.S. from investing in the development of drugs from plants. Herb companies and smaller pharmaceutical firms have been and will continue to meet the growing consumer demand for nature's remedies, however. In Japan, France, and some developing nations, drugs from herbs will become big business.

This is not to create the mistaken idea that the United States will *not* take part in the coming herb-based revolution in medicine. Currently, pharmaceuticals derived from plants are a $110 billion business in the U.S., and this is just a baseline for medicine from botanicals. By the middle of this decade, we can expect vast new markets for this class of products because over 200 research groups worldwide are engaged in creating new medicinals from nature. Surprisingly, the largest number of these research groups are based in the U.S. (97 out of a total of 209 worldwide research groups are U.S.-based).

Europeans have long been able to purchase herbal-based medicinal preparations on an OTC ("over-the-counter") basis. These remedies are utilized as a second-line treatment immediately following alterations in diet, a first-line approach. Such herbal preparations are tried before people turn to physicians for third-line treatments, the potent pharmaceuticals.

In America, our first and second lines of treating common ailments have largely disappeared. People have been taught to "see a doctor" for the smallest ache, often coming home with a potent pharmaceutical "prescription" just as likely to cause harm as to effect a cure.

With the growth of the herbal industry, Americans will join the Europeans in taking charge of their own first-symptom healthcare. The wildly escalating costs of medical care and the legion of tragic iatrogenic effects of prescription drugs have given new meaning to the old saying "Physician, heal thyself!"

When I was younger, an older, wiser man said to me, "If you don't know how to take care of your health by the time you're forty, you *deserve* the doctors!"

THE BENEFITS OF STANDARDIZATION

Natural products, either as pure compounds or as standardized plant extracts, provide extensive opportunities for new drug leads because of the unmatched availability of chemical diversity. In contrast to modern medicines, herbal medicines are frequently used to treat chronic diseases. Standardization guarantees the content of one or more active constituents and marker compounds. The plant environment and genetic factors could significantly affect the biochemical components of the plant extract. Production of botanical drugs requires genetically uniform monocultures of the source plant in fully standardized conditions to ensure the biochemical consistency and to optimize the safety and efficacy of every crop.

[Citation: Garg V, Dhar VJ, Sharma A, Dutt R. *Facts about standardization of herbal medicine: a review.* Zhong Xi Yi Jie He Xue Bao. 2012 Oct;10(10):1077-83. Doi: 10.3736/jcim20121002. PMID: 23073189.]

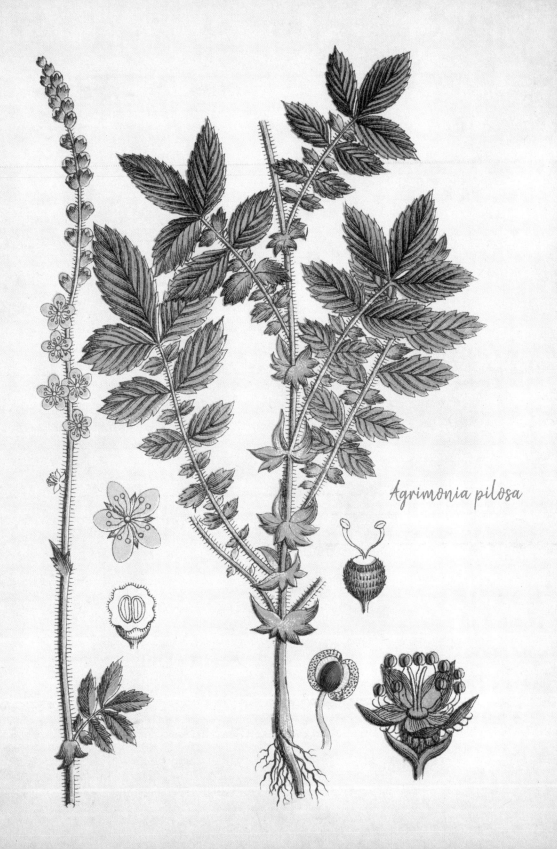

Agrimonia pilosa

ONE

HERBS & MEDICINAL PLANTS
A to Z Reference Guide

AGRIMONY
Agrimonia pilosa

Parts used: Herb, root, and fruit. *This herb has long been used in traditional Chinese medicine, and modern research is also finding this herb possesses a number of possible medicinal applications.*

TRADITIONAL USAGES

Agrimony's first recorded use dates from a Chinese book from nearly a thousand years ago. In traditional Chinese medicine, agrimony is classified among the blood-regulating drugs. It has a tendency to invigorate the functions of the stomach, liver, and bowels, eliminating foul matter from the system. It is highly recommended in the treatment of kidney and bladder stones. It is also used to stop hemorrhages. As a gargle, the decoction is considered very effective in relieving soreness and inflammation of the mouth and throat. It is also useful for diarrhea, though it needs to be used consistently for a period of time.

RECENT SCIENTIFIC FINDINGS

A member of the rose family, agrimony contains bitters, mucilage, and phytosterol, and it is rich in tannins. A study on agrimony and several other plants' effects on diabetes found that agrimony retarded the development of streptozotocin diabetes in mice. An extract has been found to have hypotensive action, and another demonstrated anti-viral activity in mice.

In other studies, agrimony exhibited a hemostasis effect, stimulating platelet formation and hastening blood coagulation. As an anticancer agent, a decoction has inhibited proliferation of certain cancer cells. Agrimony has also been found to have a cardiotonic effect. At lower doses it regulates heart rate; at high doses it slows the heartbeat.

There is a veritable treasure trove of recent work and ongoing scientific investigations regarding the potential efficacy of agrimony (Var spp) in the following ways, many of which are supported by the traditional uses:

- Astringent action in diarrheal diseases.
- Gargle for mouth sores and sore throats.
- Topical therapy for eczema and psoriasis and superficial wound healing due to its antimicrobial and antibacterial actions.
- Thought useful in treating Helicobacter pylori in conjunction with current antibiotic therapy, as well as some promising rat studies regarding blood glucose levels, which are of interest to scientists studying diabetes remedies.
- Ongoing studies concerning lowering LDL levels, hepatoprotective effects, and treatment of postmenopause symptoms continue to interest scientists, as well as investigations regarding anti-inflammatory, antioxidant, and analgesic effects that seem to point to agrimony (various species) as potentially of critical importance in future plant medicine developments.

ALOE VERA
Aloe vera

Parts used: Leaves. *Known to the ancient Egyptians as a beauty aid for the skin, this remarkable plant promotes healing from burns and wounds.*

TRADITIONAL USAGES
Ever since the age of Cleopatra, when aloe was used to treat burns, this remarkable plant has enjoyed popular acclaim and wide usage. The first known use of aloe as a medicinal came in 333 B.C. when Alexander the Great heard of this plant and sent a commission to the island of Socotra to investigate and return with samples. During

the 1800s and early 1900s, much of the aloes exported to Europe came from plants cultivated in the Dutch West Indies on the islands of Aruba and Barbados. These are variously identified as Curaçao aloe, aloe vera, and Barbados aloe. African aloe varieties are Cape aloe, Uganda aloe, and Natal aloe, collectively referred to in commerce as Zanzibar aloe.

There are about 180 aloe species of different sizes and forms. Several aloes are cultivated for ornamental purposes; with their stiffness and radial symmetry, they fit well into rock gardens, and since their home is the African desert, they grow well in direct sunlight. The true aloe (*Aloe barbadensis;* synonym *A. vera*) yields "Barbados aloes."

Along with aloe's use since ancient times as a beauty aid for the skin, externally the raw mucilage from the fresh plant has long been employed as an analgesic for burns, scrapes, sunburn, and insect bites, as well as to promote healing of such injuries. A fleshy stalk is broken off, the skin of the plant split to expose the interior, and the edges are spread apart for effective wrapping of the afflicted area. One stalk can be used piece by piece until gone since it forms its own natural container as the plant skin's surface dries and forms a seal that preserves the remainder of the stalk.

For the treatment of *chronic constipation only,* aloes were felt to be particularly effective, as their action is largely limited to the colon. However, they were not recommended as a general laxative. As the action produced by aloes often caused griping (painful muscle spasms of the bowels), it was common to include a carminative such as fennel to soothe the side effects of this purgative action. Aloes were also often utilized to treat various forms of amenorrhea (absent or suppressed menses).

RECENT SCIENTIFIC FINDINGS

I first learned of this plant's properties in 1968 when we read it was being utilized to treat radiation burns by a research group at the University of Pennsylvania. Very significantly, this university research team found the mucilaginous aloe to be the most effective treatment for minor radiation burns. Subsequent trials of my own demonstrated what folklore had long told: aloe was an effective, safe, inexpensive treatment for burns and wounds.

The leaf juice of *A. ferox* and *A. vera*, when incorporated into a water-soluble ointment base or used as the fresh juice, has well-established emollient effects on the skin. Such preparations are widely utilized to treat minor sunburn cases and also to treat burns from X-ray treatment of cancer and related diseases. The active principle has not been identified but is probably a polysaccharide that forms a protective and soothing coating when applied to the skin. If the juice is dried and then applied

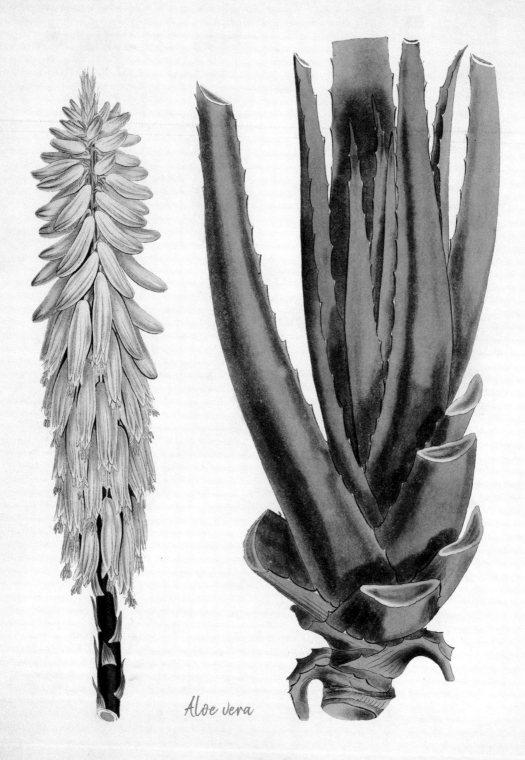

Aloe vera

to burns, it is not effective. This ancient healing plant should remain forever one of humankind's most important frontline remedies against burns and wounds.

The authors of one study wrote, "*A. vera* improves wound healing when administered either orally or topically. It not only contributes to a decrease in wound diameter but also leads to better vascularity and healthier granulation tissue. The fact that aloe is effective orally suggests that it is not broken down by the gastrointestinal tract and is absorbed into the blood. Aloe possibly improves wound healing by increasing the availability of oxygen and by increasing the synthesis and the strength of collagen. Aloe vera has become a subject of scientific study concerning inflammation and wound healing. As knowledge about aloe increases, significant benefits of a practical nature in the management of healing wounds can be expected" (Davis, et al.).

Aloe's ability to accelerate wound healing was demonstrated in a study with patients with full-face dermabrasion (surgical removal of skin imperfections, such as scars, by abrasion). One side of the face was treated with the standard polyethylene oxide gel while the other side received the standard gel saturated with stabilized aloe vera. Overall, wound healing was approximately 72 hours faster on the aloe side. The authors concluded, "This acceleration of wound healing is important to reduce bacterial contamination." One note of caution: adverse reactions to aloe have taken place following dermabrasion. It is recommended that patients refrain from using aloe vera topically in the first weeks after surgery.

In another study on aloe by a group of researchers in the Netherlands, immune-enhancing activity was discovered. Beginning with the traditional medical usages for this plant, these workers purified an aqueous gel. A highly active polysaccharide fraction was isolated from the aloe gel. This component proved active in the production of antibodies and also stimulated another aspect of the immune response (i.e., complementary activity). The authors compared the effectiveness of this gel fraction of aloe with dextran sulphate, a sulphated polysaccharide found principally in certain seaweeds. (For about 40 years, Japanese researchers have been testing dextran sulphate and ably demonstrating its antitumor and anticlotting properties.)

The known healing effects of aloe vera on infected wounds are thought to be explained by the local activation of complement, which is thought to lead to an influx of monocytes and polymorphonuclear leukocytes to the injured area. Aloe has also been found to aid in the treatment of frostbite.

In one study, an aloe extract prepared with 50% ethanol applied topically decreased inflammation by 290 percent. Another research team combined aloe with hydrocortisone and tested against acute inflammation. The authors speculated that aloe vera has significant potential as a biologically active vehicle for steroids.

If the leaves of various aloe species are extracted in a special way, and the resulting product is concentrated, a mixture of anthraquinones results. This mixture is known in the U.S. and Canada as "aloes" or "aloin," and it is well established to be an effective laxative in humans. The laxative effect is much stronger than that produced by senna or cascara products.

Another preparation from aloe, carrisyn, is a polysaccharide. It has been claimed that carrisyn directly kills various types of viruses, including herpes and measles, and possibly HIV. However, research is still in the preliminary stages.

The inclusion of aloe in varied skin remedies has exploded in recent years. Aloe is found in topical over-the-counter treatments for sunburn, rashes, cold sores, eczema, psoriasis, and wrinkles, as well as in hair shampoos, salves, and conditioners for dry hair and dry scalp issues.

We like to keep a fresh potted aloe plant at home for quick minor kitchen burns or wound emergencies, as well as for scraped knees and elbows for children. The fresh leafy stalk can be easily split open to access the healing gelatinous interior, which can be spread on the wound. The remainder of the stalk may be preserved in the refrigerator for at least a week.

This is a remarkable plant and one of our finest herbal medicines.

ANEMONE
Anemone spp.

Parts used: Root and flower. *Ancient Chinese and Greek physicians extolled these beautiful plants, which contain the compound anemonin.*

TRADITIONAL USAGES

In ancient texts of Greek and Chinese healers we find continual reference to the healing virtues of the lovely anemones. Dioscorides revered anemone in the form of external plasters or baths for skin ulcers and inflamed eyes. Pliny, the Roman naturalist and historian, advocated its use for toothaches and swollen gums. The Chinese employed *A. pulsatilla* for ailments ranging from dysentery to madness.

One type of anemone liverleaf (*A. hepatica*) is so named because its leaves resemble the shape of the liver; according to the Jakob Böhme's doctrine of signatures, a tonic of this particular anemone consequently was believed to aid liver disorders.

There are several other anemones: *A. ludoviciana* (American pulsatilla), *A. pratensis* (European pulsatilla), *A. ranunculoides* (yellow wood anemone), and *A. apennina* (blue anemone). These are also employed in folk medicines in various capacities. Some have been used as sedatives, demulcents, and vulneraries, and others were once employed as a primary treatment in early cases of tuberculosis.

RECENT SCIENTIFIC FINDINGS

Many anemone species have been studied in the laboratory, both for their chemical content and for the effects of their extracts in animals and in the test tube. They are all remarkably similar in their chemical and pharmacological properties, a majority of the effects explained by the presence of the simple chemical compound known as protoanemonin, the lactone of gamma-hydroxy-vinylacrylic acid.

Anemonin is highly active against a large number of different disease-producing microorganisms, has sedative properties, lowers blood pressure, stimulates the gallbladder, relaxes smooth muscle of the gut, allays pain, and in pure form will produce a blistering effect on the skin or mucous membranes. When a sufficiently diluted water extract of anemone is used, this blistering effect has not been observed. There is enough of this substance present to slightly irritate the mucous membranes, giving rise to an expectorant, as well as perhaps a diuretic, effect. Anemone is considered one of the most effective of all drugs for amoebic dysentery.

A 1988 analysis determined that anemonin is the primary compound responsible for the fever lowering effects, while both anemonin and protoanemonin produce a sedating effect. A 1990 study determined that protoanemonin has "in vitro" (test tube) activity against fungi.

Beyond their visual allure, anemone herbs have a long history of medicinal use in various traditional systems of medicine. Different parts of the plant, including the roots, leaves, and flowers, have been utilized to treat a range of ailments. However, it's important to note that the medicinal use of anemone herbs should be approached with caution as these are very powerful medicinal plants, and we advise the guidance

Anemone spp.

of a qualified healthcare practitioner. This is not an herb for self-treatment. Some species of anemone herbs are believed to possess anti-inflammatory properties and have been used to alleviate symptoms associated with arthritis and other inflammatory conditions. Traditional remedies have employed anemone herbs as analgesics to relieve pain, particularly joint and muscle pain. Infusions or decoctions made from anemone herbs have been used to ease respiratory issues such as coughs and bronchitis. Certain preparations of anemone herbs have been applied topically to treat skin conditions such as wounds, burns, and eczema. Clearly this is a powerful plant, and we expect research results to continue to validate the folkloric uses.

ANGELICA or Dong Quai
Angelica sinensis, A. acutiloba

Parts used: Root, herb, and seed. *It is called "the women's herb" in China, and modern research substantiates angelica's effects in regulating uterine function.*

TRADITIONAL USAGES

The Chinese name for this herb means "missing the husband" or "returned to the husband's home." It is generally employed in traditional medicine as a food (in soup) or as a tea for irregular, painful, or meek menstruation, especially when associated with the symptoms of PMS (tension, cramps, pain, weakness, etc.).

In addition, angelica has a long folkloric history as a remedy for diabetes, hypertension, cancer, angina pectoris, and nephritis. In Europe, angelica was used for infant flatulence and colic. In adults it was taken for heartburn. In the *British Flora Medica,* we find the following report:

The Laplanders considered this plant as one of the most important productions of their soil. During that part of the year which they pass in the woods, they are subject to a severe kind of colic, against which the root of Angelica is one of their chief remedies. They also frequently mix the unexpanded umbels with the leaves of the Sorrel and boiling them down in water to the consistency of syrup, mix it with reindeer's milk, and thus form a stomachic and astringent medicine.

The essential oils distilled from angelica fruit and roots are utilized in the perfumery, cosmetic, and distillery industries. The oil is found in Benedictine, Chartreuse, and gin.

RECENT SCIENTIFIC FINDINGS

Angelica contains essential oils (including ligustilide, safrole, carvacrol, and n-butylide-nephthalide); fatty acids (palmitic, linoleic, stearic, arachidonic); coumarins (bergaptene); and a host of other compounds, including beta-sitosterol and several B vitamins. These constituents are responsible for the extremely dynamic activity exhibited by this pharmacologically active herb.

Interestingly, while this herb has been shown to have genuine effects in regulating uterine function, depending upon how it is prepared, it both stimulates and inhibits uterine muscles. Here is what the *Oriental Materia Medica* advises:

Experiments indicate that its nonvolatile water-soluble compounds stimulate uterine muscle, while its volatile oil inhibits uterine muscle, producing a relaxing action. Therefore, to cause the uterus to contract the herb should be decocted for a long period of time to get rid of the volatile oil. If the uterus is to be relaxed then the herb should be put into the decoction later (that is, the other herbs should be decocted first for some time before *tang-kuei* [angelica] is added and it should be boiled over a low flame to prevent loss of the volatile oil). Animal studies show that the uterus upon being pressed will exhibit irregular contractions, but after administration of *tang-kuei* the uterus will contract regularly. This means that *tangkuei* can regulate the function of the uterus and that is most probably the mechanism of *tang-kuei*'s ability to treat menorrhalgia. Mice given feed containing 5% *tang-kuei* have higher DNA (deoxyribonucleic acid) content in their uteri, have higher glucose metabolism, and thus have a higher multiplication rate of uterine tissue.

According to extensive clinical trials, angelica has proven to be an antibacterial, antifungal, and immunostimulant (inducing production of interferon), and has exhibited antitumor activity. A study from Japan, by Dr. Yamada in 1990, suggests antitumor activity in in vitro (test tube) experiments utilizing

Angelica sinensis

> *Angelica, also known as dong quai or female ginseng, has been used in traditional Chinese medicine for more than 2,000 years.*

polysaccharide fractions from angelica. A 1991 Japanese (animal) study employed several different extracts of angelica root to test their antitumor properties. The authors concluded that two of the extracts may be useful to possibly develop an effective method of cancer prevention.

Two chalcones isolated from angelica root show antibacterial activity. A 1990 study involving two other extracts focused on anti-ulcer effects. The authors found that the derivatives "significantly inhibited acid secretion and the formation of stress-induced gastric lesions. These results suggest that the antisecretory effect is due to the inhibition of gastric H+."

Ferulic acid is a phenolic compound contained in angelica. Researchers discovered that ferulic acid showed an inhibitory effect on uterine movement and contractions. A mixture of herbal components, TS, which included angelica, hoelen, peony, alisma, and cnidum, significantly increased progesterone secretion, suggesting "an exquisitive blended effect of herbal components of TS on progesterone secretion by corpora lutea."

Two 1991 (animal) studies involved angelica's effect on arrhythmia (irregular heartbeat). The results showed that the total incidence of arrhythmia was reduced by angelica dosing, leading researchers to pursue further inquiries.

Angelica, also known as dong quai or female ginseng, has been used in traditional Chinese medicine for more than 2,000 years. It is believed to boost vitality, alleviate fatigue, relieve pelvic pain, and regulate menstrual cycles. Recent scientific research has shown that angelica may have anti-inflammatory, pain-relieving, and muscle-relaxant properties. Dong quai is commonly used as a blood tonic and is referred to as the "women's herb" due to its ability to support and maintain healthy menstrual balance in women. Both men and women can benefit from dong quai's reputed ability to balance hormones, promote circulation, and reduce inflammation, as well as seemingly calming the mind and body and assisting with equilibrium. Certainly, angelica consumption is here to stay, and we look forward to more scientific validations of the various uses of this plant.

ANISE
Pimpinella anisum

Parts used: Seed. *The aromatic seeds may also promote iron absorption.*

TRADITIONAL USAGES

The 1918 *U.S. Dispensary* says, "It is one of the oldest aromatics, having been used by the ancient Egyptians; is spoken of by Theophrastus; and was cultivated in the imperial German farms of Charlemagne."

The seeds are abundant in Malta and Spain. The Spanish seeds are smaller than the German or French and are usually preferred. Anise seeds' fragrant odor is increased by friction. They taste warm, sweet, and aromatic. These properties, which depend on a volatile oil, are imparted sparingly to boiling water, freely to alcohol. The volatile oil extract is the envelope of the seeds and is separated by distillation. Their internal substance contains a bland fixed oil. By expression, a greenish oil is obtained, which is a mixture of the two. The seeds are sometimes adulterated with small fragments of argillaceous earth. Their aromatic qualities are occasionally impaired due to a slight fermentation they undergo when collected before maturity. The seeds are the source of oil in anise, utilized extensively in flavoring.

A decoction of anise seed added to milk is used to remedy infant colic and flatulence. It also increases milk secretion for nursing mothers. Due to its pleasant aroma, it is often added to preparations to make them more palatable, mainly masking disagreeable odors.

RECENT SCIENTIFIC FINDINGS

Containing 80 to 90 percent anethole and methyl chavicol, anise seeds have been shown to be an effective expectorant (promotes discharge of phlegm from lungs).

A 1990 study tested the effect of certain beverage extracts, including anise, on the absorption of iron. The results showed that anise was the most effective of the extracts tested in promoting iron absorption.

Pimpinella anisum

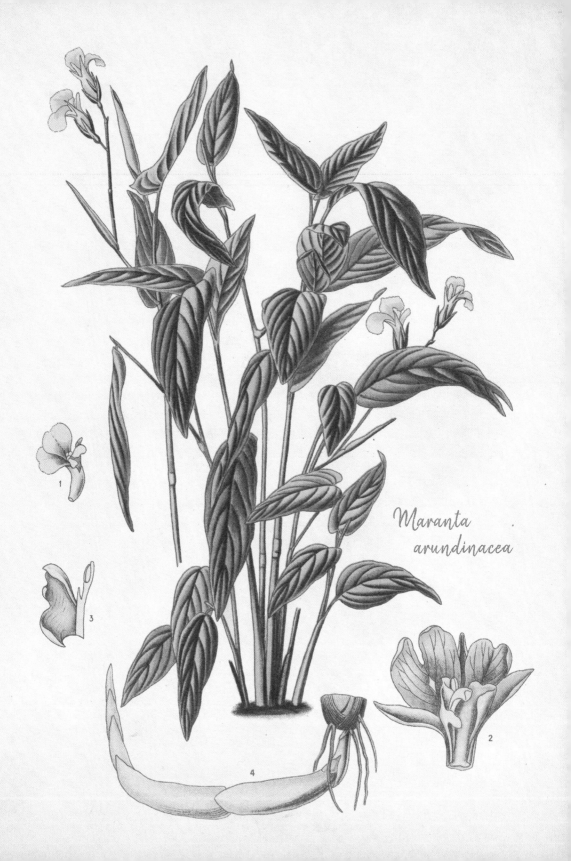

Maranta
arundinacea

The authors recommended offering beverages with anise, mint, caraway, cumin, tilia, and liquorice to children and adults as an agent to prevent iron deficiency anemia. Along with its aromatic properties, anise seeds have been shown to possess insecticidal properties.

Anise is a versatile herb that can be used in various forms to make medicine, and it can also be grown in gardens to act as a natural insecticide. Its seed (fruit) and oil are commonly used, but the root and leaf are also utilized on occasion. Anise is known for its ability to alleviate digestive problems, such as upset stomach and intestinal gas. It is also an effective expectorant that can help to increase productive cough, a diuretic that can increase urine flow, and an appetite stimulant. Anise is frequently added to over-the-counter laxative formulas to improve the taste and function. Additionally, anise may reduce the frequency and severity of hot flashes, potentially by mimicking estrogen's effects in the body.

Anise seed is a potent spice that is renowned for its strong licorice flavor. It is a popular ingredient in many liquors, including orzo and absinthe, and is commonly used in holiday cookies such as pfefferneusse and springerle. The use of anise in cooking can be traced back to ancient Egypt, but it was the Romans who enjoyed anise seed cakes after meals to help with digestion. In India, anise is traditionally used as a digestive aid and a breath freshener.

ARROWROOT

Maranta arundinacea

Parts used: Root. *The native people of Central and South America used this root as an antidote to arrow poisoning; it is now recognized as a superior carbohydrate.*

TRADITIONAL USAGES

The arrowroot plant is native to South America and to the West Indies, where it is predominantly cultivated. It also grows in Florida and has been cultivated in the southern states. The mashed rhizome of arrowroot was once used by the Indigenous people of Central and South America as an antidote for arrow poisoning, hence the plant's name. It is recorded that the Mayans utilized the root to make poultices for smallpox and, when drunk as a beverage, as a remedy for pus in the urine. This latter folkloric usage is due to the root's demulcent properties, which made it valuable for bowel complaints as well as for urinary problems.

It is probable that other plants contribute to furnish the arrowroot of commerce. It is procured in the West Indies from *M. allouya* and *M. nobilis,* beside *M. arundinacea.* Other species serve as sources of arrowroot in the East Indies.

RECENT SCIENTIFIC FINDINGS

Today, arrowroot is commonly used in baked products. It is a superior carbohydrate as well as a source of digestible calcium, which makes it a valuable element in the diet of children after weaning and for delicate people during convalescence. It can also be prepared as a jell, gruel, blancmange, or beverage.

When mixed with hot water, the root starch of this herbaceous perennial becomes gelatinous and may serve as an effective demulcent to soothe irritated mucous membranes.

Arrowroot starch has become an essential item in many West Indian and South American households due to its versatility and health benefits. This nutritious blend has soothing properties that help with gastrointestinal health. In cooking, arrowroot starch is a tasteless thickening agent that can be used to create clear sauces and glazes. It's also a gluten-free alternative to cornstarch and wheat flour, making it suitable for various dietary needs.

ARTICHOKE

Cynara scolymus

Parts used: Flowerhead bud and root. *This tasty vegetable contains flavonoids.*

TRADITIONAL USAGES

Artichokes have long been eaten as a vegetable. The leaves were used for their diuretic properties. Leaves and roots were thought to help prevent atherosclerosis and to be a diabetes treatment. Other reputed uses included assistance for jaundice, anemia, and dyspepsia.

RECENT SCIENTIFIC FINDINGS

Silymarin (flavonoid contained in artichokes) has long been thought to be useful as a benefit to people with liver disorders and as a protective compound against liver-damaging agents. Wild artichoke contains silymarin. In one study, a group of researchers pretreated rats and mice with a single dose of silymari`n isolated from artichokes. After introducing a liver toxin, they found that the silymarin completely

> *Apart from its culinary value, artichokes are packed with essential nutrients, vitamins, and minerals, making them a true powerhouse of nutrition.*

abolished the lethal effects and pathological changes, and significantly decreased the levels of serum enzymes normally induced by the toxin. These results, along with numerous other studies (see section on milk thistle), confirm, once again, silymarin's ability to protect the liver.

Recently, it has been found that globe artichokes contain the extract cymarin, which is similar to silymarin. Researchers discovered that this extract promotes liver regeneration and causes hyperaemia. It was also found that an artichoke extract caused dyspeptic symptoms to disappear. The researchers interpreted the reduction in cholinesterase levels to mean that the extract effected fatty degeneration of the liver. In another study, artichokes lowered lipids. In the 1940s, a series of experiments by Japanese, Swiss, and American researchers discovered that artichokes lowered blood cholesterol. Interestingly, in 1969 a team of French researchers patented an artichoke extract as a treatment for kidney and liver ailments.

As an interesting side note, the lead and mercury content of 20 species of edible vegetables collected in Spain was investigated. The researchers found that artichokes, along with tomatoes, cucumbers, and green beans, contained the lowest concentrations of lead and mercury, in comparison to "soft" vegetables such as lettuce, spinach, and parsley.

The artichoke is a highly versatile and intriguing plant that has been enjoyed for its delicious taste and numerous health benefits for centuries. Its distinctive appearance and delectable flavor make it a popular ingredient in the culinary world, while its medicinal properties have been recognized and valued by many. Apart from its culinary value, artichokes are packed with essential nutrients, vitamins, and minerals, making them a true powerhouse of nutrition. They are an excellent source of dietary fiber, which promotes healthy digestion and a strong gut. Artichokes are also rich in antioxidants, particularly cynarin, which helps to protect against free radicals.

In addition to their nutritional value, artichokes have been traditionally used in herbal medicine for their potential medicinal properties. They are believed to have diuretic and detoxifying effects that cleanse the body and support kidney function. Artichoke leaf extract has also been studied for its potential to aid in cholesterol regulation and support cardiovascular health. Furthermore, the mild soothing effect of artichokes on the digestive system has been used to relieve symptoms of indigestion and bloating.

ASHWAGANDHA
or "Indian Ginseng"
Withania somnifera

Parts used: Root. *In use for more than 2,500 years, this Indian shrub is proving to have adaptogenic properties, as described in ancient texts.*

TRADITIONAL USAGES

"The notion of resistance to disease and the idea that such resistance can be modified by life experience and by emotional states, forms one of the basic tenets of Ayurveda, the ancient Indian system of medicine, thus avoiding the Cartesian dichotomization of mind and body," writes Shibnath Ghosal concerning research on Ayurvedic medicines.

From antiquity to the present day, Ayurvedic medicine has employed a holistic approach to physical and mental well-being. Preserved through the ages on delicate manuscripts and scrolls, Ayurveda medicine retains a vital place in modern India. Used for more than 2,500 years, Ashwagandha is among several plants the renowned ancient texts say will, when taken with milk, oil, or water for 15 days, "impart strength for the emaciated body, as good as rain does to a crop."

Traditionally, the various preparations and forms of Ashwagandha, such as powder, decoction, oil, smoke, poultice, etc., have been utilized for a variety of conditions, including arthritis, asthma, bronchitis, cancer, candida, fever, inflammations, nausea, and rheumatism. However, its most important use is as a tonic to promote vigor and stamina.

RECENT SCIENTIFIC FINDINGS

Today's researchers continue to study and substantiate, through modern science, many traditional applications for Ayurvedic herbs. Over the last 40 years, an increasing number of studies have been conducted of Ashwagandha's constituents by scientists interested in the sedative and tranquilizing properties of Ashwagandha roots and the traditional uses of the plant in the treatment of numerous maladies. The result has been that a large number of compounds have been isolated. At present, Ashwagandha is known to contain 11 alkaloids, 35 with anolides, and several sitoindosides, a new

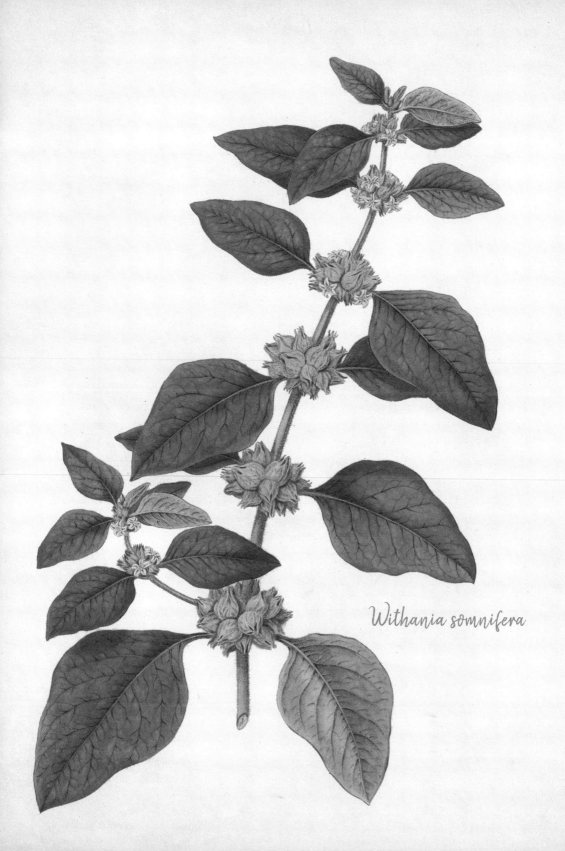

Withania somnifera

group of bioactive chemicals first isolated in the late 1980s. Yet even with all the high technology tools of modern analysis, the complexity of the plant and its constituents are not fully understood. Further studies are continuing to examine additional chemical constituents of this plant in an effort to explain and understand its unique actions.

An adaptogen is an agent that causes adaptive reactions. Adaptogenic drugs appear to increase SNIR (state of nonspecific increased resistance) in the human body, protecting against diverse stresses. Pharmacological research has shown that ashwagandha is effective for a variety of ailments, including leucoderma, bronchitis, asthma, and marasmus, and that it is also useful as a hypotensive, antispasmodic, antitumor, anti-arthritic, antipyretic, analgesic, anti-inflammatory, and antidiabetic. Because of its usefulness in diverse pathological states, it is reasonable to conclude that the herb acts by inducing SNIR in the human body.

Much of the research has concerned ashwagandha's antistress and anticancer properties. One study concluded that mice treated with ashwagandha exhibited better swimming performance, a standard means for assessing stress. The duration of swimming increased significantly in treated mice. The researchers also found ashwagandha reduced the incidence of gastric ulcers produced by high doses of aspirin and by physical stress. In a later study on albino mice, *Withania somnifera* was found to completely reverse the effects of urethane on total count, lymphocyte count, body weight, and mortality. It also afforded significant protection to the extent of 75% in the incidence as well as in the number of lung adenomas.

In studying the effects of two new sitoindosides derived from *Withania somnifera,* Ghosal found the compounds produced significant antistress activity in albino mice and rats and augmented learning acquisition and memory retention in young and old rats. These findings are consistent with the use of *W. somnifera* in Ayurveda to attenuate cerebral function deficits in the geriatric population and to provide nonspecific host defense. Ghosal concluded:

Pharmacologists have long sought a drug for the treatment of memory disorders, a drug which could enhance the acquisition, storage and retrieval of learning and memory. Most of the synthetic drugs (e.g., the nootropic agents) in use are psychostimulants which cause improved performance mainly due to improvement in attention by way of arousal induced by these agents and they have no significant effect on memory storage and retrieval. The present study suggests an opportunity for the improved use of this Ayurvedic 'Rasayan' *(Ashwa gandha)* for immunomodulation and for learning and memory.

Human studies have shown similar results. A 1965 study employed withaferin A, a compound extracted from ashwagandha leaves. Results demonstrated marked tumor-inhibitory activity when tested in vivo against cells derived from human carcinoma. In a double-blind trial conducted with children between the ages of 8 and 10, it was found that milk fortified with ashwagandha resulted in increased body weight and total protein.

In another double-blind clinical trial to study the process of aging, 101 healthy male adults between the ages of 50 and 59 were surveyed. After treatment for one year, statistically significant differences were found between the ashwagandha group and the placebo group in hemoglobin and serum cholesterol. The treated group exhibited significant increases in hemoglobin and red blood cell count. Serum cholesterol levels were much lower in the treated group. No side effects of the drug were observed.

This plant has also been shown to possess anti-inflammatory activity, making it useful for arthritis. In several animal studies, *W. somnifera* was proven to have more activity than four other herbs that were tested. Interestingly, these "others" are all respected as folkloric treatments for arthritis.

Ashwagandha's anti-arthritic activity was also demonstrated in a human clinical trial. An herbal formula consisting of ashwagandha, turmeric, and boswellin was evaluated in a randomized, double-blind, placebo-controlled study. After a one-month evaluation period, 12 patients with osteoarthritis were given the herbal formula or placebo for three months. The patients were evaluated every two weeks. Then after a 15-day wash-out period, the treatment was reversed with the placebo patients receiving the drug and vice versa. Again, results were evaluated over a three-month period. The patients treated with the herbal formula showed a significant drop in severity of pain and disability score.

As the concept of functional foods to reduce the incidence of various diseases becomes widespread in the United States, preventive herbal extracts such as ashwagandha will find a vital place among the diets of many Americans.

Commonly referred to as "Indian ginseng" or "winter cherry," ashwagandha is a small shrub that flourishes in arid regions. Ashwagandha has a rich history of traditional use as a rejuvenating and revitalizing herb. It is celebrated for its adaptogenic properties, which means it helps the body adapt to stressors and restore balance. One of the primary benefits of ashwagandha is its ability to support the body's stress response. It is said to help reduce the negative impact of stress on both the mind and body, promoting a sense of calm and relaxation. We believe this is achieved by modulating cortisol, the stress hormone. Ashwagandha reputedly aids to manage stress levels, enhance resilience, and improve overall mental well-being.

Ashwagandha is also renowned for its potential immune-boosting properties, helping the body defend against pathogens and external threats. Regular consumption of ashwagandha may enhance the body's natural defense mechanisms, reducing the risk of infections and supporting overall immune health. It is also recognized for its potential to improve cognitive function and promote mental clarity. It is believed to enhance memory, focus, and concentration, making it a valuable herb for those seeking to support their cognitive performance. We look forward to more studies in this vitally important area.

In addition to its adaptogen and immune-boosting properties, ashwagandha is valued for its potential benefits on physical performance and vitality. It is often used by athletes and fitness enthusiasts to support endurance, stamina, and muscle recovery. Ashwagandha may help increase energy levels, improve exercise performance, and reduce exercise-induced fatigue.

ASTRAGALUS
Astragalus membranaceus

Parts used: Root. *This traditional Chinese medicinal has yielded striking results in stimulating the immune system.*

TRADITIONAL USAGES

Astragalus is a commonly used traditional herb in Chinese medicine, where it is known as radix astragali, or used as part of a Chinese herbal known as "yellow leader." It is recognized for its importance as a tonic herb, and for centuries the Chinese have utilized astragalus to enhance natural defense mechanisms. Its use was first recorded in an herbal over 2,000 years ago. Astragalus is a tonic used to increase *ch'i* or "wind energy," overcome fatigue, control diabetes, lower blood pressure, and treat coronary heart disease and anemia.

RECENT SCIENTIFIC FINDINGS

Certain species of astragalus are the source of the widely used food additive tragacanth gum. *Astragalus membranaceus* has been screened for its immunomodulating activity and found to augment the proliferation of mononuclear (MNC) white blood cells (macrophages and lymphocytes) in vitro. Recent studies originating from the

MD Anderson Hospital and Tumor Institute in Houston, Texas, have yielded a stronger focus on the immunomodulating scope of *Astragalus membranaceous.*

As with many plant extracts, certain fractions may possess biological activities that are in direct contrast with those of other fractions. Doctors performed several extraction procedures and manipulations on air-dried roots of astragalus, ultimately producing eight different fractions, fraction 7 being the original crude extract. The authors used a testing model developed in their laboratory, designed to evaluate the competence of human T-lymphocytes in attacking foreign cells (rat skins). The animals were rendered immunosuppressed, due to the administration of cyclophosphamide, a potent immunosuppressive agent routinely used in human organ transplantation procedures. This minimized the influence of the animal's immune system upon the actions of the implanted human cells.

Individuals with various types of cancer and "normal" controls served as blood donors for the MNCs. MNCs were treated with one of the eight fractions derived from the original roots of astragalus. Fractions 2, 3, 7, and 8 displayed significant immunomodulating activity in cells from controls in this system. Fractions 3, 7 (the original crude extract) and all produced a significant increase in the immunocompetence of the animals. However, fraction 2 led to a further reduction of immune function, indicating this fraction to have immunorestorative effects.

The treatment of MNCs from cancer patients revealed additional striking result. Only fractions 3, 7, and 8 were used in this part of the study. Five of the 13 cancer patients' MNCs experienced immune restoration in their T-cell activity. The MNCs from the remaining eight patients had intact T-cell function before incubation with the fractions; following incubation T-cell function was actually increased.

The authors pointed out that the immune responsivity seen in most of the astragalus-treated cells from cancer patients was greater than that observed in the cells from untreated "normal" donors. Cancer patients' cells treated with fractions 3 and 8 displayed the greatest degree of immune restoration, being significantly greater than that of untreated normal control values. Treatment with fraction 7 did not produce a significantly greater response.

Comparison of the stimulating effects of fractions 3, 7, and 8 on MNCs from both cancer and normal donors revealed fraction 3 to possess a higher stimulating activity in cancer patients than in normal patients. No difference existed between the two groups for the other two fractions. Fraction 3 also proved to have superior immunorestorative actions in cancer patients alone, relative to the crude extract (7) and the extract derivative (8).

A companion study evaluated the ability of immunosupressed animals treated with fraction 3 to generate an immune response against untreated human MNCs. This is similar to a reversal of the previous experiments, where the animal T-cells are tested in their capacity to attack human T-cells. They found fraction 3 to completely reverse the effects of cyclophosphamide-induced immunosuppression upon their test system. Although fraction 3 was administered intravenously, it is very likely that oral administration of a carefully fractioned Astragalus preparation would also exert significant immunorestorative activity in such conditions as cancer and AIDS.

A third subfractionation was performed, using AR-4E as the parent fraction. This step produced four more subfractions (AR-4El to AR-4E4), with AR-4E2 having the greatest antitumor potential. This third-generation fraction was composed of 87% hexose-type sugars (e.g., galactose, arabinose, and rhamnose). The authors performed extensive analysis of the chemical properties of this latter fraction, leading them to conclude that the structure of the side chain of the polysaccharide fraction determines its antitumor activity, but not its anti-complementary activity.

These structure-activity relationship studies are crucial to the understanding of the specific component(s) responsible for the biological effects of a given plant extract and in the development of powerful plant drug extracts with a high degree of specificity. Reducing a plant extract to a single molecule or compound does indeed lead one into the world of conventional medicine, as many drugs currently used were once derived from plant sources. However, this process also provides a marker, or series of markers, whereby crude plant extracts can be objectively assessed for their content of active principles.

Several new studies focusing on the whole plant also demonstrate the immune-enhancing properties of this remarkable plant. Extracts of Astragalus injected into mice were seen to increase the T-cell activity in both normal and immunodepressed mice. Even an oral dose of an ethanol extract of the root of this herb was shown to alleviate liver injury that had been experimentally induced in mice and also to protect mouse liver cells from pathological changes.

Astragalus membranaceus

In a study of chronic cervicitis, it was found that this disorder was associated with three types of virus: papillomavirus type 16, herpes simplex virus type 2, and cytomegalovirus (CMV). Treatment with recombinant interferon alpha 1 improved clinical symptoms in 93.8% of cases. The study authors then added *A. membranaceus* to the therapy and concluded it was "synergistic to interferon therapy." Perhaps the future of medicine will show that a combination of ancient and modern therapies will offer the best hope for medical treatment.

Within the last 10 or 20 years, interest in *A. membranaceus* for immune enhancement has moved from its home (in China) to the U.S. and Japan. An Italian study found that astragalus extracts were immunostimulatory on mononuclear cells from normal healthy donors and cancer patients. The authors believe that the observed enhancement of Th cell activity results from increased induction of these Th cells, both in normal mice or immunodepressed mice. Perhaps most interestingly, the biological activity of astragalus extracts were found to depend on the carbohydrate content, lending support to the continued use of the whole plant in herbal medicine.

As we have illustrated, the astragalus plant, scientifically known as *Astragalus membranaceus*, is a remarkable herb deeply rooted in traditional Chinese medicine. Revered for its potent immune-boosting properties, this herb has gained widespread recognition for its ability to support overall health and well-being.

One of the key benefits of astragalus is its profound impact on the immune system. It is renowned in Chinese medicine for its ability to enhance immune function and promote a robust defense against infections and illnesses. Astragalus contains a variety of active compounds, such as polysaccharides and saponins, which stimulate and modulate the immune response. Regular consumption of astragalus might indeed help strengthen the immune system, reduce the frequency of infections, and promote overall immune health.

In addition to these reported immune-boosting properties, astragalus has been revered for its potential to support cardiovascular health. It is believed to have cardioprotective effects, helping to maintain healthy blood pressure levels and promote optimal heart function. Astragalus may also contribute to the management of cholesterol levels, thereby supporting a healthy cardiovascular system.

Astragalus has also been studied for its potential anti-inflammatory and antioxidant effects. The herb's active constituents have been shown to possess anti-inflammatory properties, which may help mitigate chronic inflammation and support overall wellness. The antioxidant compounds found in astragalus help protect the body against oxidative stress and damage caused by free radicals.

BARBERRY
Berberis vulgaris

Parts used: Root bark and berries. *Used by the ancient Egyptians, this plant is rich in the astringent berberine.*

TRADITIONAL USAGES

Barberry is noted throughout herbal literature for its important economic and medicinal properties. The ripe fruit is eaten as a preserve; the roots yield a yellow dye that at one time was utilized in the dyeing of wool, cotton, and flax.

In ancient Egyptian medicine, syrup of barberry combined with fennel seeds was reputedly of value in warding off the plague. This possibility is not to be laughed off since the ancient Hebrews relied on hops for the same purpose. Hops contain effective antibacterial principles and were in fact valuable against the infectious agent *Yersinia pestis,* the plague bacillus. In exploring the possible validity of barberry and fennel seed for the same purpose, we would have to evaluate potential antibacterial properties.

Soon after barberry's introduction to North America, several tribes employed it for medicinal purposes. The Penobscots of Maine pulverized the roots or bark in water and applied them to mouth ulcers or to relieve sore throat. The Catawbas drank a tea of the boiled roots and stems for stomach ulcers. Since barberry was employed in Europe for similar purposes, it is safe to assume that the Native Americans borrowed these uses from the early settlers.

The fruits of this shrub were formerly used in England to reduce fevers, while the bark was employed as a purgative and as a diarrhea treatment. During the early part of the 19th century, the acidic berries were also used in Egypt to reduce fevers. Throughout other traditional herbal literature we find patterns of usage surrounding high fevers, jaundice, and chronic dysentery.

RECENT SCIENTIFIC FINDINGS

The most credible medicinal uses are centered in the herb's strong purging effects and as a gargle for sore throats. While the root bark, rich in berberine, is used for the former effect, the barberry fruit itself is crushed for that latter; it also finds application as a mouthwash.

Barberry owes virtually all of its effects to its high content of the alkaloid berberine, which is present in all parts of the plant. Berberine, when applied externally, causes an astringent effect, and if placed in the eye will reduce the "bloodshot" appearance, since the blood vessels are constricted by the alkaloid. Due to the berberine, barberry berries would be useful as a mouthwash and gargle for their astringent effect and some local anesthetic effect. It has also been studied for its antimicrobial, anti-inflammatory, and antioxidant effects, making barberry a valuable herb for overall health.

If the correct amount is used, barberry roots will act as a purgative. Barberry root preparations are even more useful, however, to halt diarrhea. Such preparations are well established as effective in stopping diarrhea in cases of bacterial dysentery. Since berberine is not very well absorbed if taken by mouth, the risk of any possible toxic effects is reduced.

Barberry, scientifically known as *Berberis vulgaris*, is a versatile herb that has been valued for its medicinal properties and culinary uses throughout history. It has caught the attention of herbalists, chefs, and health-conscious individuals due to its striking appearance and numerous health benefits.

Berberis vulgaris

Barberry is particularly well-known for its traditional use in promoting digestive health. It has been used to stimulate appetite, improve digestion, and relieve gastrointestinal discomfort. The antimicrobial properties of barberry's berberine content may help combat harmful bacteria, parasites, and fungi in the digestive system.

Moreover, barberry is recognized for its potential to support liver health. It has traditionally been used to promote liver function and aid in the detoxification process. The antioxidant compounds found in barberry, including berberine, may help protect the liver from oxidative stress and enhance its ability to eliminate toxins.

Barberry has been studied for its potential cardiovascular benefits. It may help maintain healthy cholesterol levels and promote optimal heart function. Berberine's presence in barberry has been linked to its ability to support healthy blood pressure and improve lipid profiles.

BAYBERRY

Myrica cerifera

Parts used: Bark. *At one time the bark was a popular drug in domestic American medicine.*

TRADITIONAL USAGES

Bayberry bark was popular in domestic American medicine for its astringent and tonic properties. A decoction was used in cases of diarrhea, dysentery, dropsy, and uterine hemorrhage, and as a gargle for sore throat. A poultice was applied to sores and ulcers. The root bark was official in the *National Formulary* for only twenty years, from 1916 to 1936.

The wax that forms around the berries was also used medicinally. It was boiled "to an extract [as] a certain cure for the most violent cases of dysentery." Some physicians of the 18th century even considered this wax a narcotic!

Native American use of the plant was quite limited. Only one tribe, the Louisiana Choctaws, employed it as a fever remedy. They boiled the leaves and stems and drank the resulting tea.

RECENT SCIENTIFIC FINDINGS

Bayberry's use in modern medicine continues to be limited, as there are other more effective astringent and tonic herbs.

Interestingly, the extract has proven to be useful as an insect attractant, particularly for male Mediterranean fruit flies. Thus, it may become of importance as a natural means of controlling fruit fly infestations.

Bayberry has a long history of traditional use in herbal medicine, particularly among Native American tribes and early settlers. The bark of the bayberry plant is known for its astringent properties, which have been utilized to support various aspects of health.

One of the primary uses of bayberry is its potential to aid in respiratory health. It has been traditionally used to alleviate symptoms of congestion, coughs, and sore throats. Bayberry's astringent properties may help reduce excessive mucus production and provide relief from respiratory discomfort.

Furthermore, bayberry is valued for its potential as a digestive aid. It has been used to support healthy digestion, alleviate indigestion, and improve appetite. The astringent nature of bayberry may help tone the digestive system and promote proper functioning.

In addition to its respiratory and digestive benefits, bayberry has been studied for its potential antimicrobial and anti-inflammatory effects. It contains bioactive compounds, such as tannins and flavonoids, that may help combat harmful bacteria and reduce inflammation in the body.

Bayberry is also recognized as a natural adjunct for oral hygiene, as it may help reduce plaque formation, alleviate gum inflammation, and freshen breath.

BEARBERRY or Uva Ursi
Arctostaphylos uva-ursi

Parts used: Leaves. *The leaves of this evergreen shrub have a long history of use as a diuretic.*

TRADITIONAL USAGES

It appears that the medicinal properties of bearberry were discovered independently by Native Americans and white settlers. The Thompson tribe of British Columbia drank a tea of steeped bearberry leaves to promote the flow of urine and to strengthen the bladder and kidneys. The Menominees added the leaves to their menstrual remedies. The Cheyenne and Sioux used bearberry to promote labor contractions. The early fur traders of the Scottish Northwest Company reported that many tribes used the leaves with honey, pollen, and other herbs as a longevity elixir.

Although this evergreen shrub was used in ancient medicine, it was not popularly employed for kidney disorders until the mid-18th century. From that time on, bearberry leaf was a recognized diuretic. The *London Pharmacopoeia* admitted it in 1763, and it was included in the *U.S. Pharmacopoeia* from 1820 until 1936.

The strong astringent properties of the leaves have led to usage as a diuretic and tonic. Inflammation of the urinary tract, especially in

Arctostaphylos uva-ursi

acute cystitis, was formerly treated with a decoction of these leaves. (Patients were forewarned to expect a sharp greenish color of their urine during treatment.) Bearberry leaves, prior to the discovery of synthetic diuretic and urinary antiseptic drugs, were the major medicine available to physicians for these purposes.

RECENT SCIENTIFIC FINDINGS

We have known for a number of years that the diuretic, astringent, and urinary antiseptic value of bearberry leaves can be accounted for by the fact that they contain the active principles hydroquinone and arbutin. In the body, arbutin is rapidly converted to hydroquinone, which is what causes the harmless effect of changing the color of the urine.

A study examined the combined effect of arbutin isolated from bearberry leaves and indomethacin on immuno-inflammation, edema, and arthritis. When arbutin and indomethacin were administered simultaneously, the inhibitory effect was more potent than indomethacin alone. The authors stated that these results suggest that arbutin may increase the inhibitory action of indomethacin on edema and arthritis.

A similar 1990 series of studies by a Japanese research group employed a 50% methanolic extract from bearberry leaf with prednisolone to determine its effect on immuno-inflammation. Like the indomethacin research, the authors found that when simultaneously administered, the inhibitory effect was more potent than that of prednisolone alone. They also isolated arbutin from the methanolic extract and found similar results.

Additionally, bearberry leaves contain allantoin, a substance that is known to soothe and accelerate the repair of irritated tissues.

A liquid extract of bearberry given in the form of a chamomile tea was reported to be useful in the treatment of cystitis in paraplegics. Unlike nitrofurantoin, bearberry did not cause gastric irritation. Experiments conducted by Romanian scientists in 1980 proved bearberry exhibits antitrichomonal activity in in vitro tests. Current pharmacology indicates bearberry demonstrates antiviral (particularly strong against herpes and flu) and antibacterial action, enhances cytotoxic activity, and exhibits antifungal and antiplaque action.

A dietary study involving an herbal mixture containing bearberry, goldenseal, mistletoe, and tarragon found significant effects on the symptoms of diabetes without affecting glycemic control.

Bearberry is a remarkable plant found in North America, Europe, and Asia. This low-growing evergreen shrub has glossy leaves and vibrant red berries and has been treasured for centuries for its medicinal properties.

Bearberry has been utilized as a natural remedy for urinary tract infections and bladder-related issues. It contains arbutin, a compound believed to have antimicrobial properties that help combat harmful bacteria and maintain a healthy urinary tract.

Bearberry is also valued for its potential diuretic properties, which aid in flushing out toxins and reducing water retention. This makes it a popular herb for supporting kidney health and addressing mild edema. It has also been studied for its potential anti-inflammatory benefits. Its constituents have shown anti-inflammatory activity, which may help reduce inflammation in the urinary tract and other areas of the body.

BEE POLLEN
Entomophilous spp.

Parts used: Plant pollen collected by bees, mixed with honey and nectar, and then fermented in the hive. *Pollen extracts have been shown to increase stamina.*

TRADITIONAL USAGES

Pollen extracts are a highly concentrated energy source for protein and carbohydrates. They are often taken as a food supplement. Among athletes, pollen has a reputation for increasing stamina and, in general, improving athletic ability. More recently, in Eastern Europe and Russia, pollen has been used to treat a variety of ailments, including anemia, diarrhea, mental illness, obesity, rickets, and skin problems.

Royal jelly is the larval bee food produced from saliva of the honeybee *(Apis mellifera)*. It is the sole food of bee larvae for the first three days of life. It is also the continued food for the queen bee. This food is what causes queen bees to differentiate and develop. In folk medicine, royal jelly has been used as a youth enhancer, hair restorer, and fertility aid.

RECENT SCIENTIFIC FINDINGS

Animal studies of pollen extract have demonstrated remarkable lipid-lowering effects. Researchers found that rats fed an atherogenic (i.e., causes atherosclerosis) diet consisting of a high saturated fat content and concurrently fed pollen extract attained a lowered total cholesterol content and a rise in serum HDH cholesterol.

At Pratt Institute in New York, bee pollen was shown to improve endurance and speed. This finding was substantiated by a study in which four groups of rabbits were fed differing diets. (The rabbit was chosen by this group of Polish scientists owing to

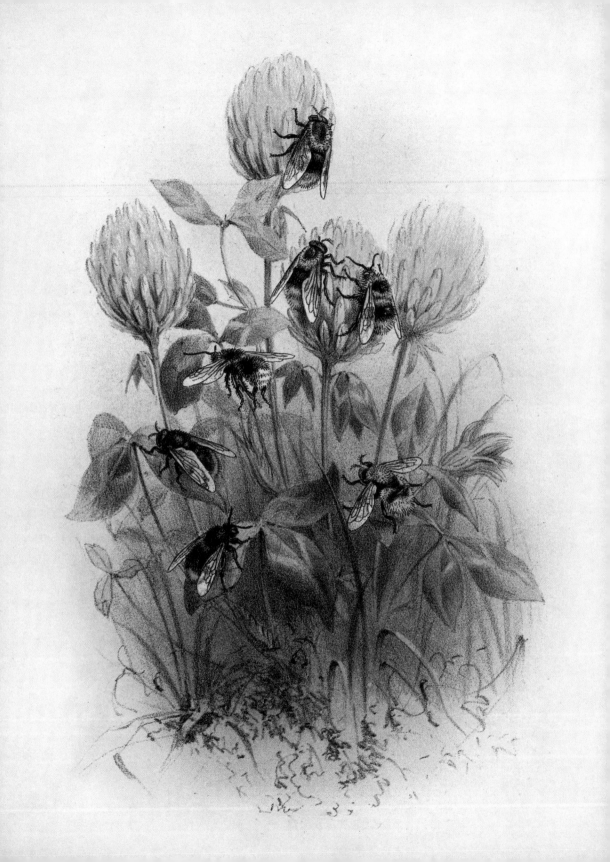

Bee pollen, a natural superfood created by honeybees from collected pollen grains, may work similarly to anti-inflammatory drugs by relieving inflammation.

its susceptibility to atherosclerosis and its similarity to man in bile acid metabolism. While I strongly *oppose* most animal experimentation, we feel it would be a double tragedy *not* to report on valuable work already completed.)

The study showed that the pollen extracts not only significantly lowered blood lipid levels, but they also suppressed the development of atherosclerotic plaque formation.

These effects are thought to be due to the known constituents of pollen extract, such as polyunsaturated fatty acids (23% linolenic acid) and sterols, 21 amino acids, all known vitamins, enzymes and coenzymes, minerals, and trace elements. The researchers utilized a pollen extract that is a trademarked product derived from six plant species: rye grass, maize, timothy grass, pine, alder flower, and orchard grass. These extracts (Cernitin T60 and Cernitin GBX, also known in the industry by the names AB Cernelle, Vegeholm, Sweden) are uniquely treated. Pollen grains have their membranes removed with a solvent and are then flushed out through the hila. The solvent is later removed, and the pollen extract digested microbiologically. This process transforms the difficult to absorb high-molecular weight material to low-molecular weight substances that are easily absorbed in the GI tract. Because the final product is free of antigens and other high-molecular weight substances, it ought not produce allergic reactions in humans.

There has been no evidence to support the folkloric uses of royal jelly. However, it has exhibited anti-inflammatory action and analgesic activity in mice and rat experiments.

In regard to allergy, an interesting 1991 paper proposed that mammals evolved allergic reactions "as a last line of defense against the extensive array of toxic substances that exist in the environment in the form of secondary plant compounds and venoms." The authors stated that allergic responses, such as sneezing, coughing, diarrhea, and scratching, help the body expel the toxic substance that triggered the response. Since toxic substances also bind to the DNA of target cells, they are potentially mutagenic and carcinogenic as well. Thus, by protecting against acute toxicity, allergies may also defend against mutagens and carcinogens. This fascinating hypothesis explains why allergies occur to many foods, pollens, etc.; why allergic cross-reactions occur to allergens from unrelated botanical families; why allergies appear to be so capricious and variable; and why allergies are more prevalent in industrial societies.

Bee pollen, a natural superfood created by honeybees from collected pollen grains, may work similarly to anti-inflammatory drugs by relieving inflammation. It acts as an antioxidant, is thought to boost liver health, strengthens the immune system, eases menopause symptoms, reduces stress, and helps speed up the healing process. Due to its dense nutrient composition, bee pollen is often referred to as nature's nutritional powerhouse and provides a concentrated source of nourishment for the body. It is rich in vitamins, minerals, enzymes, amino acids, antioxidants, and phytonutrients.

Caution: People with pollen-sensitive allergies may find bee pollen aggravating.

BILBERRY
Vaccinium myrtillus

Parts used: Fruit. *Modern research is finding a variety of promising applications, including for atherosclerosis and ulcers.*

TRADITIONAL USAGES
Traditionally, both the leaves and berries of this shrub have been used as an astringent. A decoction of the berries was employed for fevers. The juice of the berries was used as a gargle and mouthwash for catarrh.

RECENT SCIENTIFIC FINDINGS
Extracts of bilberry have been found to be antiviral in cell cultures for herpes simplex virus II, influenza, and vaccinia viruses. In vitro testing of bilberry extracts for antimicrobial activity is encouraging. Extracts have been found to kill or inhibit growth of fungi, yeasts, and bacteria. They have also been shown to kill protozoans such as *Trichomonas vaginalis.* Anthocyanins in bilberry act to prevent capillary fragility and inhibit platelet aggregation. Bilberry is therefore demonstrated to be an anti-inflammatory herb. Anthocyanins stimulate the release of vasodilator prostaglandin in vitro. These compounds, therefore, have potential for the prevention of thrombosis. They also cause coronary vasodilation in animals, which would reverse attacks of angina. Moreover, they prevent atherosclerosis in cholesterol-loaded animals.

Since bilberry extracts reduce capillary permeability, there is antihistamine activity, too. Many clinical tests have shown that bilberry anthocyanosides given orally to humans improve vision in healthy people and also help treat people with eye diseases such as pigmentary retinitis.

Toxicology reports are especially promising regarding the anthocyanins. Tests in rats, mice, and rabbits showed no abnormalities or toxicity. Even pregnant women who were given extracts of bilberry (and vitamin E) were seen to have fewer varices and various blood problems. The study author concluded that the extract "was well tolerated and no side effects were found in either the mother or the infant."

A 1988 research project indicated that one bilberry extract possesses a promising anti-ulcer activity. The researchers speculated this was probably due to the extract potentiating the defensive barriers of the gastrointestinal mucosa. In experiments with rats, bilberry proved to exert a significant preventive and curative anti-ulcer activity.

Bilberry extracts have been found to have anticancer activity with certain cancer cell strains in laboratory tests.

Bilberry extracts administered in controlled experiments, conducted with people suffering from diabetes, exhibited resulting normalization of capillary collagen thickness and reduced blood sugar levels in humans and animals.

Royal Air Force (RAF) pilots in World War II, who reported improved night vision after consuming bilberry jam before their missions, theoretically enabling them to hit their targets more effectively, sparked scientific research into the herb's benefits for eye ailments. This research continues to this day.

The phytochemicals anthocyanosides are in high quantity in bilberry extract. The anthocyanosides are responsible for the regeneration of rhodopsin, a purple pigment in the eye that is responsible for night vision. In 2005, Russian scientists conducted a rat study that proved conclusively that

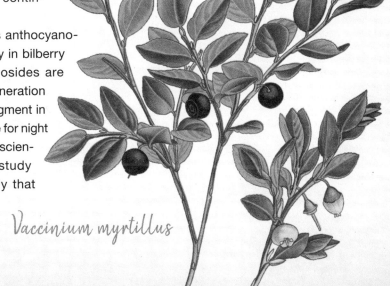

Vaccinium myrtillus

"bilberries pose a viable complement in the venue of treating ocular disease and conditions." These rats were fed very high doses of bilberry extract composing 25% of their diet. This lends credence to the RAF pilot claims.

Further, the anthocyanins in bilberry are powerful free radical scavengers. The result is protecting cells from oxidative stress and neutralizing free radicals, which cause cellular damage.

More research is needed; however, there is much interest in bilberry for heart health, specifically its use to prevent oxidation of LDL cholesterol, which is a major risk factor for atherosclerosis.

Bilberry contains vitamins E, C, and K. Minerals contained are copper, manganese, calcium, phosphorus, and iron.

BIRCH
Betula spp.

Parts used: Leaves and bark. *This tree's marvelous bark was once a common remedy.*

TRADITIONAL USAGES
This tree's beautiful distinctive bark was commonly boiled and used as a poultice for minor wounds. The leaves and bark, both separately and together, were steeped to make a tea drunk for a variety of ailments, including fevers, rheumatism, and abdominal complaints. A tea from the boiled fruit was used during menstruation. The smoke from the burning fruit was inhaled to treat respiratory problems. White settlers also used birch as a mouthwash and to treat intestinal worms. Indeed, in some regions of the U.S. the twigs are still chewed as a dentifrice.

RECENT SCIENTIFIC FINDINGS
Unfortunately, there is little research to confirm or deny birch's folkloric claims. Birch contains methyl salicylate, which is often used in ointments and liniments for conditions such as rheumatism.

Birch trees are naturally found in Europe and some parts of Asia. The tree's leaves, bark, and buds are commonly used for medicinal purposes. Birch has been known to help with joint pain, kidney stones, bladder stones, urinary tract infections (UTIs), and other health conditions. Birch oil was also touted for treating rheumatism, arthritis, calcium spurs, heart and kidney edema, and chronic cystitis, as well as for treating high cholesterol. Additionally, the astringent properties of birch make it effective in treating skin eruptions and wet eczema. This is due no doubt mainly to the constituent mentyl salicylate as an external ointment.

BLESSED THISTLE

Cnicus benedictus

Parts used: Herb. *Human experiments have confirmed this herb's folkloric use as a gastrointestinal remedy.*

TRADITIONAL USAGES

Blessed thistle has been recorded as a medicinal since the first century A.D. Credited with the medical virtues of a diuretic, diaphoretic, febrifuge, and cholagogue, it has been used to treat a variety of ailments. It is a bitter tonic and a good appetite stimulant and is still utilized today to treat indigestion. At one time this herb was ascribed the nearly supernatural qualities of a "cure all." The Zuni used blessed thistle to treat venereal disease and to lower fever.

Blessed thistle was considered an excellent appetite stimulant. It was also taken to relieve flatulence and indigestion, as well as to treat liver and gallbladder disorders.

RECENT SCIENTIFIC FINDINGS

Although this herb, at one time, was considered a "cure all," current knowledge yields no evidence to support such a belief. On the other hand, the use of leaf decoctions as a bitter tonic is well founded. The bitter principle in this plant is known to be cnicin, and human experiments have shown that extracts of blessed thistle stimulate the production of gastric juices, confirming its folkloric use as a gastrointestinal aid.

Cell cultures have shown cytotoxicity against cancer cells using extract of blessed thistle and antitumor activity in mouse cancer (sarcoma) as well.

In vitro studies with extracts of blessed thistle have shown considerable antibacterial activity against a wide variety of organisms, including *Mycobacterium phlei.* Anti-yeast activity against *Candida albicans* has been found in vitro using extract of blessed thistle.

Blessed thistle is a type of herb that is known to stimulate the production of bile, which helps detoxify the liver. This can lead to a reduction in symptoms associated with poor liver function, such as fatigue, loss of appetite, nausea, and brain fog. Additionally, this herb can also help stimulate the production of gastric juices and saliva, which can improve digestion and reduce cholesterol, ultimately helping to prevent gallstones. Blessed thistle is also rich in sesquiterpene lactones, such as cnicin, which can help increase the secretion of digestive enzymes, leading to improved digestion and appetite. Studies have also shown that two compounds present in blessed thistle, polyacetylene and cnicin, can help fight bacterial infections. This herb also has anti-inflammatory properties and can help remedy infections. Additionally, blessed thistle is known to stimulate milk supply.

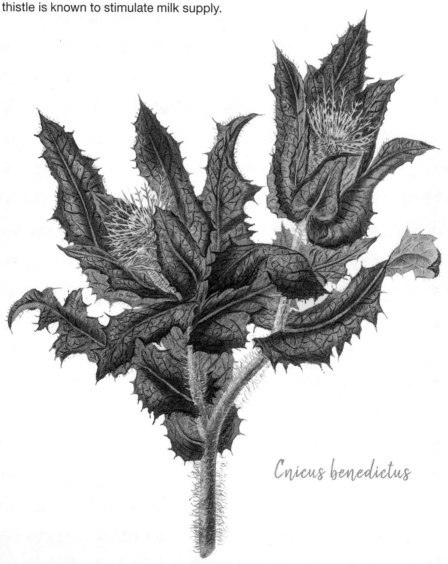

Cnicus benedictus

BLOODROOT
Sanguinaria canadensis

Parts used: Root. *Once a common Native American medicine for rheumatism, this root's alkaloid extract prevents cavities and plaque.*

TRADITIONAL USAGES

Bloodroot owes its name to the red juice in the roots and stems, which was used as a facial dye by North American tribes. Among Native Americans of the Mississippi region, bloodroot was a favorite remedy for rheumatism. The Rappahannocks of Virginia also made a tea from the root that they drank for rheumatism.

The Iroquois used bloodroot to treat ringworm. The Pillager Ojibwas squeezed the root juices on a piece of maple sugar and held the astringent lump in their mouth to cure sore throat.

Bloodroot became popular in domestic American medicine for its ability to remove mucus from the respiratory mucous membranes and was official in the *U.S. Pharmacopoeia* from 1820 to 1926. A powder was also applied externally to skin eruptions, nose polyps, ulcers, and badly healing sores.

RECENT SCIENTIFIC FINDINGS

An aero-narcotic poison on overdose, the plant has been reported to cause death. It is one of the 27 plants included in the USFDA unsafe herb list, published in March 1977.

Bloodroot contains tormentil, which contains high amounts of tannic acid, explaining the plant's astringent properties. The root is emetic and purgative in large doses; in smaller doses it is a stimulant, diaphoretic, and expectorant.

Experimentally, bloodroot preparations are known to induce emesis, have expectorant properties, and be an irritant. These activities are all due to the presence of the toxic alkaloid sanguinarine. Topically, sanguinarine and/or bloodroot preparations have been helpful in the treatment of eczema and most probably would give a mild local anesthetic effect. Mausertre commends an external application of the powder for nose polyps, ulcers, and bad sores, stating that it encourages new and healthy tissues.

Several recent studies, including a long-term clinical evaluation, have found that an extract of bloodroot in toothpaste and mouth rinses helped prevent cavities and destroy plaque.

It is a very powerful plant and we do not recommend its use internally. It may also cause skin irritations when topically applied.

Bloodroot is a fascinating herbaceous perennial plant that holds both medicinal and cultural significance. With its vibrant flowers and potent properties, bloodroot has been used for centuries in traditional medicine and herbal remedies.

One of the primary uses of bloodroot is as a topical remedy. The sap of bloodroot contains several bioactive compounds, including alkaloids such as sanguinarine, which have demonstrated antimicrobial and anti-inflammatory properties. Bloodroot preparations have been applied topically to address skin conditions such as warts, skin tags, and fungal infections. However, bloodroot can be highly potent and may cause skin irritation if not used properly.

Bloodroot has also been valued for its potential in supporting oral health. The antimicrobial properties of its constituents may help combat oral bacteria and contribute to maintaining a healthy mouth. Historically, bloodroot has been used in oral care products, such as toothpaste and mouthwash, for its potential to promote gum health and freshen breath.

Sanguinaria canadensis

In addition to its topical and oral uses, bloodroot has been studied for its potential anti-inflammatory and antioxidant effects. These properties may contribute to its traditional use in supporting respiratory health and soothing coughs. Bloodroot has also been explored for its potential in supporting cardiovascular health and promoting normal blood flow.

BONESET
Eupatorium perfoliatum

Parts used: Tops and leaves. *In the late 19th century, this plant was extensively used in American medical practice.*

TRADITIONAL USAGES

Boneset was a favorite remedy of North American tribes. The Menominees used it to reduce fever, the Iroquois and Mohegans for fever and colds, the Alabamas for upset stomachs, and the Creeks for body pain. Among settlers, boneset soon became a very popular remedy for fever and colds; it was in use at least 100 years before it was listed in any American medical text. In 1887, Dr. Charles Millspaugh wrote, "There is probably no plant in American domestic practice that has more extensive or frequent use than this [boneset]."

The plant derives its common name from its usefulness in treating a kind of influenza prevalent in the United States in the 19th century known as "break-bone fever," which was characterized by pains that felt as if all the bones of the body were broken. The plant has also been used in the treatment of intermittent fevers, although its action was acknowledged to be inferior to that of quinine. As a mild tonic, it was given in cases of dyspepsia and as an aid to indigestion in the elderly. Boneset is said to act as a mild tonic and diaphoretic in moderate doses and as an emetic and purgative in larger doses. Drunk as hot as possible, it was given to induce vomiting and the evacuation of the bowels; when drunk at warm temperature, the action was somewhat milder, producing increased perspiration and somewhat later a mild evacuation of the bowels. Boneset's ability to produce perspiration made it useful in catarrhal conditions, especially influenza; the administration of a warm infusion would produce perspiration and sometimes vomiting, often arresting the complaint. Of this numerous genus, comprising not less than 30 species within the limits of the United States, most of which probably possess analogous medical properties, three have found a place in the *Pharmacopoeia* of the United States: *E. perfoliatum, E. teucrifolim,* and *E. purpureum*, the first in the primary, the last two in the secondary list. *E. cannabinum* of Europe, the root of which was formerly used as a purgative, and *E. Aya-pana* of Brazil, the leaves of which at one time enjoyed a very high reputation as a remedy for numerous diseases, have fallen out of use.

RECENT SCIENTIFIC FINDINGS

The leaves contain several sesquiterpene lactones that stimulate the appetite. In sufficient amounts, they would have anthelmintic effects. Toxic relatives of boneset, such as white snakeroot *(E. rugosum)* have been responsible for numerous cases of agricultural animal poisonings, as well as human poisonings.

Researchers experimenting with a sesquiterpene lactone from boneset, EVP, concluded that EVP may possess antitumor activity in vivo.

Boneset is a remarkable herbaceous perennial plant renowned for its historical use in supporting whole body health. With its unique

Eupatorium perfoliatum

appearance and potential medicinal benefits, boneset has captured the attention of herbalists and individuals seeking natural remedies.

Eupatorium perfoliatum is native to North America and can be found growing in wetlands, meadows, and woodland areas. It derives its common name from its historical use in treating dengue fever. Dengue is known as "break-bone fever," due to the severe joint and bone pain associated with the illness. It is unfortunately making a comeback.

In traditional folk medicine, boneset is used to address symptoms associated with viral infections and fevers, including colds, flu, and respiratory ailments. Boneset contains bioactive compounds, such as sesquiterpene lactones and polysaccharides, which may help promote overall immune health.

Boneset is also recognized for its potential diaphoretic properties, meaning it can induce sweating. Sweating is considered a natural mechanism for cooling down the body and eliminating toxins. Traditionally, boneset has been used to help break fevers and promote sweating to support the body's natural healing process.

Furthermore, boneset has been studied for its potential anti-inflammatory effects. Its constituents may help reduce inflammation and alleviate pain associated with conditions such as arthritis and muscle aches.

BOSWELLIN
Boswellia serrata

Parts used: Gum resin. *Known as Indian frankincense, a purified compound from its gum resin has been found to have beneficial effects on rheumatic disorders.*

TRADITIONAL USAGES

There are many medicinal plants of great therapeutic value referred to in the ancient treatment systems of Ayurveda. The two important Ayurveda treatises, *Sushruta Samhita* and *Charaka Samhita,* describe the antirheumatic activity of guggul (gum resins of certain trees), especially those of the tree *Boswellia serrata,* whose extract the ancients claimed to have potent anti-inflammatory and anti-arthritic properties.

Boswellia serrata is a moderate to large branching tree generally found in dry hilly areas of India. The tree exudes a gummy oleo-resin when it is tapped by scraping away a portion of the bark. The chemical constituents of the gum resin include essential oils, terpenoids, and gum. Also known as Indian frankincense, *Boswellia serrata*'s essential

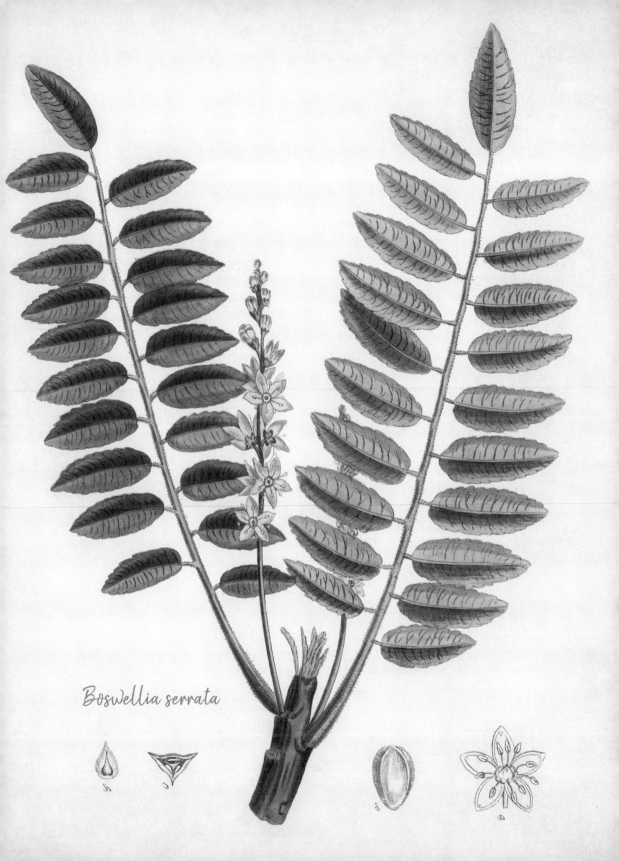

Boswellia serrata

oil is an ingredient in many Oriental perfumes and is closely related to the incense of Biblical renown. Along with its aromatic properties, the gummy exudate is lauded by the Ayurvedic texts as a remedy for diarrhea, dysentery, pulmonary diseases, boils, ringworm, and other afflictions, as well as rheumatoid arthritis.

RECENT SCIENTIFIC FINDINGS

To verify the Ayurvedic claims, the Regional Research Laboratory in India undertook a series of studies. The researchers hoped "to discover herbal-based anti-inflammatory products having beneficial effects on rheumatic diseases without any adverse and undesirable side effects." Rheumatic disorders affect people throughout the world and are a major cause of disability. It is not usually possible to cure the disease. However, through proper treatment, it is possible to alleviate pain, prevent further tissue injury, and increase mobility.

By means of a chemical process of defattening and extracting, the Indian researchers derived a purified compound from the gum resin exudate of *Boswellia serrata.* The researchers found this extract to be more beneficial, less toxic, and more potent than the standard "drug of choice," ketoprofen (benzoyl hydrotropic acid). In turn, ketoprofen is preferred over other anti-inflammatories such as indomethacin, phenylbutazone, or acetylsalicylic acid.

Researchers concluded that boswellic acids (BAs), as nonsteroidal, anti-inflammatory agents, are beneficial because they suppress the proliferating tissue found in inflamed areas and also prevent the breakdown of connective tissue. "It appears from the experimental studies done so far that it acts by a mechanism similar to nonsteroidal groups of anti-arthritic drugs with the added advantages of its being free from side effects and gastric irritation and ulcerogenic activity."

Because of the success of these studies, Indian authorities approved the marketing of a product made from the purified compound under the trade name Sallaki. Since then, in several other acute and chronic experimental test models of inflammation, *Boswellia serrata* has shown potent anti-inflammatory and anti-arthritic activity. In animal studies, Boswellin was also seen to promote a reduced rate of body weight loss associated with inflammatory disorders, to reduce secondary lesions, and to be free from any effect on the central nervous system and cardiovascular system. In human studies, Boswellin has been found to improve blood supply to the joints and restore integrity of vessels weakened by spasm. In one clinical trial conducted for four weeks on early cases of osteoarthritis of the knee, 26 patients showed a good response. The researchers concluded, "If the drug had been continued for a longer period, they would have shown excellent results." In another clinical trial in the orthopedic department of Government Medical College, Jammu, India, 122 out of 175 rheumatoid arthritis patients who were either bedridden or incapacitated from doing normal work and suffered from morning stiffness showed an abatement of symptoms two to four weeks after the initiation of therapy. None of these patients complained of any undesirable side effect. The authors concluded, "All these patients were happier with this therapy than with any other drugs given previously."

Boswellin's anti-arthritic properties were demonstrated in a human clinical trial. An herbal formula consisting of Boswellin, ashwagandha, and turmeric was evaluated in a randomized, double-blind, placebo-controlled study. After a one-month evaluation period, 12 patients with osteoarthritis were given the herbal formula or placebo for three months. The patients were evaluated every two weeks. Then after a 15-day wash-out period, the treatment was reversed with the placebo patients receiving the drug and vice versa. Again, results were evaluated over a three-month period. The patients treated with the herbal formula showed a significant drop in severity of pain and disability score.

Boswellia serrata is proving to be a potent addition to the drugs physicians may use to deal with rheumatoid arthritis. And, as the Regional Research Laboratory researchers concluded, physicians "may in due course be convinced of its superiority over the conventional drugs as it is a plant product being used since the ages and is absolutely free from any toxic and side effects."

BROOM
Sarothamnus scoparius

Parts used: Tops and seeds. *This beautiful shrub contains an alkaloid that appears to regulate the heart.*

TRADITIONAL USAGES

This familiar and beautiful shrub is a plant of many uses. The seeds, dried and roasted, have been used as a coffee substitute. The twigs have been employed as a fiber, to make brooms, and as a substitute for jute.

Medicinally, broom was used for urinary tract disorders, especially in cases where urination is scanty or painful. It was also employed to increase the flow of urine in dropsical conditions and relieve bladder spasms. It was believed to have a tonic effect on the heart.

RECENT SCIENTIFIC FINDINGS

Collected before blooming, the flowering tops are a source of sparteine sulfate. The medicinal action of the plant, which has a most disagreeable taste in decoction, is diuretic and cathartic, while it is emetic in large doses. It has been especially valued in treating dropsical conditions, particularly those associated with heart diseases, as it is efficacious in acting on the kidneys to produce urine flow. Because of its action on the kidneys, it is contraindicated in acute renal disease.

Recent research has uncovered possible effects on heart arrhythmia. Since broom contains no glycosides, it is not one of the plants with digitalis properties (such as foxglove). Instead, broom contains sparteine, an alkaloid that appears to regulate the action of the heart.

Traditionally, broom has been used as a diuretic and a mild laxative. It has been employed to support kidney and bladder health, aiding in the elimination of excess fluid and waste from the body. Broom is believed to stimulate urine production and promote the removal of toxins, which may be beneficial for individuals with water retention or mild edema.

Broom has also been utilized for its cardiotonic properties. It has been suggested that certain compounds present in broom may help strengthen and regulate heart function.

People taking kidney or blood pressure medication should speak to their doctor before taking broom or butcher's broom, as it may interact with these medicines.

BUCHU

Agathosma betulina, A. crenulata (Plant family: *Rutaceae*)

Parts used: Leaves. *Used for centuries in South Africa, the leaves are rich in volatile oils.*

TRADITIONAL USAGES

Buchu has been used in South Africa since long before colonization. Its name is a Hottentot word. These native South Africans used the dried leaves for various urinary disorders. Early in the 1800s, the leaves' medicinal qualities were introduced in Europe. In South Africa, buchu is still commonly employed as a tincture for a variety of ailments, especially urinary, kidney, and prostate problems.

Buchu was used to relieve catarrhal conditions and inflammation in the kidneys and cramps in the bladder. It has also been recommended for kidney and bladder stones. Its soothing and strengthening effect on the urinary organs has been highly praised.

RECENT SCIENTIFIC FINDINGS

Buchu is one of the best and most useful herbs in urinary tract diseases that are coupled with increased uric acid. Its effect is due to its volatile oils, including limonene and diosphenol (a phenolic ketone), as well as glycosides and flavonoids, which all contribute to its reputed medicinal properties.

Buchu is not as strong as some diuretics but is sometimes blended in conjunction with stronger agents due to buchu's overall effects and restorative properties. Several proprietary drugs commonly used in South Africa for urinary disorders still contain buchu leaves as a major ingredient.

The leaves of the buchu plant are the most commonly used part and are known for their strong aromatic scent.

Buchu has traditionally been used as a diuretic and urinary antiseptic. It is believed to have a cleansing and soothing effect on the urinary system, helping to alleviate symptoms of urinary tract infections, cystitis, and inflammation. It is also thought to assist in flushing out toxins and impurities from the body.

Agathosma betulina

In addition to its urinary tract benefits, buchu has been employed as a digestive aid. It has been used to relieve stomach discomfort, bloating, and indigestion. Buchu is thought to possess mild antispasmodic and anti-inflammatory properties, which may help soothe the digestive system and promote healthy digestion.

BUCKBEAN
Menyanthes trifoliata

Parts used: Leaves, root, and rhizome. *At one time, this plant was considered a panacea in Western European countries.*

TRADITIONAL USAGES

The buckbean, or marsh trefoil, was formerly considered a medicinal of great value in Europe, and in some countries it was regarded practically as a panacea. According to strength and dosage, its action ranges from that of a bitter tonic and cathartic all the way to purgative and emetic effects. In earlier times, buckbean was employed in the treatment of dropsy, catarrh, scabies, and fever. Early modern physicians used the plant for rheumatic complaints and skin diseases, and also to reduce fever. Buckbean is also reportedly excellent for relieving gas and excess stomach acid.

In domestic American medicine, a tonic was prepared consisting of 1.3 to 2.0 grams of the powdered leaves or root. While all parts of the plant are medicinally active, only the leaves were officially listed in the *U.S. Pharmacopoeia* from 1820 and 1842 and in the *National Formulary* from 1916 to 1926.

RECENT SCIENTIFIC FINDINGS

This perennial herb contains a bitter glucoside, menyanthin. Due to its tart taste, it is an ingredient in beer (Scandinavia) and is also a substitute for tea. Buckbean leaves contain a number of alkaloids, especially gentianine and gentianadine. In animals, gentianine shows analgesic and tranquilizing effects; gentianadine lowers blood pressure and has significant anti-inflammatory activity.

One of the primary traditional uses of buckbean is as a bitter tonic. The plant's bitter compounds stimulate the digestive system, promoting the production of digestive enzymes and enhancing appetite. It has been used to alleviate digestive complaints such as indigestion, bloating, and loss of appetite.

Some studies have suggested that certain compounds found in buckbean may exhibit antimicrobial activity against certain bacteria and fungi.

BUCKTHORN

Rhamnus cathartica, R. frangula

Parts used: Bark and berries. *Buckthorn has been used since the Middle Ages, and research reveals that extracts of it may have antiviral properties.*

TRADITIONAL USAGES

Esteemed for its purgative powers, the freshly powdered bark of buckthorn is highly irritating to the gastrointestinal mucous membrane, causing violent catharsis coupled with vomiting and pain. The dried bark is much milder. Buckthorn has been utilized as a medicinal since the Middle Ages, when it was called waythorn or hartsthorn. It appeared in the *London Pharmacopoeia* in 1650.

The tribes of southern Vancouver Island prepared a decoction from the bark to treat digestive tract ailments. A European variety (*R. bulbosus*) was official in the *U.S. Pharmacopoeia* from 1820 to 1882. It was used as a counterirritant and to promote blistering of pimples. In 1887, a report stated that "violent attacks of epilepsy are recorded

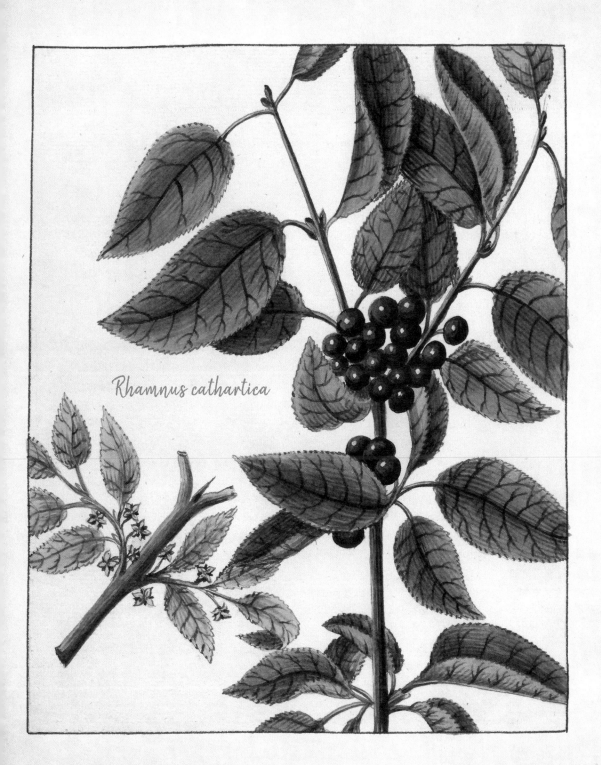

Rhamnus cathartica

as having been induced by this plant, a sailor who inhaled the fumes of the burning plant was attacked with this disease for the first time in his life, it returned again in two weeks, passed into cachexia, nodous gout, headache, and terminated in death." Interestingly, a related species (*R. acris*) was crushed and the vapor inhaled as a cure for headaches by the Montagnais of Newfoundland and Nova Scotia.

RECENT SCIENTIFIC FINDINGS

The berries of *Rhamnus cathartica* are known to contain anthraquinone glycosides, which are responsible for the cathartic effect attributed to them. Similarly, buckthorn bark (*R. frangula*) is used widely in Europe as a cathartic in the same way that *R. purshiana* (cascara sagrada) is utilized in North America. The active principles in buckthorn bark and cascara sagrada bark are similar, with buckthorn the mildest anthraquinone herb and cascara the next mildest. For additional information, see the entry for cascara sagrada.

Buckthorn extract has been found to kill several species of fungi, including *Aspergillus*, *Trichophyton*, and *Fusarium*. In some studies, external applications of buckthorn extract were found to be active against herpes simplex virus I and II in adult humans. In cell culture, buckthorn extract was found to be an antiviral agent against influenza virus A2 and vaccinia virus. Moreover, in cell cultures, it was found to have cytotoxic activity toward HELA cancer cells.

In a 1991 study, the authors found that aqueous extracts from buckthorn showed significant activity against staphylococcus and candida. Antitumor activity of buckthorn extract was found in mice with sarcoma 37 and leukemia P388. Another study found that an extract of buckthorn lowered arterial blood pressure in rats.

Buckthorn has been traditionally used as a natural laxative due to its cathartic properties. The bark, leaves, and berries contain anthraquinone compounds, such as emodin and frangulin, which have a stimulating effect on the intestines. These compounds can help promote bowel movements and relieve constipation. Care must be used as this can be highly purgative in too high dosages.

Aside from its laxative effects, buckthorn has also been used in traditional medicine for other purposes. It has been employed to support liver and gallbladder health. Some studies suggest that certain components of buckthorn may have hepatoprotective properties and help with liver detoxification processes.

It is important to exercise caution when using buckthorn as an herbal remedy. The plant contains compounds that may cause cramping, diarrhea, and electrolyte imbalances if consumed in excessive amounts.

More research needs to be done in the areas that have shown promise.

BUPLEURUM or Chai Hu

Bupleurum falcatum, B. chinense, B. longiradiatum

Parts used: Root. *Long an integral part of Oriental medicine, a mixture containing the root shows promise as an adaptogen and in treating Alzheimer's disease.*

TRADITIONAL USAGES

Also known as hare's ear, chai hu is the dried root of certain members of the Umbelliferae family. Traditionally, the species used have been *B. chinense* in China, *B. falcatum* in Japan, and *B. longiradiatum* in Korea.

In Oriental traditional medicine, certain herbal mixtures containing the plant have long been used for the treatment of chronic inflammatory and autoimmune diseases, as well as the management of certain neurological disorders. Bupleurum is classified as sudorific, meaning it was used to dispel and disperse "surface" problems.

Bupleurum was given to treat malaria, as well as for blackwater fever and as a liver "sedative."

RECENT SCIENTIFIC FINDINGS

Stress can be of a nonspecific origin or can involve specific physical or psychological factors capable of producing a disease state. The ability of stress to cause disease may be related to its suppression of the immune system. Numerous plant extracts have been described as having powerful antistress activity (adaptogenic).

Shosaikoto is an extract containing *Bupleurum falcatum*. The extract also includes *Pinellia ternata* (21%), *Scutellaria baicalensis*, *Zizyphus vulgaris*, Korean ginseng (12.5% each), licorice root (8%), and ginger root (4%). Experiments have found that shosaikoto possesses immunomodulating activity, stimulating immune cell activity in immunesuppressed or normal mice, and suppressing immune responsivity in hyperimmune rats.

Recent studies have evaluated the effect of shosaikoto on stress-induced immunosuppression in mice. It was found that shosaikoto stimulated the pituitary-adrenal cortex axis, leading to elevations in blood corticosterone levels and increases in adrenal gland weight in normal mice.

Adrenal gland enlargement is one of the hallmarks of continuous exposure to a significant stressor. Indeed, adrenal glands from stressed rats in this study increased in weight by approximately 13%. However, two different shosaikoto oral dosing schedules (equivalent to two and ten times the normal human dose) had no effect upon adrenal gland weight.

Shosaikoto was able to restore the immunosuppression resultant to the physical stress, although only at the lower dosage. These animals showed a significantly enhanced immune response to foreign red blood cells, relative to the untreated or high dose shosaikoto groups. Conversely, only the higher dosage of the plant extract combination was able to restore rectal temperature to normal following the final exposure to the stress. The authors concluded that shosaikoto may act as an immuno-restorative agent via its direct immunomodulating and/or antistress activities. Additionally, they suggested that shosaikoto also acts upon the central nervous system in a manner similar to that of Valium.

A companion paper by the same authors tested the effects of shosaikoto upon age-induced amnesia in rats. Shosaikoto-treated animals displayed learning response times significantly lower than those of the control group of old animals, and equal to those of the young animals. Additionally, shosaikoto appeared to reduce age-related memory loss, preserving memory function virtually identical to that seen in the young animals.

Analyses of neurochemicals from the brains of the various groups indicated that shosaikoto-treated animals had higher levels of dopamine, found to be low within the brains of Alzheimer's disease patients. The authors suggested that the reputed beneficial effects of shosaikoto in Alzheimer's may be due to its ability to elevate brain dopamine levels, possibly leading to improved memory and cognitive processing.

A detail meriting attention is the amount of shosaikoto fed to the animals in this study. These animals received only half of the low dose, and one-tenth of the high dose of shosaikoto given to the animals in the stress study described previously. The effects of higher doses upon neurological function chemistry warrants further investigation.

These results show that the components of shosaikoto act as biological response modifiers in the immune and central nervous systems. Their promise as immunomodulating and neuroactivating agents awaits further studies.

Bupleurum falcatum

In traditional Chinese medicine, bupleurum has been highly regarded for its medicinal properties and has been used for centuries as an herbal remedy. The roots and aerial parts of bupleurum plants are commonly utilized for their therapeutic benefits.

Bupleurum is known for its hepatoprotective (liver-protecting) properties. Bupleurum is often included in traditional Chinese medicine formulas for liver-related conditions, such as liver congestion, hepatitis, and jaundice.

Bupleurum is used in traditional Chinese medicine to address imbalances in the body's energy systems, specifically the "shaoyang" meridian. It is believed to have a regulating effect on this meridian, which is associated with symptoms like alternating chills, fever, irritability, and digestive disorders.

Bupleurum has also been studied for its potential anti-inflammatory and immune-modulating effects. Some research suggests that certain compounds found in bupleurum may inhibit inflammation and modulate the immune response, making it a subject of interest for conditions related to immune dysregulation, such as allergies and autoimmune disorders.

Clearly this herb warrants examination and further studies as it shows enormous promise in several arenas of human health.

BURDOCK
Arctium lappa

Parts used: Root. *Long used as a vegetable and medicinal, the root of this weed has shown antibacterial and antifungal properties.*

TRADITIONAL USAGES

This common weed is native to Europe and is abundant in the United States. The root, which should be collected in spring, loses four-fifths of its weight by drying. The root's odor is weak and unpleasant, the taste mucilaginous and sweetish with a slight tinge of bitterness and astringency.

Widely eaten as a vegetable, burdock has also been praised for its medicinal virtues since antiquity. A root decoction has been reported useful in the treatment of gout, rheumatism, and dropsy. In Japan, the tender leaf stalks and roots are boiled in two changes of water to remove the tough fibers, and then eaten. The Iroquois and other Native American tribes learned how to prepare burdock from colonial settlers. The dried roots of young plants were added to soups, while the leaves were cooked and included in their diet as greens.

In his *Travels into North America*, the Swedish naturalist Peter Kalm wrote about burdock in a 1772 visit to Ticonderoga, New York: "And the governor told me that its tender shoots are eaten in spring as radishes, after the exterior part is taken off." According to William Woodville, an 18th-century writer on medical botany, the plant was very useful as a diuretic, and it effects cure without increased irritation and nausea as side effects.

Externally, the leaves have been applied to benign skin tumors as well as in the treatment of knee joint swellings unresponsive to other medicines. A poultice was made by boiling the leaves until most of the liquid was boiled off, then applying the hot, wet mass to the affected area. In tandem with the drinking of the root decoction, this same poultice was applied in the treatment of gout. Burdock poultices were also used to treat severe, bloody bruises and burns.

RECENT SCIENTIFIC FINDINGS

Burdock root extracts have been shown experimentally to produce diuresis and to inhibit tumors in animals. Extracts also lower blood sugar and have estrogenic activity. In test-tube experiments, extracts show antibacterial and antifungal properties.

These experiments indicate potential use of burdock for dysmenorrhea, in diabetes, and for bacterial or fungal infection.

Throughout history, burdock has been valued for both culinary and medicinal purposes. Its roots, leaves, and seeds are all used for various applications.

In traditional herbal medicine, burdock root is commonly used for its purifying and detoxifying properties. It is believed to support liver function by assisting in the elimination of waste and toxins from the body. Burdock root is often used as a gentle diuretic and blood purifier, promoting the excretion of waste products through the urine.

Burdock root is also known for its potential anti-inflammatory and antioxidant effects. It contains compounds such as inulin, flavonoids, and lignans, which contribute to its therapeutic properties. These compounds may help reduce inflammation, support healthy skin, and scavenge harmful free radicals in the body.

Arctium lappa

Additionally, burdock root has been traditionally used to support digestive health. It is believed to stimulate digestive juices and enhance appetite, making it beneficial for individuals with poor digestion or loss of appetite.

Beyond its medicinal uses, burdock has culinary applications as well. The young leaves can be cooked and eaten as greens, while the roots can be used in various dishes, including soups and stir-fries. Burdock root is often described as having a slightly sweet and earthy flavor.

BUTCHER'S BROOM
Ruscus aculeatus

Parts used: Rhizome. *Modern research is confirming ancient Mediterranean healers' use of this plant as an anti-inflammatory agent.*

TRADITIONAL USAGES

This member of the lily family has very active chemical constituents, saponins, similar to those found in licorice and sarsaparilla. That this evergreen shrub, native to the Mediterranean region, has been found to contain highly active chemical constituents would not come as a surprise to ancient peoples. While the stiff, leaf-like twigs were once used by butchers to whisk scraps from their cutting blocks, ancient Mediterranean healers utilized the rhizome for a wide variety of circulatory and inflammatory disorders. Varicose veins were cured with this species according to the Roman scholar Pliny the Elder (c. A.D. 60), while in more ancient years, Greek doctors reported curing "swelling" with "the miracle herb."

RECENT SCIENTIFIC FINDINGS

Beneath the stiff twigs of this plant long employed for mundane purposes courses chemical constituents with profound effects. Oral contraceptives are made from steroids derived in large part from the plant kingdom. So, too, are other important steroids, such as cortisone, testosterone, and estradiol. Thanks to the pioneering efforts of many scientists who investigated the plant world for starter compounds, these synthetic drugs are now available at very low prices.

The saponin glycosides found in some plants are the basis for the production of many useful steroid pharmaceuticals. During the course of investigations into finding new saponins, two new sapogenins were discovered in the rhizomes of butcher's broom. These were named ruscogenin and neo-ruscogenin and are chemically similar to diosgenin, the principle steroid starter compound found in Mexican yams (various species of *Dioscorea*).

Relatively recent pharmacological findings indicate vasoconstrictive and anti-inflammatory properties. Tests conducted on animals by Capra showed that the ruscogenins have good anti-inflammatory activity. As for toxicity, tests in mice and rats showed that when administered orally, these compounds from butcher's broom were well tolerated.

The saponins it contains constricts the veins and decreases the permeability of capillaries. Consequently, several writers state that this so-called "phlebotherapeutic agent" is utilized to treat disorders of circulation, such as varicose veins and hemorrhoids.

A venotropic drug (RAES) composed of an extract of butcher's broom along with hesperidin and ascorbic acid was examined in a 1988 clinical trial. Four patients between the ages of 28 and 74 suffering from chronic phlebopathy of the lower limbs were evaluated in the double-blind, cross-over trial. The authors undertook two periods of treatment of two months with RAES or a placebo. They concluded that symptoms "immediately changed significantly in correspondence with the administration of RAES. The biological and clinical tolerability were excellent."

Another randomized double-blind study of 50 patients suffering from varicose veins employed a commercial preparation of butcher's broom extract. The research indicated improvement in those treated with the extract.

The root of butcher's broom is the most commonly used part for its medicinal properties. It has a long history of traditional use in herbal medicine, particularly for its potential effects on blood circulation and vascular health.

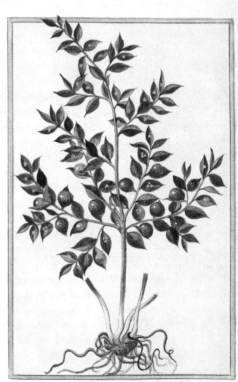

Ruscus aculeatus

One of the key traditional uses of butcher's broom is for venous insufficiency and related conditions. It is believed to strengthen and tone blood vessels, particularly those of the lower extremities. Butcher's broom is often used to alleviate symptoms associated with poor circulation, such as gout, leg swelling, varicose veins, and heaviness or discomfort in the legs. Some studies suggest that certain compounds in butcher's broom, such as ruscogenins, may have vasoconstrictive and anti-inflammatory effects, which could contribute to its therapeutic benefits.

Butcher's broom is also used for its potential diuretic properties. It has been traditionally employed to support urinary tract health and relieve water retention. By promoting diuresis, it may help reduce swelling and assist in the elimination of excess fluid from the body.

Butcher's broom has also been explored for its potential anti-inflammatory and antioxidant effects. It contains various bioactive compounds, including steroidal saponins and flavonoids, which are believed to contribute to its pharmacological properties.

People taking kidney or blood pressure medication should speak to their doctor before taking broom or butcher's broom, as it may interact with these medicines.

CASCARA SAGRADA
Rhamnus purshiana

Parts used: Bark. *The bark of this tree remains the world's most popular laxative.*

TRADITIONAL USAGES

The bark of cascara sagrada has been called the most widely used cathartic on earth. Traditionally employed as a remedy by Native Americans, the bark became known to settlers and eventually passed into use by the medical profession. The pharmaceutical house of Parke, Davis, and Co. first marketed cascara sagrada in 1877, although the plant did not become official in the *U.S. Pharmacopoeia* until 1890.

This tree is native to the northwest Pacific Coast, ranging from British Columbia to California. Various tribes throughout this range utilized cascara sagrada for its laxative effects. The Thompson tribe of British Columbia boiled a small amount of the bark or wood in water. This was a standard method of preparing plant medicines and consistently reappears throughout the literature on Native American remedies.

The early Spanish priests of California most probably learned of this "sacred bark" from the native people of Mendocino County. In 1877, Dr. J. H. Bundy "rediscovered" this plant, probably through Native Americans, and introduced cascara into medicine. It quickly became a favorite laxative throughout the world.

Indiscriminate cutting destroyed great stands of these trees. In 1909, the botanist Alice Henkel wrote:

Many trees are annually destroyed in the collection of cascara sagrada, as they are usually peeled to such an extent that no new bark is formed. It has been estimated that one tree furnishes approximately 10 pounds of bark, and granting a crop of 1,000,000 pounds a year, 100,000 trees are thus annually destroyed.

RECENT SCIENTIFIC FINDINGS

No synthetic substance can equal the mild and speedy action of the "holy bark"; it is marketed in pills, powders, and fluid extracts by many pharmaceutical companies. The basis of cascara's laxative effect is the presence of a mixture of anthraquinones, either free (e.g., aloe emodin) or as sugar derivatives (glycosides). The free anthraquinones remain in the intestines and cause catharsis by irritating the intestinal wall. Those anthraquinones present in the plant as sugar derivatives are largely absorbed from the intestine, circulate through the bloodstream, and eventually stimulate a nerve center in the lower part of the intestine, which causes a laxative effect.

Though its effectiveness has been proven, research continues. A 1991 study involving 271 human patients compared a Cascara-Salax laxative with two other regiments, a senna and saline laxative as well as a polyethylene glycol electrolyte lavage solution (Golytely). The researchers found no differences between the regimens, either in the patients' impressions or for the convenience of the preparation.

Cascara bark should always be aged for at least one year before being employed as a laxative. During this period of time, certain chemical changes occur in the bark that reduce the "griping" effect that often accompanies the use of a laxative preparation of this type.

Aqueous extracts of cascara have been found to be antiviral against herpes simplex virus II and vaccinia virus in cell culture.

Cascara sagrada is primarily valued for its effects on the digestive system. In herbal medicine, cascara sagrada is often used as a gentle and natural alternative to conventional laxatives. It is believed to have a regulating effect on bowel movements, helping to establish a regular and healthy pattern. Unlike some harsher laxatives, cascara sagrada is thought to be less likely to cause dependence or disrupt the natural functioning of the digestive system.

Cascara sagrada is commonly available in various forms, including dried bark, capsules, tablets, and liquid extracts.

CATNIP
Nepeta cataria

Parts used: Leaves and flowering tops. *This feline favorite also has a long history of use as a domestic remedy.*

TRADITIONAL USAGES

This plant was originally distributed in Europe, Siberia, and western Asia to the Himalayas. Introduced in North America, the weed now grows in dry soil from Canada to Minnesota and south to Virginia and Arkansas. It flowers June to September, and when utilized medicinally, the leaves and flowering tops are collected and then dried.

The Mohegans made a tea of catnip leaves for infantile colic. This became a popular domestic remedy and is still used today in some regions of the United States. Catnip was also used to induce sweating to cure colds. At the beginning of this century, the leaves and flowering tops were widely utilized in medicine as a stimulant or to promote suppressed menstruation. The plant was also thought to have a sedative effect. It was official in the *U.S. Pharmacopoeia* from 1842 through 1882 and in the *National Formulary* from 1916 to 1950.

RECENT SCIENTIFIC FINDINGS

Surely a plant that has such a powerful impact on our feline friends, causing them to "roll upon, chew, and tear to bits any withered leaf till nothing remains," could not be destitute of medicinal value in humans. Catnip has been reported efficacious in the treatment of iron-deficiency anemia, menstrual and uterine disorders, and dyspepsia, and as a gentle calmative. It has been administered in a variety of forms, including infusion, injection, lavement, and in the bath. It has been drunk as a treatment for chronic cough and chewed for relief of toothache. Extract of catnip has been found to be cytotoxic to HELA-S3 cancer cells in cell culture.

Catnip has a long history of traditional use in herbal medicine, particularly for its calming and soothing properties. Catnip contains a compound called nepetalactone, which is responsible for its effects on both cats and humans.

Nepeta cataria

In herbal medicine, catnip is often used to promote relaxation and relieve nervous tension. It is believed to have mild antianxiety and stress-reducing effects, making it a popular choice for individuals seeking natural remedies for relaxation. Catnip is commonly prepared as an herbal tea or included in herbal blends for its calming properties.

Catnip is considered a diaphoretic, which means that it can cause sweating without increasing body temperature. This can help alleviate a fever, which, in turn, helps a quicker recovery.

Catnip has a long-standing reputation for relieving indigestion, bloating, and mild gastrointestinal issues.

For cats, catnip is a well-known stimulant that triggers a euphoric response. The scent of catnip can induce various playful and energetic behaviors in cats, such as rolling, rubbing, and jumping. It is often used as an enrichment tool or to encourage exercise in feline companions.

CAYENNE
Capsicum frutescens

Parts used: Fruit. *This condiment is producing surprising results as a short-term anti-inflammatory agent.*

TRADITIONAL USAGES
The stimulant effect of the common chili pepper is reflected in its use as a condiment in foods, with a resulting promotion of digestion. As a medicine, cayenne pepper is a general stimulant and has been reported of value in the treatment of dyspepsia, diarrhea, and prostration. It has been used as a remedy for nausea from seasickness.

As a gargle, the seeds are valued as a treatment for sore throat and hoarseness. In the treatment of ague (painful swelling of the face due to decayed or ulcerated teeth or a cold), inhalation of the steam of cayenne and vinegar, coupled with a small mouth poultice containing one teaspoon of cayenne pepper, will reportedly afford relief by producing a free discharge of saliva.

RECENT SCIENTIFIC FINDINGS
Cayenne pepper acts as a rubefacient when applied externally, and as a stimulant internally, due to the presence of capsaicin, which is the "hot principle" in the fruit of this plant.

Oleoresin of *Capsicum* is still used in the preparation of a number of popular proprietary products to be applied locally for the relief of sore muscles, and it produces the

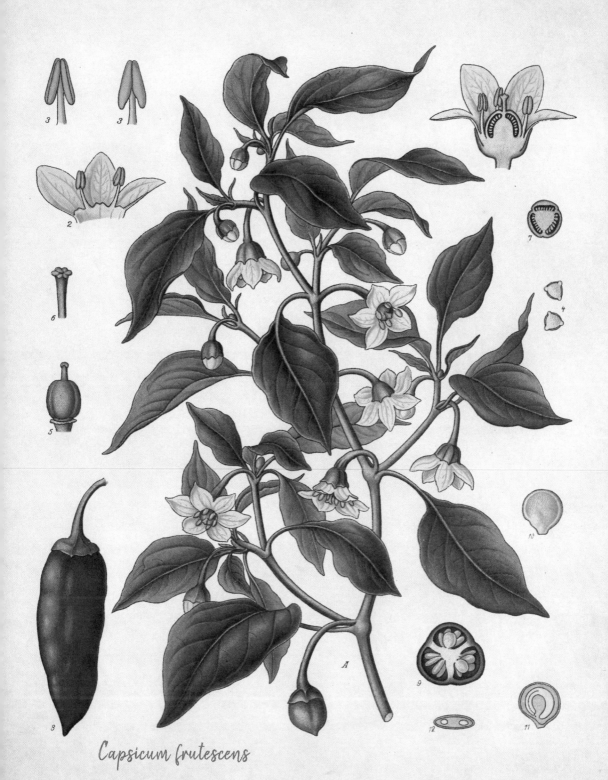

Capsicum frutescens

desired effect by mildly irritating the surface of the skin, which causes an increased blood flow to the area of application. The increased blood flow reduces inflammation of the affected area. Capsaicin, a phenol present in cayenne pepper, has shown a variety of medicinal benefits. In a recent letter to *The Lancet,* it was reported that topical applications of capsaicin cream completely alleviated the severe stump pain experienced by a middle-aged female diabetic. This double-amputee patient subsequently underwent a placebo trial, where it was proved that while this cream completely relieved the pain, the placebo had no effect. Given the successful outcome of this extreme example, it would be reasonable to expect capsaicin creams to yield beneficial topical results when applied to various painful neuropathies.

Further information regarding the anti-inflammatory property of capsaicin is revealed in the paper "Direct Evidence for Neurogenic Inflammation and Its Prevention by Denervation and by Pretreatment with Capsaicin," as quoted in Dr. J. Garcia-Leme's book *Hormones and Inflammation* (1989). In studies with rats given capsaicin systemically, the results proved that "sensory nerve endings became insensitive to chemical pain stimuli for a long time. Neurogenic inflammation cannot be elicited in animals pretreated with capsaicin."

Additionally, two Indian scientists recently reported that long-term treatment with capsaicin "desensitizes" the membrane against various gaseous irritant-induced free radical damage. They found that this compound protects lung tissue (in experiments with rats) by increasing superoxide dismutase (SOD), catalase (CAT), and peroxidase (POD) activities. In as yet unpublished studies by the same authors, pretreatment with capsaicin also protected the lungs of rats from nitrogen dioxide and formaldehyde-induced free radical damage.

Two double-blind studies with human patients investigated a capsaicin-based pharmaceutical's effect on the daily activities of patients suffering from the nerve pain associated with diabetes. Such neuropathy usually interferes with the ability to work, sleep, walk, eat, use shoes and socks, and enjoy recreational activities. This complication of diabetes often reduces the overall quality of a patient's life with the pain usually lasting for many years.

On July 23, 2020, it was announced that the FDA approved a capsaicin patch as a treatment for diabetic neuropathy, with potential benefits for millions of diabetic patients suffering with burning or stinging pain in their hands or feet. This can be viewed as "fighting fire with fire" as the active principle of the patch is capsaicin, which is the spicy substance that makes chili peppers hot! The capsaicin acts on pain receptors in the skin by desensitizing and numbing nerve endings. A note of caution: This therapy

> *Cayenne is also known for its potential pain-relieving properties. Capsaicin, the active component in cayenne, has been extensively researched for its pain-relieving effects.*

must be administered by health professionals and closely monitored. There can be some skin burning in some cases, and the frequency of treatments must be carefully adjusted per individual.

The failure of drugs such as tricyclic antidepressants, anticonvulsants, narcotic analgesics, and phenothiazines for this condition led to the search for safer, more effective alternatives.

Researchers at the prestigious Scripps Clinic and Research Foundation in La Jolla, California, enrolled 277 men and women with this painful condition and followed them for eight weeks in this double-blind study. The capsaicin cream was tried against a neutral cream and applied to the painful areas four times daily. Statistically significant differences were observed, with improvement in favor of the capsaicin cream. Such a natural-based medicine is now being utilized to improve the lives of thousands. The marvelous benefits of capsaicin were reported earlier by a group from Henry Ford Hospital in Detroit, Michigan. This double-blind study tested 15 patients with diabetes mellitus suffering from neuropathy. The authors concluded that this plant-derived compound is "potentially effective when burning pain is a major symptom of PDN [painful diabetic neuropathy]. The side effects of capsaicin were limited and minimal. This agent should be considered by clinicians for treatment of PDN."

Also, human studies have been done on capsaicin's effectiveness in treating rhinitis. Capsaicin was given to patients three times daily for three days. The patients' symptoms were recorded over a one-month period. The results indicated that the capsaicin treatment markedly reduced nasal obstruction and nasal secretion.

Interestingly, both cayenne pepper preparations and the active principle capsaicin have been shown in humans and in animals to stimulate the production of gastric juices, resulting in improved digestion.

Cayenne has been used for centuries as both a culinary spice and a medicinal herb. The active compound responsible for its heat is capsaicin, which gives cayenne its hot spicy flavor.

Cayenne pepper can both prevent and ease the pain of ulcers by regulating stomach secretions. The main cause of peptic ulcers is *Helicobacter pyloria*, according to the Mayo Clinic website. Capsaicin, the compound that gives cayenne pepper its heat, can promote healing of peptic ulcers and act as a natural pain reliever. The compound can also stop your stomach from producing acid, which can irritate an ulcer. Cayenne pepper also tells your stomach to produce more protective juices, which may prevent an ulcer from forming in the first place. Capsaicin also stimulates blood flow to the stomach lining and enhances the release of mucus in the stomach, all of which aid in healing, in addition to active antibacterial properties.

In herbal medicine, cayenne is commonly used to support cardiovascular health. It is believed to have vasodilatory effects, meaning it helps widen blood vessels and improve blood flow. Cayenne may also assist in maintaining healthy blood pressure levels. Additionally, it is thought to help lower LDL cholesterol levels and reduce the risk of blood clots.

Cayenne is also known for its potential pain-relieving properties. Capsaicin, the active component in cayenne, has been extensively researched for its pain-relieving effects. It is commonly used topically in the form of creams, ointments, or patches to provide temporary relief from muscle and joint pain, including arthritis and neuropathy. Capsaicin works by desensitizing nerve receptors, reducing the perception of pain.

Moreover, cayenne is believed to possess digestive benefits. It can stimulate saliva production, promote healthy digestion, and increase gastric acid secretion, aiding in the breakdown of food. It may also have a mild laxative effect, supporting regular bowel movements.

CHAMOMILE

Matricaria chamomilla (German), *Anthemis nobilis* (Roman)

Parts used: Flowers. *This is one of nature's safest and most effective sedatives.*

TRADITIONAL USAGES

There are two major types of chamomile; they should not be confused. Roman chamomile is derived from the flowers of *Anthemis nobilis,* whereas German, or Hungarian, chamomile makes use of the flowers of *Matricaria chamomilla.* The Greek name for German chamomile signifies "ground-apple" and is appropriate. The whole plant when bruised affords a pleasant aromatic smell very similar to that of apples. German chamomile is an annual herb.

German chamomile, a showy annual cultivated in Europe, has long been taken in home remedies for anthelmintic and antispasmodic effects. The dried flower heads are known to stimulate the digestive process and are equally well established for their mild relaxing properties. It was a popular remedy for gas and cramps of the stomach.

Externally, an infusion was applied in compresses to relieve pain and swelling. The flowers have been used extensively as a rinse to keep the hair golden. This chamomile species is also used for flavoring liqueurs and in perfumes, shampoos, and special tobaccos.

Also known as English chamomile, Roman chamomile flowers are an excellent stomachic in indigestion, flatulent colic, gout, and headaches in moderate doses. A strong infusion acts as an efficient emetic (try it combined with ginger!). The oil has stimulant and antispasmodic properties; it is useful in treating flatulence and is added to purgatives to prevent griping pain in the bowels.

A related species, *A. cotula*, known as stinking chamomile or may weed, was once widely used in the United States to promote sweating in chronic rheumatism and was recommended by Tragus, a 16th-century herbalist, in the form of a decoction as a remedy for hysteria.

Chamomile has been safely utilized for thousands of years in folk remedies, chiefly for female hysteria, dyspepsia, fever, anxiety, depression, insomnia, indigestion, constipation, diarrhea, hemorrhoids, and painful menstruation, amongst dozens of conditions cited in literature. Chamomile is found in the writings of early Greek botanists/ physicians Hippocrates (fifth century B.C.) and Dioscorides (first century A.D.), and the Roman physical Galen (second century A.D.). It is a valuable herb with many medicinal benefits. Known to help with anxiety, as well as for calming upset stomachs, chamomile is found useful as a sleeping aid and assists with alleviation of gas and diarrhea symptoms. When applied topically,

Anthemis nobilis

The dried flower heads are known to stimulate the digestive process and are equally well established for their mild relaxing properties.

chamomile might also promote wound healing, particularly for mouth sores. Chamomile flowers remain one of the most "in demand" medicinal plants in global trade. Increasing demand for sustainable (organic and fair trade) chamomile has caused a new emphasis on cultivation to catch up with the needs of consumers.

RECENT SCIENTIFIC FINDINGS

Chamomile's mild sedative effects have been well documented. In 1973, a study was carried out in the United States in which 12 hospitalized patients having various types of heart disease were administered chamomile tea in order to determine its effect. Each patient was given a six-ounce cup of hot tea prepared from two commercial chamomile tea bags. Approximately 10 minutes after the ingestion of the tea, 10 of the patients fell into a deep sleep. They could be aroused but immediately fell again into a deep sleep. The sleep lasted approximately 90 minutes. The only other effect seen in the patients was a small but significant increase in arterial blood pressure. In the years since, hundreds of studies have showed similar effects.

Experimentally in animals, the volatile oil from chamomile flowers was given orally to rabbits with impaired kidney function, so the amount of urea in the blood was increased. In all cases, the uremic condition in the rabbits normalized. This indicates a possible usefulness in regard to impaired kidney functions.

Another study in animals, using a flavonoid found in chamomile flowers (apigenin), showed that this substance had antihistaminic effects. When administered orally to arthritic rats, chamomile's essential oil reduced the inflammation markedly. It was further shown that the constituents in the oil responsible for most of this effect was a substance known as alpha-bisabolol. In test-tube experiments, chamomile oil has also been shown to relax smooth muscle of the intestine.

Chamomile has also been a popular eyewash for treating conjunctivitis and other reactions. It has also been found to promote wound healing. A double-blind study with 11 patients found that chamomile's effect was statistically significant in decreasing the wound area as well as the drying tendency.

With the exception of an occasional allergic response, there have been no adverse effects for humans reported in the literature for chamomile. Thus, here is another safe sedative from nature's garden.

CHASTEBERRY
Vitex agnus-castus

Parts used: Fruit. *This was called monk's pepper during the Middle Ages, and modern research has found that it reduces or eliminates premenstrual symptoms.*

TRADITIONAL USAGES

Chasteberry has been used since ancient times as a female remedy. One of its properties is reducing sexual desire, and it is recorded that Roman wives whose husbands were abroad with the legions spread the aromatic leaves on their couches for this purpose. It became known as the chasteberry tree.

During the Middle Ages, chasteberry's supposed effect on sexual desire led to it becoming a food spice at monasteries, where it was called monk's pepper or cloister pepper.

In tradition, it was also known as an important European remedy for controlling and regulating the female reproductive system. Long used to regularize monthly periods and treat amenorrhea and dysmenorrhea, it also helped ease menopausal problems and aided the birth process.

The fruit's peppermint-like odor comes from its volatile oils.

Nowadays, it is believed to help relieve premenstrual symptoms such as breast pain. Some studies have shown that the use of chasteberry extract may also help with the symptoms of perimenopause (the earliest stage of menopause). This herb is commonly prescribed in Germany to treat menstrual cycle irregularities, period related breast pain, and premenstrual syndrome (PMS).

Chasteberry might help reduce menopausal symptoms by reducing the frequency of hot flashes and night sweats due to the phytoestrogen content. Studies on chasteberry for infertility are promising but still in progress.

RECENT SCIENTIFIC FINDINGS

Chasteberry has not been significantly investigated for its therapeutic effects. Preliminary investigations do indeed show the presence of compounds that are able to adjust the production of female hormones. It is thought to contain a progesterone-like

During the Middle Ages, chasteberry's supposed effect on sexual desire led to it becoming a food spice at monasteries, where it was called monk's pepper or cloister pepper.

compound and is now thought to be useful in the following conditions: amenorrhea, dysmenorrhea, PMS, endometriosis.

The chemical constituents are the monoterpenes agnuside, eurostoside, and aucubin. Chasteberry also contains the flavonoids casticin, chrysosplenol, and vitexin. While it is not known which constituent is responsible for its beneficial effects, it has been shown in laboratory animals in German experiments that extracts of *Agnus castus* can stimulate the release of leutenizing hormone (LH) and inhibit the release of follicle stimulating hormone (FSH). This hormonal effect has been confirmed in another laboratory report, which suggests that the volatile oil has a progesterone-like effect.

Interest in this plant as an aid in PMS has arisen as a result of a clinical study carried out by Dr. Alan Stewart, who heads a clinic in a London hospital specializing in the treatment of premenstrual problems. Dr. Stewart's study indicated a 60% group reduction or elimination of PMS symptoms such as anxiety, nervous tension, insomnia, or mood changes, from subjects who were taking dried *agnus castus* capsules.

This trial studied the premenstrual symptoms reported by 30 women who took 1.5 gm/day dried agnus castus tablets, and 80 women who took a placebo. The symptoms were classified into groups and assessed by a daily symptomatology diary and by a questionnaire. Nearly 60 percent of the women reported that the symptoms were all or practically all gone, a much higher score than the placebo. Symptoms such as anxiety, nervous tension, insomnia, or mood changes were most reduced.

Vitex agnus-castus

Employing an aqueous extract from the fruit, a 1979 study reported good results on premenstrual water retention. Another study discovered that women were able to sustain a good level of milk production for breast feeding. While it took some time for the drug to take effect, the women were able to continue use of the drug for months without harmful side effects.

CHERRY (Wild)
Prunus virginiana

Parts used: Stem and bark. *A Cherokee tea of the inner bark has remained in the U.S. Pharmacopoeia since 1820.*

TRADITIONAL USAGES
The Mohegans allowed the ripe wild black cherry to ferment naturally in a jar for about one year and then drank the juice to cure dysentery. The Meskwakis made a sedative tea of the root bark, and this drink has long been popular in domestic American medicine. Cherokee women were given a tea of the inner bark to relieve pain in the early stages of labor. This preparation was soon adopted by the early settlers, and in 1820 it became official in the *U.S. Pharmacopoeia,* where the bark is still listed for its sedative properties.

The most widespread popular use of wild cherry bark is as a cough sedative. It acts as a tonic and calms irritation, diminishing nervous excitability. It has been employed in the treatment of bronchitis, and because it slows heart action, it has been used in heart disease characterized by frequent, irregular, or feeble pulse. It has also been considered a good remedy for weakness of the stomach or of the system coupled with general or local irritation.

When used in medicine, the bark is collected in autumn when it contains the greatest concentration of precursors to hydrocyanic acid. Alice Henkel, an early expert on medicinal plants, cautioned against storing the bark for longer than one year, stating that it deteriorates with time. She added that young, thin bark was preferred and that bark from small or old branches was discarded.

RECENT SCIENTIFIC FINDINGS
The *Prunus* genus includes plums, almonds, peaches, apricots, and cherries. All these possess to some degree the glycoside amygdalin, which when combined with water reacts to form hydrocyanic acid.

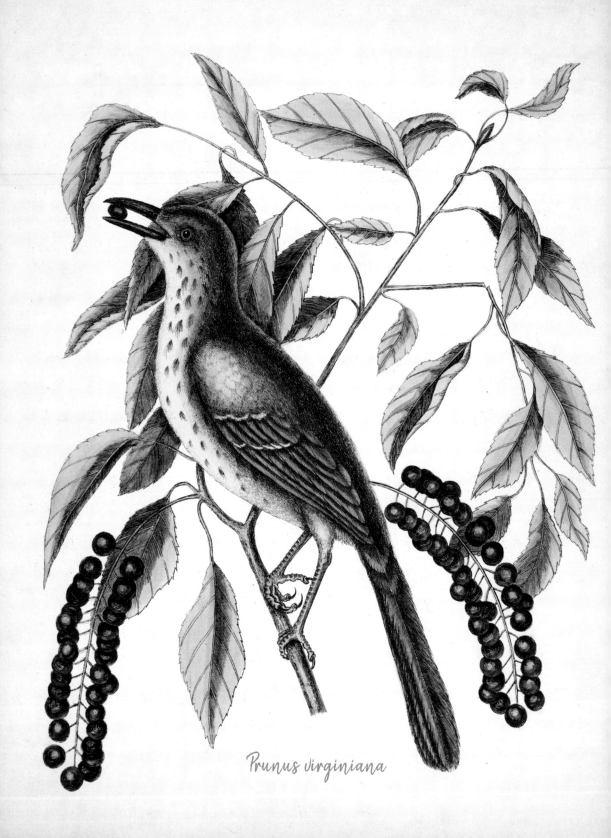

Prunus virginiana

Both hydrocyanic acid and benzaldehyde, formed during the water extraction of the bark, contribute to the pleasant characteristic odor of wild cherry preparations. It should be pointed out that heat should be avoided during the preparation of wild cherry extracts, since both hydrocyanic acid and benzaldehyde are very volatile and would be lost if heat is applied.

Hydrocyanic acid is toxic in sufficient dose, and there are many reports of animals being poisoned fatally by eating the leaves or fruits of many *Prunus* species. The degree of toxicity depends on a number of factors, and it is generally agreed that the wilted leaves are the most toxic.

CHESTNUT (Spanish)
Castanea sativa

Parts used: Leaves and bark. *These tasty nuts were at one time a common remedy for bronchitis and whooping cough.*

TRADITIONAL USAGES

Chestnuts are, of course, better known for their edibility. As well as being eaten roasted or boiled, they have traditionally been ground into flour in order to make breads and cakes, and to thicken soups. Eating too many can result in constipation, due to tannin content. Being astringent, the bark and leaves were used to make a tonic that was also reportedly useful in the treatment of upper respiratory ailments such as coughs, and particularly whooping cough.

The American chestnut was utilized as a remedy for whooping cough by the Mohegans. They learned to use a tea of the leaves from European settlers, who derived the remedy from an unknown source. Dr. Charles Millspaugh wrote that chestnut leaves were used for whooping cough. However, the 1942 *Dispensatory of the United States* characterized this belief as a superstition, declaring, "There is...no sufficient reason to believe them to possess any therapeutic value except that of a mild astringent." As an astringent, the leaves were official in the *U.S. Pharmacopoeia* from 1873 to 1905.

RECENT SCIENTIFIC FINDINGS

The bark of Spanish chestnut is known to contain high concentrations of tannins, which explains the astringent effect claimed when water extracts of this plant are applied externally.

Although there is no direct experimental evidence to corroborate claims that the leaves of this plant have value in treating coughs, they are rich in polysaccharides. If taken orally in a water infusion, polysaccharides would produce a demulcent and soothing effect on the irritated mucous membranes and hence tend to lessen the symptoms of cough.

Spanish chestnuts are a rich source of carbohydrates, dietary fiber, and essential minerals such as potassium and magnesium. They are relatively low in fat compared to other nuts and contain various vitamins, including vitamin C, vitamin B6, and folate. Chestnuts are also gluten free, making them suitable for individuals with gluten sensitivities or celiac disease.

CHINESE CUCUMBER

Trichosanthes kirilowii

Parts used: Root and tubers. *Used for centuries in traditional Chinese medicine, this is the source of the drug Compound Q.*

We do not recommend home use of this plant. This entry is written to give the consumer an overview of this herb.

TRADITIONAL USAGES

In Oriental medicine, root preparations have been utilized for centuries to induce abortion and treat certain cancers. This drug is also employed (again in China) as a treatment for choriocarcinoma, a cancer found in the uterus. Apparently, trichosanthin is either selectively absorbed by these cancer cells or it has selective antiviral activity.

In traditional Chinese medicine, each part of the plant has been employed for various other ailments. The roots were also utilized to treat jaundice, diabetes, hemorrhoids, and sore throats. The first recorded use of the seeds dates from the fifth century A.D. Along with the same ailments as the roots, the seeds also were used as a laxative and to reduce phlegm.

RECENT SCIENTIFIC FINDINGS

Chinese cucumber became the hottest herb of the past 40 years because it is the source of the drug GLQ223, or "Compound Q." Early findings suggested this drug may work on HIV. Not since *Rauwolfia* (Indian snakeroot) was introduced from Ayurvedic medicine as an antihypertensive in the 1950s under the name reserpine has an herbal remedy generated so much hope and hype.

The plant itself is not being tested for anti-AIDS activity. GLQ223 is a highly purified version of trichosanthin, which is a protein isolated from root tubers of *T. Kirilowii* from southern China.

T. kirilowii contains compounds with antibacterial activity, anti-yeast activity, gallstone inhibitory activity, oestrogenic activity, uterine relaxant activity, and white blood stimulant activity (from sitosterol). The plant also contains alpha-spinasterol, which is anti-inflammatory and antipyretic. Other of its compounds kill tumor cells and increase prostaglandin levels (PG72A), to mention only a few of the documented actions.

Exciting preliminary results show that GLQ223 selectively destroys macrophages infected with the human immunodeficiency virus type 1 (HIV-1). Such infected T cells are thought to be the major sites of the virus in the human body. In addition, the CD4 T cells have been found to be a reservoir for latent HIV-1 viruses.

As testing of this promising drug continued, people wanted to know if they can take the plant itself, as a hot-water infusion of the root? Is it safe and effective, and will this plant work against other viral infections? Does Chinese cucumber somehow stimulate the immune system? All very good questions. First, it is important to emphasize here that Compound Q is very dangerous! It must *not* be utilized without strict and expert medical supervision owing to potential side effects and toxicity. Some doctors have observed severe anaphylactic reactions in their patients. Other effects include flu-like symptoms such as fevers, as well as seizures, stupors, and even coma.

It is easy to kill infected monocytes with many different compounds. Chloroquine, an antimalarial, for example, is an effective agent. St. John's wort (*Hypericum perforatum*) has also been shown to be active against the AIDS virus in test-tube experiments. To be effective against the virus *in a human,* relatively high concentrations of hypericin, the active ingredient, would be required, perhaps at a toxic level. At this time, we do not know if GLQ223 is any more effective than chloroquine or hypericin. Further, Compound Q may prove to be too large to reach the infected cells, its potency has not been established, and it may also kill healthy cells.

To develop an immunotoxin for an HIV infected cell, highly specialized procedures are required. The envelope glycoproteins, GP160, for example, are found on the surface of HIV cells and are the target receptors for immunotoxins. We do not know, however, if GLQ223 reaches these receptors.

Moreover, it has not yet been determined if trichosanthin is even extracted when Chinese cucumber roots are boiled. So, we do not yet know if a "tea" of this interesting species would have any medicinal properties, let alone be capable of killing viruses or stimulating immunity.

Further, assuming that small quantities of trichosanthin were found to occur in a hot-water extract, as an herbal tea, we do not know if this agent would be *absorbed* from the gastrointestinal tract. (It may prove to work only via the injectable route.)

For these reasons, we *cannot* recommend the self-administration of extracts of this species. Only careful human trials of the drug will answer the many questions that remain outstanding.

One peer review study involved 18 patients receiving various doses of tricosanthin. Those patients who received the highest doses exhibited *in vitro* antiviral effects. However, the researchers felt these effects did not have therapeutic value, though they did declare the drug safe for further study.

A subsequent study involving 51 patients relied on higher doses. The researchers reported significant decreases in p24 antigen levels with an overall reduction of 67%. Those patients who received the full course of three infusions of the drug showed the best results. The researchers stated, "A picture is forming of a drug which seems to have at least some benefit for some patients, and on which a handful of patients have done extremely well while others appear to have shown little or no benefit and a few have suffered catastrophic side effects."

As of this writing, we have discovered no new studies that would lead to a belief that this plant is useful for AIDS treatments.

CINCHONA

Cinchona spp.

Parts used: Bark. *The alkaloid distilled from the bark of the tree is the source of the malarial cure quinine.*

TRADITIONAL USAGES

Cinchona bark was first brought to Europe in 1640 through the auspices of the Countess of Chinchon of Peru. However, it was not until 97 years later while journeying in the Loxa province of Peru that a French naturalist identified the tree from which the bark was obtained. Once cinchona became popular as a cure for intermittent fevers, it was distributed and sold by the Jesuit fathers, who maintained missions in the area. It was so popular that it became known as Jesuit's bark or Peruvian bark. Because it was used to cure King Charles II of malaria, it became popular in London during his reign. In the late 18th century, other sources of the bark were discovered in Columbia, central Peru, and Bolivia.

At one time, the Peruvian government outlawed the export of cinchona seeds and saplings to control its monopoly. There is a record of an illegal sale of seeds to the Dutch government, which led to the death of the perpetrator of the theft. The Dutch grew the plants in Indonesian plantations and became the main suppliers of the bark. By the 1930s, Dutch Javanese plantations were producing 97% of the world's quinine. Due to German and Japanese controls during World War II, the Allies were cut off from their supply of quinine and many thousands of troops died in Africa and the South Pacific due to malaria.

According to tradition, because of the bitter taste of the antimalarial quinine tonic, British colonials in India mixed it with gin to make it more palatable, thus creating the gin and tonic cocktail, which is still popular today. Other countries, such as France and Spain, created their own versions of alcohol and tonic (quinine).

Quinine has been recognized as one of nature's most important medicinal gifts to the human race, for it has been instrumental in relieving great suffering from malaria and other intermittent fevers.

RECENT SCIENTIFIC FINDINGS

The alkaloid quinine is derived from cinchona bark and is well known for its antimalarial properties. Besides its antiperiodic action against intermittent fever, cinchona bark has tonic, antiseptic, and astringent properties.

Although quinine and preparations containing quinine are relatively safe, one must be cautious of the amounts used. Excessive doses of cinchona can lead to a condition known as cinchonism or quinism, marked by buzzing in the ears, deafness, headache, vertigo, and nausea. While these effects generally disappear within a few hours, they are a warning signal regarding dosage.

Nature, as in many cases, has provided a built-in warning to notify us when the safe limit of these preparations is approaching. When one experiences a ringing in the ears, the amount being taken should be reduced, and the sounds will disappear.

Cinchona spp.

Recent research has only confirmed cinchona's effectiveness against malaria and its superiority to synthetic pharmaceuticals. During the Vietnam War, a strain of malarial parasite developed that was highly resistant to both well-established and new synthetic antimalarial drugs. It was soon found, however, that most cases of malaria caused by the new parasite could be effectively treated with the centuries-proven drug quinine. In recent years, cases such as this have led to increased use of quinine in place of synthetic drugs.

In addition to its antimalarial effects, cinchona bark and its extracts have also been studied for other potential health benefits. The alkaloids present in cinchona have proven to have fever-reducing, pain-relieving, and anti-inflammatory properties.

It is worth mentioning that cinchona trees are now considered endangered in the wild due to overharvesting for their medicinal properties. Efforts are being made to sustainably cultivate cinchona and protect its natural habitats to ensure the preservation of this valuable plant species.

There is a narrow difference between therapeutic and toxic effects of quinine and it must be used carefully even when consumed in common beverages that can be purchased at any supermarket. People with existing known heart issues should avoid quinine containing beverages, such as tonic waters. Quinine may potentiate the anticoagulant effects of warfarin, and other common adverse effects involve a group of symptoms called cinchonism. Symptoms are headache, nausea, sweating, vertigo, vomiting, and blurred vision. Clearly, this strong medicine should be discontinued with any of these symptoms.

CINNAMON
Cinnamomum zeylanicum, C. cassia

Parts used: Bark, leaves, and roots. *Cinnamon is a well-loved herb famous for its unique fragrance and delightful, warm, and sweet taste. It is extracted from the bark of trees that belong to the Cinnamomum genus, and its use has been widespread in various cultures for centuries, both in cooking and medicine. Apart from being a common ingredient in baking, where it enhances the taste of cakes, pastries, and cookies, cinnamon has also been acknowledged for its potential health benefits. It contains several compounds, including polyphenols, with antioxidant and anti-inflammatory properties, which may positively affect health. More recent research has revealed that it may also be an effective antibacterial agent.*

TRADITIONAL USAGES

Cinnamon trees have been extensively cultivated in the tropics for the dried bark, which is a common spice. Cinnamon's use as medicinal also goes back to ancient times; it is mentioned in both early Chinese herbals and Egyptian texts. The Greeks used cinnamon as a treatment for bronchitis. In his writings, Galen mentions that he employed five different types of cinnamon.

Cinnamon has long been a popular carminative. It was commonly employed for most gastrointestinal problems. Most often, cinnamon was used in conjunction with other herbs in the treatment of a variety of ailments, including respiratory issues and dysentery.

RECENT SCIENTIFIC FINDINGS

Various parts of this plant have been so widely used throughout the world and have been so extensively tested that only a brief summary will be possible. The leaves, bark, stems, and roots contain several essential oils that are used as a flavoring in food and gum as well as in perfumes and incense. In these formulas, the essential oil from the flowers is used.

This essential oil has been found to stimulate the gastrointestinal tract, supporting cinnamon's traditional use. Cinnamon also has been found to dilate blood vessels. This may explain cinnamon's folkloric use in conjunction with other herbs since increased blood circulation may enhance the delivery of the herb's effects.

Mitogenic activity occurred in cell culture experiments as well as antifungal activity against *Aspergillus flavus.* An estrogenic effect in animals has been demonstrated. Anti-yeast activity also took place in agar plate experiments, especially against *Candida, lipolytica,* and another yeast known as *Kloeckera apiculata.* Many other types of yeast have been destroyed in agar plate experiments by extracts of the essential oil of this species.

A commercial sample of the bark has been tested in Japan and found to have anesthetic activity in animal experiments. Numerous experiments with extracts of this plant showed wide antibacterial activity against various species of bacillus. Dried bark has been tested in Japan as a decoction and found to possess anticonvulsant activity in experiments with mice. Again, antibacterial activity of the essential oil of the bark has been shown to kill *staphylococci* and other kinds of bacteria, including *Staphyloccus aureus.* Interesting experiments in India showed the essential oil to have insect repellent activity and also to have spermicidal effects. Most interestingly, extracts of the leaf juice in agar plate experiments had strong activity against *Mycobacterium tuberculosis,* the bacteria found in tuberculosis.

Finally, cinnamon is high in polyphenols, which are of benefit for their antioxidant properties.

Some studies suggest that cinnamon may help regulate blood sugar levels, improve insulin sensitivity, and lower cholesterol. Traditionally, it has been used for its antimicrobial, antifungal, and digestive properties. Additionally, cinnamon is associated with potential benefits for heart health and cognitive function. There are ongoing research studies regarding potential reduction of triglycerides, LDL (bad cholesterol), and blood sugar, which are all associated as risk factors for heart disease. Furthermore, there are concurrent research studies illustrating potential beneficial effects on neurodegenerative diseases in humans that require further study.

CITRUS
Various species

Parts used: Essential oils extracted from peel of lemons and oranges. *Citrus contains limonene, which may both prevent and treat cancer.*

TRADITIONAL USAGES

Citrus is most well-known historically as a treatment for scurvy. Though used in folk medicine for some time, it was James Lind who in 1753 conducted his renowned experiment that proved citrus fruits cured scurvy. The British navy's requirement that ships carry limes or lemons led to the epithet Limey.

The name "citrus" was first used by Pliny. Lemon juice was employed as a diuretic and astringent.

RECENT SCIENTIFIC FINDINGS

In recent years, research has uncovered reputed anticancer properties in certain essential oils. Limonene is the major component of the essential oil of orange and other citrus fruits. It also occurs widely in the plant kingdom, particularly in those species producing essential oils, flavors, and spices. This compound belongs to a class of natural compounds known as terpenes, soon to equal the bioflavonoids and carotenoids in their applications.

About 10 animal studies have been published that show that dietary limonene (the d-isomer or l-limonene) lowers the incidence of chemically induced cancers as well as delaying their appearance. Elson and colleagues at the University of Wisconsin are currently the leaders in this field. In one study, they demonstrated that dietary d-limonene markedly reduced dimethyl benzanthracene–induced mammary cancers. The dosage used in this study was 1,000 parts per million, or 1 gram per kg of diet. (Note: humans eat about 1/2 kg per day, which translates to about 500 mg of d-limonene per day.)

Using this same model system, they subsequently showed that the essential oil of orange (85% d-limonene) was more effective than pure d-limonene in preventing tumor formation. Thus, naturally occurring terpenes in orange oil other than d-limonenes also possess anticancer activity. Further investigations by this group revealed that dietary d-limonene is effective in reversing preformed tumors, as evidenced by an increase in the tumor regression rate. Finally, Elson and associates recently observed that dietary d-limonene was effective in reducing the number of chemically induced mammary tumors in rats when provided either during the initiation phase or during the promotion/progression phase.

The mechanism(s) of action of d-limonene against cancer is not well understood but may involve the enhancement of drug-metabolizing systems such as glutathione S-transferases. The ability of d-limonene to reverse preformed tumors and to inhibit tumor growth during the promotion/progression phase of cancer suggests an immunostimulating action, and some recent evidence does support this concept. As an added benefit, limonene is a potent, natural cholesterol-lowering compound. It acts by inhibiting the same enzyme (HMG-coenzyme A reductase) that is the target of many prescribed cholesterol-reducing drugs, such as lovastatin. If these actions were not sufficient, limonene is also a powerful agent for dissolving gallstones.

Researchers at the University of Wisconsin, Madison, confirmed d-limonene's antitumor potential. In a series of animal experiments, up to 90% of tumors completely disappeared in mice fed this compound, whereas only 15% of tumors spontaneously diminished in size in animals not given the compound. Human cancer cells have also been shrunk with d-limonene in laboratory experiments.

In another study of d-limonene it was found that gallstones were dissolved by this "simple, safe, and effective solvent."

Citrus fruits are not only delicious, but they also have many health benefits. They contain high amounts of vitamin C, a powerful antioxidant that supports the immune system and promotes healthy skin. Additionally,

Citrus Medica

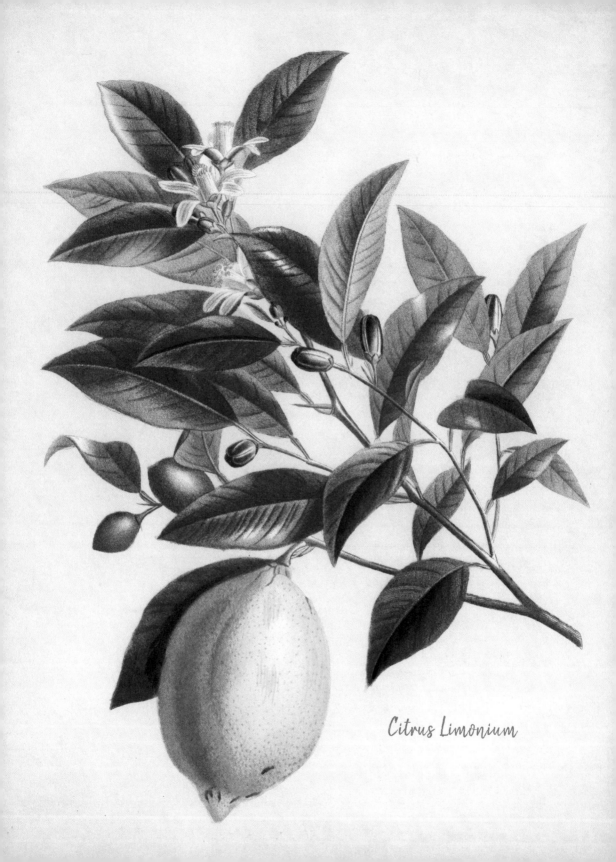

Citrus Limonium

they provide dietary fiber, which aids digestion and helps maintain a healthy weight. Citrus fruits are also a rich source of essential minerals, such as potassium, which can improve heart health.

Research has shown that citrus fruits are packed with nutrients, including flavonoids, vitamin C, and fiber, which can protect blood vessels, reduce inflammation, improve gastrointestinal function, and prevent diseases such as cancer, diabetes, and neurological disorders.

Studies have also found that citrus flavonoids can protect cells from free radical damage and reduce inflammation. As a result, these anti-inflammatory pathways can provide therapeutic benefits against diseases such as cancer, cardiovascular disease, and diabetes. Flavonoids may also prevent atherosclerosis and improve arterial blood pressure by scavenging free radicals, inhibiting LDL cholesterol oxidation, and reducing oxidative stress and inflammation.

Additionally, citrus flavonoids can improve glucose tolerance, increase insulin secretion and sensitivity, and decrease insulin resistance. They may also play a significant role in the development of anti-obesity agents, reducing obesity and inflammation in adipose tissue.

A mouthwash containing grapefruit, lemon, and orange juices is thought to be healthy for the gums and tongue.

CLOVE

Syzygium aromaticum

Parts used: Flower bud. *The essential oil of this common spice has shown promising anti-inflammatory effects in recent experiments.*

TRADITIONAL USAGES

Cloves are aromatic flower buds known for their strong, sweet, and spicy flavor. They are used in various cuisines globally and are especially popular in Asian, Middle Eastern, and Indian dishes. Beyond their culinary uses, cloves have been valued for their medicinal properties in traditional medicine.

The dried flower buds of cloves are well known as the source of this common spice. Oil of cloves has long been employed as a mild anesthetic as well as a stimulant and carminative. Clove oil was used to alleviate nausea and stop vomiting. It has especially been used for toothaches, with drops of the oil placed on a cavity. Clove tea was used to relieve nausea.

In traditional Chinese medicine, cloves are a common digestive remedy, used for vomiting, diarrhea, and pains in the chest and abdomen.

Overall, cloves are a versatile spice with a rich history in both culinary and traditional medicinal practices, and they continue to be appreciated for their unique flavor and potential health advantages. However, it is essential to use cloves in moderation as excessive consumption of clove oil or supplements may have adverse effects.

RECENT SCIENTIFIC FINDINGS

Clove's essential oil has exhibited much promise in recent research. Anti-inflammatory activity of clove extract has been demonstrated in rats and adult humans.

Essential oil of clove has been shown to kill (in vitro) the pathogenic yeast *Candida albicans* and many other species of yeasts, including *Trichophyton.* The essential oil also inhibited prostaglandin production and is therefore an anti-inflammatory. Antifungal activity against *Trichophyton rubrum* has been shown in humans.

Clove oil demonstrated in vitro antibacterial activity against *Bacillus subtilis* (one causative agent of food poisoning). Other susceptible organisms are *E. coli, Pseudomonas aeruginosa,* and *Staphylococcus aureus.* Clove oil was also active against *Mycobacterium tuberculosis* in vitro. Antiviral activity has been shown against herpes simplex virus.

Extract of clove suppresses dental plaque formation, specifically by being active against *Streptococcus mutans,* a causative agent in dental cavity formation. Test-tube studies have demonstrated eugenol (found in cloves) in concentrated amounts caused cell death in esophageal and cervical cancers. Ongoing studies are needed to confirm these effects. Eugenol in high amounts is toxic to the liver, even though there have been ongoing animal studies for liver protection benefits, such as reducing fatty liver disease. The studies are few and far between, and it must be emphasized that eugenol is not for amateurs. This is a serious compound and must be treated with caution.

Syzygium aromaticum

CLOVER (Red)

Trifolium pratense

Parts used: Blossoms. *An extract is marketed in Europe as a treatment for diarrhea.*

TRADITIONAL USAGES

Red clover was used for female complaints, as an anti-diarrhetic, and to treat dysentery.

RECENT SCIENTIFIC FINDINGS

An extract of red clover, uzarin, paralyzes smooth musculature. It is marketed in Europe under the name Uzara in the form of drops and tablets and is recommended as an antidote to diarrhea.

The isoflavone biochanin A is another extract of red clover. It has been found to be a potent carcinogenic inhibitor.

Red clover is a short-lived perennial plant with a fibrous root system. The leaves are trifoliate, consisting of three oval leaflets with characteristic white V-shaped markings. The flowers are borne in dense, globular clusters at the end of the stems and have a sweet fragrance.

One of the primary bioactive compounds found in red clover is a group of plant chemicals called isoflavones. The most prominent isoflavone in red clover is called biochanin A, followed by formononetin and genistein. These compounds are classified as phytoestrogens, as they have a chemical structure similar to the hormone estrogen found in the human body.

Red clover is often used as a natural remedy to ease menopausal symptoms in women, such as hot flashes, night sweats, and mood swings. The isoflavones in red clover may act as weak estrogen-like compounds, binding to estrogen receptors in the body and providing mild hormonal support.

Topical formulations containing red clover extracts have gained attention for their potential skin benefits. The isoflavones in red clover may promote collagen synthesis and inhibit enzymes that degrade collagen, contributing to improved skin elasticity and a more youthful appearance.

Apart from menopause and skin health, red clover has been studied for its potential in supporting respiratory health, promoting cardiovascular well-being, and even showing anticancer properties in some research.

Osteoporosis is a condition in which your bones exhibit low bone mineral density (BMD) and have become weak. This condition affects women after menopause due to the decline of estrogen. Red clover contains isoflavones, which are a type of phytoestrogen. In 2015, a study of women taking red clover extracts showed promise, yet another study that same year showed no positive results. Likewise, there have been other conflicting studies, so the evidence is not yet there that this plant is of assistance for osteoporosis. Concurrently, there have been numerous other studies regarding menopausal symptoms such as anxiety, depression, vaginal dryness, and hair and skin texture losses, and there are no conclusive positive results gleaned from these studies. Evidently more research is needed.

COHOSH (Black)
Cimicifuga racemosa

Parts used: Rhizome and root. *Used for centuries by Native Americans, an extract of black cohosh has also been used as a central nervous system tonic and as a treatment for high blood pressure.*

TRADITIONAL USAGES

Native American tribes used this plant for "women's problems," hence the Anglicized named "squawroot." The black cohosh, or black snakeroot, is native to the United States, growing in shady and rocky woods from Canada to Florida, and flowering in June and July.

Collected in the autumn, particularly in the Blue Ridge Mountains, this interesting root has been used as a relaxant, an antispasmodic, and a sedative. In the course of its employment as a treatment for chorea, or St. Vitus' dance, it was reported to have the undesirable side effects of inducing vomiting, giddiness, headache, and prostration. Between 1820 and 1936, when the plant was official in the *U.S. Pharmacopoeia,* the rhizome and root were utilized in the U.S. as a sedative, for rheumatism, and to promote menstruation. It is thought to reduce muscle aches and body pains associated with menopause, perimenopause, hot flashes, and postmenopausal complaints. Studies show that black cohosh binds to your body's opiod receptors, giving it a "painkilling effect."

RECENT SCIENTIFIC FINDINGS

Acetin, one of black cohosh's active principles, has been shown to lower blood pressure in experiments with rabbits and cats, and experiments with dogs have shown significant peripheral vasodilation. Furthermore, black cohosh extracts have been proven antimicrobial in in vitro experiments. This bacterial and yeast-killing activity

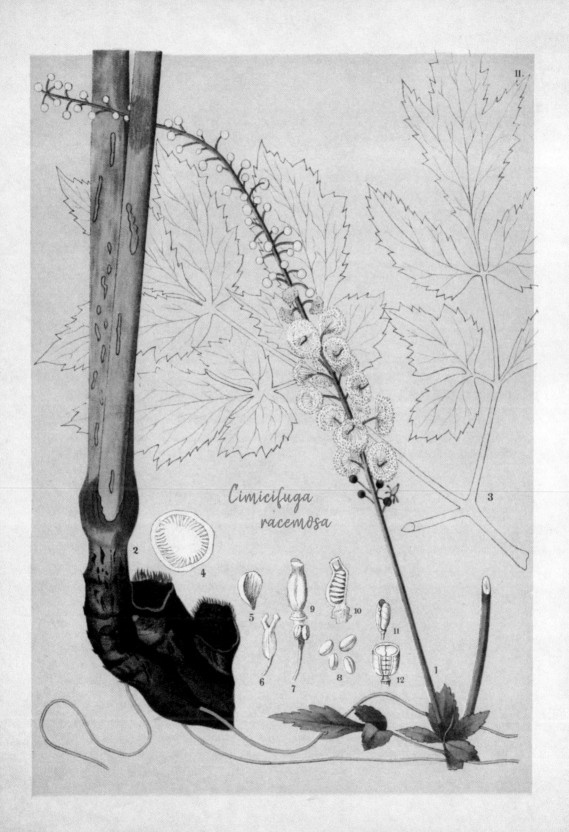

Cimicifuga racemosa

may support the folkloric use of black cohosh for a myriad of "women's complaints," most importantly hot flashes. Both traditional Chinese medicine and Western herbal traditions have long used black cohosh to reduce pain and calm the nervous system.

Extracts of black cohosh rhizomes and roots have been shown to decrease experimental inflammation by one-third in laboratory animals, although the constituents responsible for this effect have not yet been identified. Thus, it appears that the use of this plant for neuralgia and rheumatism has a rational basis.

Extracts of black cohosh also have been tested for estrogenic effects in mice and are devoid of this activity. Since this type of biological test is most always predictive for humans, it must be presumed that the use of black cohosh for dysmenorrhea cannot be based on an estrogenic effect. Other experiments have shown that black cohosh reduces hypertension and acts as an anti-inflammatory and hypoglycemic. In one experiment, it was found that black cohosh had a hypotensive effect.

Investigations have also verified the use of black cohosh as a smooth muscle and nerve relaxant. Recently, the Russians approved an extract of black cohosh as a central nervous system tonic and as a treatment for high blood pressure.

Caution: People taking other drugs of either pharmaceutical or herbal origin to lower their blood pressure are warned against the use of black cohosh concurrent with these other medications.

Cimicifuga racemosa is a flowering perennial plant native to North America. It belongs to the buttercup family, Ranunculaceae, and has a long history of traditional use by Native American tribes for various medicinal purposes.

Black cohosh gained popularity in modern herbal medicine for its potential to alleviate menopausal symptoms, including hot flashes, night sweats, and mood swings. It contains bioactive compounds such as triterpene glycosides and phytoestrogens, which are believed to provide hormonal support and help balance estrogen levels.

COHOSH (Blue)
Caulophyllum thalictroides

Parts used: Rootstock. *This plant is potentially unsafe and is known to have caused a number of adverse side effects in pregnant women, including birth defects, heart disease, and strokes. We do not recommend the use of this plant for any purpose.*

TRADITIONAL USAGES

Like the Mayapple, this plant is quite bitter, and is therefore avoided by grazing animals. The thickened rootstocks have been used in medicine. Some people are susceptible to irritation by handling the plant and have developed dermatitis.

Blue cohosh was widely utilized as an aid to parturition, first by Native Americans and then by the early white settlers, who called it squawroot and papoose root. To promote a rapid delivery, an infusion of the root in warm water was drunk as a tea for a week or two prior to the expected delivery date. Various tribes took this same preparation for other purposes as well. The Menominees, Ojibwa, Meskwakis, and Potawatomis used it for "female troubles." The Omahas boiled a decoction of the root as a fever remedy.

Reportedly, blue cohosh has also been employed to purge the intestinal tract of infestations of worms. The root is a diuretic as well, promoting urination; it has also been used medicinally for its ability to produce sweating.

The dried root was official in the *U.S. Pharmacopoeia* from 1882 to 1905, when it was used for antispasmodic, emmenagogue, and diuretic purposes. At the turn of the century, blue cohosh root was actively collected and traded, bringing a wholesale price between two and one-half to four cents a pound. One clinician found that an extract of the root has a pronounced stimulating effect on the uterine muscle.

COLTSFOOT

Tussilago farfara

Part used: Leaves. *For centuries, this has been a respiratory remedy.* **Caution: Coltsfoot preparations should be approached cautiously.**

TRADITIONAL USAGES

Coltsfoot has been recognized as a remedy for coughs and respiratory ailments since antiquity. An external emollient and internal demulcent, coltsfoot has been considered very helpful in relieving the coughs of colds and was applied externally as a poultice for relief of chest congestion. In traditional Chinese medicine, coltsfoot has long been used to treat various respiratory conditions. Hippocrates recommended mixing the root with honey for ulcerations of the lungs, while other classical Greek physicians reported that the smoke of the leaves was helpful for coughs and difficulty breathing. Reportedly, the fumes of the burning leaves relieved toothache.

Containing an acrid essential oil, a bitter glucoside, a resin, and gallic acid, the leaves are often used as a tobacco substitute and are sometimes smoked in an herbal blend for asthma.

Amongst Native American tribes in Northern California, sweet coltsfoot was a salt substitute that became so important that it led to intertribal warfare.

RECENT SCIENTIFIC FINDINGS

Test-tube and culture studies have shown coltsfoot extracts to have anti-inflammatory, antispasmodic, and anti-tuberculosis properties. In a mixture with other plants, coltsfoot leaves, when smoked by human subjects, had anti-asthmatic activity. However, it is not known whether it was the coltsfoot or other plants in the mixture that accounted for these results.

In animal studies in China, coltsfoot flowers, when added to the diet, were observed to be strongly active in producing liver tumors in rats. Because of this finding, coltsfoot should probably not be used internally until further research has been done on its possible carcinogenic properties.

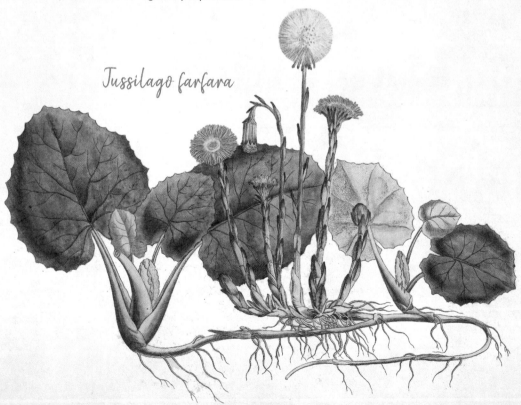

Tussilago farfara

Recently, an extract of coltsfoot has been found to be a potent cardiovascular and respiratory stimulant. In animal experiments, its effect has been similar to dopamine without tachyphylaxis.

Coltsfoot contains mucilage, flavonoids, and other compounds that are believed to have expectorant and anti-inflammatory properties. These properties may help alleviate coughs and promote the expulsion of mucus from the respiratory tract, making coltsfoot a popular remedy for various respiratory issues.

Coltsfoot, with its distinctive appearance and historical significance in traditional medicine, holds a special place as an herbal soother for sore throats, coughs, and respiratory ailments. Its traditional use for respiratory health has contributed to its continued interest.

COWSLIP
Primula officinalis, P. veris

Parts used: Flowers, roots, and leaves. *Once a renowned remedy for paralysis and headache, now the leaves are used to make a pleasant relaxing tea.*

TRADITIONAL USAGES

Once highly renowned as a narcotic and sedative, by 1837 cowslip had ceased to be much more than a rustic remedy. Linnaeus deemed it useful as an analgesic and as a sleep inducer, as did many of the old herbalists.

At one time, cowslip was the chief plant employed to treat paralysis and headache. All parts of the plant were used, but the dried flowers were believed to be the most potent.

In some countries, fermented beverages are made from the flowers with sugar, honey, and lemon juice, while the roots are also put into casks of wine or beer to enhance the strength and flavor of those beverages.

From all accounts it appears that cowslip was an extremely gentle pain reliever and sleep inducer, which caused none of the undesirable side effects that are encountered in some other such remedies.

RECENT SCIENTIFIC FINDINGS

Containing primulin and cyclamen, cowslip leaves are a good substitute for tea used to improve various nervous conditions.

Cowslip, with its graceful appearance and historical significance in traditional medicine, remains a delightful herbal treasure. While it is less commonly used today, its traditional uses for respiratory, skin, and digestive health have contributed to its herbal legacy. Throughout history, cowslip has been admired for its various medicinal properties. Different parts of the plant, such as the flowers, leaves, and roots, were utilized in traditional herbal preparations.

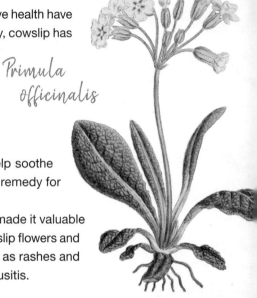

Primula officinalis

Cowslip was often employed as an expectorant to ease respiratory congestion and coughs. Its flowers were infused into teas or syrups to help soothe and clear the airways, making it a popular herbal remedy for colds and respiratory discomforts.

Cowslip's soothing and emollient properties made it valuable in topical applications. Infusions or extracts of cowslip flowers and leaves were used to alleviate skin irritations, such as rashes and mild inflammations. It is particularly useful for sinusitis.

CRAMP BARK
or Highbush Cranberry
Viburnum opulus

Parts used: Bark. *True to its name, this bark has been found to be a uterine relaxant.*

TRADITIONAL USAGES

Indigenous to southern Canada and the northern United States, highbush cranberry was a popular remedy among the tribes of those regions. The Malecites and the Penobscots drank an infusion of an unnamed part of the plant as a treatment for mumps. Since the bark most clearly holds the medicinal properties, one can assume that these people discovered this remedy through their own methods. One early 20th century writer stated that Native Americans used cramp bark as a diuretic, which is interesting since the excretion of liquids is desirable during mumps.

From 1894 to 1916, cramp bark was listed in the *U.S. Pharmacopoeia.* It was popularly employed as a sedative and antispasmodic. It was believed that its use during pregnancy tended to diminish miscarriage, especially if used with equal parts of button snakeroot.

RECENT SCIENTIFIC FINDINGS

Research supports cramp bark's folkloric reputation. Test-tube studies have shown cramp bark to have both uterine-stimulant and uterine-relaxant properties. Other studies show cramp bark to be active as a smooth muscle relaxant and as a cardiotonic.

Animal studies have shown *Viburnum* species extracts to reduce blood pressure in dogs and lower body temperature in mice. Cardio activity (strengthening heart muscle contraction) of aqueous extract was observed in both the dog and frog model.

Antiviral activity of aqueous extract of cramp bark was observed in cell culture against influenza virus. Cytotoxic activity of aqueous extract was observed in cell culture against the HELA cancer cell line.

This herbal remedy has been cherished for centuries for its potential to ease muscle cramps and spasms, hence its name. Native American tribes and European herbalists recognized the beneficial properties of cramp bark and have long used it in traditional medicine. The bark of the shrub, as well as the flowers and berries, were utilized to address various health issues, primarily those associated with muscle cramps and spasms.

Cramp bark is renowned for its muscle-relaxing properties. It contains compounds like valerenic acid, which have antispasmodic effects, making it useful in easing menstrual cramps, stomach cramps, and muscle tension. It is often used as a natural alternative for those seeking relief from muscle discomfort. Cramp bark's ability to alleviate menstrual cramps has earned it a special place in women's health remedies. It is believed to help relax the uterine muscles and ease the pain associated with menstrual cycles.

Due to its antispasmodic properties, cramp bark has also been used to support digestive health by easing stomach cramps and discomfort.

Viburnum opulus

CRANBERRY
Vaccinium macrocarpon

Parts used: Berries. *This common berry has shown remarkable properties in combating urinary tract infections.*

> *One of the key attributes of cranberries is their high content of antioxidants, which are responsible for many of their health-promoting properties.*

TRADITIONAL USAGES

One of the key attributes of cranberries is their high content of antioxidants, which are responsible for many of their health-promoting properties. These antioxidants help protect the body against oxidative stress and inflammation. One well-known benefit of cranberries is their potential for urinary tract health. Cranberries contain a compound that can help prevent certain bacteria from adhering to the urinary tract walls, thereby reducing the risk of urinary tract infections. Cranberry juice is rich in B vitamins, vitamins A and E, calcium, magnesium, quercetin, vitamin C, and potassium. An antioxidant in cranberry juice, A-type proanthocyanidins, can help prevent the growth of bacteria. Cranberry has also been used for dissolving kidney stones and gallstones.

RECENT SCIENTIFIC FINDINGS

The folkloric claims of cranberry's effectiveness against urinary tract infections have been confirmed by several studies. In one study, cranberry juice was given to a group of people with urinary tract infections. After drinking the juice for 21 days, 70% of the individuals improved.

Cranberry's chemical constituents are anthocyanins, catechin, and triterpenoids. Cranberry contains 10% carbohydrate, protein, fiber, vitamin C, and citric acid. The high acid content also increases urine's acid content, killing the bacteria that cause urinary infections. Interestingly, cranberry also prevents the bacteria from adhering to cells, allowing the bacteria to be flushed from the system. Dr. Anthony Sobota discovered this property of cranberry when he observed this effect under the microscope. He even found that commercial cranberry juice was strong enough to achieve this effect. Sobota also analyzed the urine of individuals after having them drink cranberry juice. The amount of antibacterial chemical present in the urine *was* significantly higher. Though further research continues on the specifics of cranberry's properties, it appears that this common drink is a simple and effective means for combating urinary infections.

DAMIANA

Turnera diffusa

Parts used: Leaves. *This is one of the most popular and safest of the plants claiming to be aphrodisiacs.*

TRADITIONAL USAGES

About 60 species of damiana occur mainly in tropical and subtropical America. The two *Turnera* species that yield damiana are small shrubs indigenous to Southern California, Mexico, and Antilles. The leaves are reputedly aphrodisiac and have also been utilized as a tonic stimulant and for laxative purposes.

Damiana acquired a reputation for curing sexual impotence; however, in these treatments it was generally administered in conjunction with a more powerful stimulant, such as strychnine or phosphorous, and so it is difficult to assess the degree to which damiana alone contributed to the results.

In Mexico, the leaves are used as a substitute for Chinese tea and also to flavor liqueurs.

RECENT SCIENTIFIC FINDINGS

Damiana is one of the most popular and safest of all plants claimed to have an aphrodisiac effect. Although some sources claim that caffeine is present in this plant, we have been unable to substantiate this claim from an exhaustive search of the literature. In fact, there are no animal experiments that have been reported that would lead one to believe that damiana has an aphrodisiac effect, and no chemical compounds have been found in this plant that would be expected to cause such an effect. Clearly this is a plant that needs and deserves a careful chemical and pharmacological study.

Apart from its potential aphrodisiac properties, damiana is also used as a mild relaxant and is believed to have calming effects on the nervous system. Some people use it as an herbal remedy for anxiety and stress.

Turnera diffusa

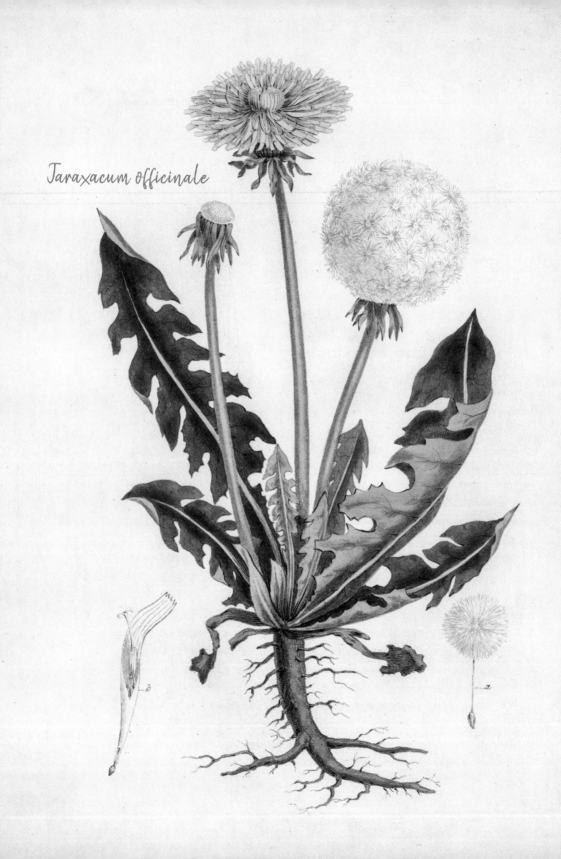

Taraxacum officinale

Damiana can be prepared and consumed in various ways, such as teas, tinctures, or capsules. It is readily available in health food stores and herbal shops.

DANDELION
Taraxacum officinale

Parts used: Rhizome and root. *A German over-the-counter preparation containing this common weed has been found effective against gallstones.*

TRADITIONAL USAGES

This species grows spontaneously in most parts of the globe. It is abundant in the U.S., adorning our grass plots and pasture grounds with its bright yellow flowers. All parts of the plant exude a milky, bitter juice when they are broken or wounded.

Although introduced to North America from Europe, many tribes soon learned to enjoy eating dandelion. The Iroquois preferred the boiled leaves with fatty meats. It was used in Native American medicine soon after it was introduced to this country. No doubt Native Americans got the recipes for this plant from colonial settlers.

A tea made from the roots was drunk for heartburn by the Pillager Ojibwas, while the Mohegans and other tribes drank a tea of the leaves for their tonic properties. Kiowa women boiled dandelion blossoms with pennyroyal leaves and drank the resulting tea to relieve cramps and pain associated with menstruation. The dried rhizome and roots were official in the *U.S. Pharmacopoeia* from 1831 to 1926.

RECENT SCIENTIFIC FINDINGS

Best prepared by boiling in water and then chilling, the leaves are used throughout the world as greens. They are rich in vitamins A and C and should be considered an important survival food. To verify the value of this common weed, we are told that many of the inhabitants of Minorca, one of the Balearic Islands in the Mediterranean, subsisted on dandelion roots after their staple harvest had been entirely destroyed by locusts.

A mild laxative and tonic medicine, dandelion is commonly administered as a home remedy for mild constipation and stomachache. Dandelion leaf tea, drunk often, is recommended as an aid for promoting digestive regularity. The plant was noted to have an almost specific affinity for the liver, modifying and increasing its secretions; hence it has been used in chronic diseases of the digestive organs, especially hepatic disorders, including jaundice and chronic inflammation and enlargement of the liver.

> *The root of the dandelion plant is rich in the carbohydrate inulin, a type of soluble fiber found in plants that supports the growth and maintenance of healthy gut bacteria*

The young leaves of dandelion, collected in the spring, make a healthful and tasty addition to salads. The root, dried and powdered, may be added to coffee for its medicinal value or used as a coffee substitute.

Experimentally, extracts of dandelion rhizomes and roots have been shown to increase the bile flow in animals when administered orally, and thus might have beneficial effects in hepatic disorders. The specific substance responsible for this reported cholagogue effect has not yet been identified, but it is known that the roots contain inulin, an essential oil, and a bitter compound.

The German over-the-counter preparation Hepatichol, which contains dandelion and other herbs, has proven effective against gallstones. Further testing found the preparation significantly enhanced the concentration and secretion of bilirubin.

Dandelion has also been found effective in relieving chronic arthritis. Although some herbalists have claimed that the plant has diuretic effects, we are unable to confirm that dandelion has such properties on the basis of laboratory research.

Dandelion leaves, roots, and flowers are all edible and have been used in traditional medicine for various purposes. Dandelion leaves are rich in vitamins and minerals, particularly vitamin A, vitamin C, vitamin E, and vitamin K. Dandelion greens contain several minerals, including iron, calcium, magnesium, and potassium. They are often used in salads or cooked as greens and are considered a nutritious addition to a balanced diet.

The root of the dandelion plant is rich in the carbohydrate inulin, a type of soluble fiber found in plants that supports the growth and maintenance of healthy gut bacteria in your digestive tract and is commonly used in herbal remedies and traditional medicine. It is believed to have diuretic properties, which means it can increase urine production and help with water retention and bloating. Dandelion root is also thought to support liver health and aid in digestion.

Some herbalists and natural health practitioners suggest that dandelion may have additional benefits, such as supporting the immune system and acting as an antioxidant due to its phytochemical content.

DEVIL'S CLAW

Harpagophytum procumbens

Parts used: Tuber and root. *Modern research confirms this South African plant's effectiveness against arthritis and rheumatism. The plant contains compounds known as iridoid glycosides, which have been shown to suppress inflammation in test-tube and animal studies.*

TRADITIONAL USAGES

For more than 250 years, decoctions of the roots of this plant were popularly embraced by various cultures in South Africa, including the Hottentots, Bantus, and Bushmen. The claims for devil's claw root are as a tonic and for arthritis and rheumatism. To reduce fevers, an infusion of the roots is employed, while an ointment is applied to ulcers, sores, and boils.

RECENT SCIENTIFIC FINDINGS

Devil's claw root has been introduced into North America as an herbal remedy during recent years. It is also currently very popular in Europe. This plant has been found to contain at least three bitter principles, the main one being an iridoid glucoside named harpagide. In animal studies, harpagide has shown anti-inflammatory activity in a number of different types of animal models in which inflammation was induced by the injection of various types of agents.

Harpagide and other extracts of devil's claw have been evaluated in recent times in clinical trials involving human subjects with arthritis and have shown a beneficial effect. Inflammatory responses have been shown to be curbed. There have been no adverse effects published for extracts of devil's claw root; thus the folkloric claims seem to be justified.

In many excellent animal studies, devil's claw has shown analgesic activity, anti-inflammatory activity, smooth muscle relaxant activity, and antihypertensive activity. In rat and rabbit studies, cardiac effects included antiarrhythmic

Harpagophytum procumbens

activity. However, the plant may interfere with heart medications and possibly worsen some health conditions such as diabetes. Care must be used when taking this plant.

One study treated patients with metabolic diseases with a tea of devil's claw root. Cholesterol and neutral fat levels were lowered. Currently the drug is quite popular in Europe.

Devil's claw is primarily known for its potential anti-inflammatory and analgesic properties. It has been used in traditional African medicine for centuries to alleviate pain, particularly associated with joint and musculoskeletal conditions such as arthritis, back pain, and tendonitis. Currently the herbal supplement is used as a treatment for gout (reduction of uric acid levels) and may also support weight loss.

The active compounds in devil's claw, including harpagosides and other iridoid glycosides, are believed to be responsible for its therapeutic effects. These compounds may help reduce inflammation and provide pain relief, making it a popular herbal remedy for individuals seeking natural alternatives to manage discomfort.

Today, devil's claw is commonly available in various forms, including capsules, tablets, tinctures, and topical preparations. It is often used as a complementary approach to support joint health and manage mild to moderate pain.

DOGWOOD

Cornus spp.

Parts used: Bark. *The bark of this lovely tree was once a common substitute for cinchona. Flowering dogwood has potent antipyretic, anti-inflammatory, analgesic, and antimalarial properties.*

TRADITIONAL USAGES

In folk medicine, dogwood is esteemed for its tonic properties. Numerous Native American tribes used dogwood for fevers. The Delawares called the tree *Hat-ta-wa-no-min-schi* and boiled the inner bark in water to make a fever-reducing tea. Flowering dogwood bark was similarly utilized by the Alabamas and the Houmas. Young branches were stripped of their bark and used to clean teeth.

During the last century, dogwood bark was often substituted for cinchona bark. When the alkaloid quinine was successfully isolated from cinchona and administered as a sulfate, the use of both cinchona and dogwood for intermittent fevers ceased almost completely. Up until that time, dogwood bark had also been given for typhoid fever and other disorders.

RECENT SCIENTIFIC FINDINGS

Dogwood bark contains cornin, a bitter principle, and high concentrations of tannin, which explains its astringent effect.

Cornus florida

The *Cornus florida* tree not only has an attractive appearance but also holds cultural significance in certain regions. Native American tribes have traditionally used the bark and root of the tree for medicinal purposes, such as treating fever, pain, and other ailments. The flowering dogwood was widely used by Indigenous North American tribes for its astringent and antiperiodic properties. Although it is not commonly used in modern herbalism, the dried root bark is still recognized for its antiperiodic, astringent, diaphoretic, mildly stimulant, and tonic properties. The flowers are believed to share similar properties. A tea or tincture of the astringent root bark has been used as a substitute for quinine to treat malaria and chronic diarrhea. The bark has also been used as a poultice on external wounds and ulcers. The glycoside cornin found in the bark has astringent properties, and the inner bark was boiled and consumed as a tea to reduce fevers and restore lost voices. A combination infusion of the bark and root has been used to treat childhood diseases such as measles and worms, often in the form of a bath. Additionally, the fruits are used as a bitter digestive tonic.

ECHINACEA
Echinacea angustifolia, E. purpurea, E. pallida

Parts used: Root and rhizome. *Native Americans believed this plant possessed almost magical healing properties; recent scientific documentation reveals startling immune-enhancing effects.*

The most commonly used species of echinacea in herbal medicine are *Echinacea purpurea*, *Echinacea angustifolia*, and *Echinacea pallida*. The plant is characterized by its distinctive pink to purple flowers surrounding a spiky, cone-shaped center.

Echinacea is believed to possess immune-enhancing properties and is commonly used to support the body's natural defense mechanisms, especially during the onset of colds, flu, or other respiratory infections. Some studies suggest that echinacea may stimulate certain immune cells, helping to combat infections and reduce the severity and duration of cold and flu symptoms.

TRADITIONAL USAGES

Sometimes known as coneflower, this perennial grows from the prairie states north and eastward to Pennsylvania. Its distinctive spiny appearance led the German botanist Conrad Moench in 1794 to name the *purpurea* species of this plant *Echinacea—echinos* is the Greek word for sea urchin or hedgehog. Native American tribes considered echinacea a panacea and utilized it to treat abscesses, boils, gangrenous wounds, septicemia, scarlet fever, ivy poisoning, spider bites, and ulcers. The tribes of the Western Plains applied echinacea to insect bites, stings, and snakebites. A piece of the plant was used for toothache and mumps. The Sioux drank a root decoction as a remedy for hydrophobia and snakebites. By the 1880s, it had become the most widely prescribed agent among American medical practitioners for infections and inflammations. Echinacea was used to treat common fevers and minor infections, as well as to treat typhoid, meningitis, malaria, and diphtheria.

In 1906, a report was published by Hewett describing several case reports on the treatment of various conditions, such as abscesses, boils, gangrenous wounds, septicemia, scarlet fever, ivy poisoning, spider bites, and ulcers. The dried roots and rhizome of the coneflower were official in the *National Formulary* from 1916 to 1950.

RECENT SCIENTIFIC FINDINGS

This plant of the Western Plains will serve mankind well into the future, based on recent scientific documentation of its immune-enhancing effects. Current pharmacology indicates echinacea is antitumor, antiviral, and an immunostimulant. It also is effective against herpes and influenza, is used for wound healing, has been proven to activate the reticulo-endothelial layer to increase alpha, beta, and gamma globulin (which is the formation of antibodies), and increases the rate of phagocytosis.

In 1972, an extract of echinacea root was shown to possess significant antitumor activity in experiments with rats. Antiviral activity was reported in 1978, showing that a root extract

Echinacea angustifolia

was effective in destroying herpes influenza viruses. Work in the previous decade (1956) demonstrated the powerful antibacterial properties of coneflower. By adding an aqueous extract of the root to suspensions of penicillin, activity levels of the drugs were increased.

In Germany in the 1980s, Wagner and coworkers reported on immunologically active polysaccharides derived from tissue cultures of this beautiful plant. Other European laboratories reported the activation of human lymphocytes, increased rate of phagocytosis, and macrophage activation. An extract of echinacea also revealed antiviral activity. In extensive experiments, the extract exhibited an action similar to interferon except, unlike interferon, the drug remains active even when stored at room temperature. Since interferon is difficult to obtain, echinacea could prove to be a very important aid in increasing immunoproduction.

Echinacea may help treat common skin concerns and is thought to be a mild antianxiety aid, and additionally contains anti-inflammatory properties. As echinacea stimulates the immune system, people taking immunosuppressive drugs should avoid this herb.

This is a biologically active plant, known to the Native Americans to possess almost magical healing properties and now proving itself worthy of acceptance as a world-class medicine.

EPHEDRA or Ma-Huang
Ephedra spp.

Parts used: Branches. *This has been used in Chinese medicine for over 5,000 years, and modern medicine continues to find both synthesized compounds and the natural herb beneficial. Known as Mormon tea in the United States, ephedra was commonly used by Western Plains practitioners of herbal remedies as a bronchodilator for asthmatic conditions.*

TRADITIONAL USAGES

The genus *Ephedra,* of which there are approximately 40 species all over the world, may be one of the most effective of all plants used to treat allergy. The plant's yellow color and its numbing of the tongue led the Chinese to name it *ma-huang.* Ephedra has been in use in Chinese medicine as a crude drug for over 5,000 years. It was recommended by herbalists as a bronchodilator, especially for conditions such as bronchial asthma (but *not* as a "simple nonspecific bronchodilator"). In China it has also been employed to relieve cough and reduce fevers, and even allergic skin reactions. Widely utilized for pain or inflammatory conditions, the herb was never given alone but always in combination with other herbs. Topically, ephedra has been used as an eyewash.

RECENT SCIENTIFIC FINDINGS

The interest in Oriental herbal medicine is most readily traced to the story of ephedrine from the ephedra herb. During his investigation of the pharmacological mechanisms of herbal medicines, N. Nagamine isolated the alkaloid ephedrine from the herb ephedra in 1885. Three years later, Takahasi and Miura discovered the mydriatic action (i.e., it dilates the pupil) of this chemical extract. At the University of California, San Francisco, School of Medicine, in 1924, Chen and Schmidt demonstrated that ephedrine had powerful bronchodilatory activity. Finally, in 1927, ephedrine was synthesized and rapidly accepted by Western physicians as a new pharmacologic agent. Both ephedrine and pseudoephedrine (e.g., Sudafed) are still widely utilized for their anti-asthmatic and anti-allergic properties.

Modern research has tried to elucidate the varied actions of "Ephedrae Herba," but its complete profile is still undefined. Many compounds are found in this genus, most notably ephedrine and pseudoephedrine. The ephedras contain 0.5–20% alkaloids, with most *Ephedra* species containing the alkaloid ephedrine in all parts of the plant. Ephedrine may account for 30–90% of this alkaloid content. Some plants also contain pseudoephedrine, which is an isomer of ephedrine. Pseudoephedrine and ephedrine may be naturally derived or produced synthetically. Ephedrine and pseudoephedrine are potent sympathomimetics, which means they excite the sympathetic nervous system, causing the vasoconstriction of the nasal mucosa, dilation of the bronchioles, and cardiac stimulation.

Other compounds found in ephedra include phenylalanine, ascorbic acid, catechin, cinnamic acid, quercetin, leucodelphinidin, rutin, tannic acid, tannin, and terpinen-4-ol. All of these compounds exhibit anti-inflammatory or anti-allergic activity.

Ephedrine produces many effects when taken orally by humans, the most important being dilation of the lung bronchioles and an increase in blood pressure. Ephedrine is employed as a vasoconstrictor and cardiac stimulant and as a bronchodilator in the treatment of hay fever, asthma, and emphysema. It should be noted that the effects of either alkaloid last a few hours and that side effects may appear, including nervousness, insomnia, and vertigo.

We have all heard of pseudoephedrine because it is often in over-the-counter products. Some confusion surrounds this alkaloid; people are unsure if it is made in the laboratory or extracted from ephedra. Both may be so! Pseudoephedrine may have certain advantages. Compared to ephedrine, it causes fewer heart symptoms, such as palpitation, but is equally effective as a bronchodilator.

This is but one example of the transition of a "folk-remedy" into the annals of world medicine. There are dozens of other current prescription and over-the-counter drug preparations that a succession of investigators have defined, but all leading to their original usage as herbal treatments. The story is simple enough, but subtle clinical twists explain why the herbs themselves are still used today, *not* having been rendered obsolete by their modern, synthesized cousin compounds. If ephedrine produced all the effects associated with Ephedrae Herba, then Ephedrae Herba would have fallen out of use; however, this has not happened. These natural substances produce effects similar to epinephrine (adrenaline) but are, of course, *less* stimulating to the central nervous system than amphetamine. This is why ephedra is such a useful plant. When properly utilized, it is extremely effective without being too strong in its actions.

Ephedra has also been found to promote weight loss due to its thermogenic and fat-metabolizing effect. Ephedrine also exhibits anorectic properties (reducing the desire for food). The alkaloid is thought to activate both alpha and beta adrenoceptors, which elevate metabolic rate, increase calorie expenditure, and result in weight loss. When combined with caffeine, a synergism results, yielding greater increase in metabolic rate than ephedrine or caffeine alone. For those interested in increased energy, endurance, alertness, and weight loss, this ancient remedy from China may hold the key.

Warning: Do not use if you have high blood pressure, heart or thyroid disease, or diabetes, or if you are specifically taking an MAO inhibitor or *any* prescription drug. Do not use if you are pregnant or nursing. Not for children under 18. Do not take after 4:00 p.m., as this herb may cause sleeplessness.

Due to its stimulant effects, ephedra has been used to treat conditions such as asthma, bronchitis, and nasal congestion. It was also commonly used in various weight loss and athletic performance supplements because of its potential to increase metabolism and energy levels. The abuse of ephedra products has led to regulations involved with over-the-counter access.

ERGOT

Claviceps purpurea

Parts used: Sclerotium of fungus. *This fungus was used by midwives to promote contractions during birth; however, the risks were high for both mother and infant and often resulted in harm. There are modern medications that* *contain ergot compounds (ergotamine) to treat migraine headaches, which may only be safely prescribed by a physician familiar with the attendant risks.*

TRADITIONAL USAGES

The word "ergot" is derived from the French word *argot*, meaning "spur," due to the resemblance of the fungus to a spur or elongated seed. This product is most frequent in rye, *Secale cereale,* and from that grain it was adopted in the first edition of the *U.S. Pharmacopoeia* under the name of *Secale cornutum*, or spurred rye.

In the Middle Ages, epidemics of ergotism from eating contaminated rye flour were characterized by both gangrenous and convulsive symptoms. Ergot's principal uses were as a uterine stimulant and a vasoconstrictor.

It was long used by midwives to promote contraction of the uterus during labor, particularly at the end of the second stage, as well as to speed childbirth and prevent possible postpartum hemorrhage. Ergot was also utilized in the nonpregnant uterus to check excessive menstrual bleeding or other uterine hemorrhaging. A common belief was that ergot extracts when taken orally were useful to induce abortion.

RECENT SCIENTIFIC FINDINGS

Investigation has revealed that ergot is not the diseased grain of rye, but the sclerotium of a fungus, the *Claviceps purpurea.* This fungus has three stages in its life history.

The sclerotium of ergot contains a number of complex and potent alkaloids, some of which have the lysergic acid (LSD-like) basic skeleton. There are two major indole alkaloids. The first, ergonovine, acts primarily to contract uterine muscle and to constrict blood vessels of the endometrium of the uterus. The second, ergotamine, acts primarily on the blood vessels of the brain, with minimal effects indicated here for ergonovine. This explains why ergot (or ergonovine) has been an indispensable drug for centuries in obstetrics. It initiates contractions of the pregnant uterus, primarily at the time of delivery, and is used to aid difficult deliveries. Of great importance is the fact that ergot constricts blood vessels of the endometrium and prevents the hemorrhaging that often accompanies childbirth.

There is no evidence that supports the belief that ergot induces abortion, since ergot only acts in the terminal stages

Claviceps purpurea

> *The word "ergot" is derived from the French word argot, meaning "spur," due to the resemblance of the fungus to a spur or elongated seed.*

of pregnancy, when abortion is not desired. Thus, ergot preparations do not usually induce abortion, but were thought useful to aid in term delivery of the fetus, to expel the placenta, and to prevent hemorrhage after delivery. Maximum labor-induction effect was attained only by injection of ergot extract or ergonovine.

The other useful alkaloid of ergot, ergotamine, is used extensively to relieve the symptoms of migraine headaches. Ergot itself is not utilized for this purpose.

It must be pointed out that regular use of ergot preparations must be avoided, since the blood vessels of the extremities, i.e., fingers and toes, will be constricted. This constriction restricts the blood supply to the extremities, and the end result would be gangrene.

As with any drug plant, when used properly and in the correct amount, its virtues are an asset. When misused, the attributes are changed to the detriment of the health and well-being of the user.

Ergotamine poisoning results from the fungus growing on rye, and it caused havoc and death during the plague in Europe and is thought to be responsible for the young girls of Salem, Massachusetts, in 1692 becoming "bewitched," exhibiting skin lesions, hallucinations, and convulsions. Fourteen people were executed as witches as a result of this unhappy phenomenon.

EUCALYPTUS
Eucalyptus globulus

Parts used: Leaves, also oil distilled therefrom. *The essential oil of the leaves can be toxic if consumed. Eucalyptus oil can be inhaled through the nose and offers some cold system and decongestant relief. The main ingredient is eucalyptol, also known as cineole.*

TRADITIONAL USAGES

Eucalyptus was commonly used to treat respiratory ailments. The leaves were smoked for relief of bronchitis and asthma. A mixture of a few drops of the oil to a gallon of water was boiled and the steam inhaled as a stimulating expectorant to treat chronic bronchitis and tuberculosis as well as asthma.

The volatile oil, distilled from the leaves, has also been used as a germicide and has been applied locally as an antiseptic; in this connection, it has been employed to topically treat skin diseases.

Eucalyptus oil was sometimes utilized as a substitute for quinine in the treatment of malaria and other intermittent fevers. The leaves have a characteristic aromatic odor that is due to an essential oil made up almost entirely of a monoterpene compound known as eucalyptol.

RECENT SCIENTIFIC FINDINGS

Human and animal testing has shown that eucalyptus essential oil and eucalyptol both dilate the bronchioles in the lungs and have antiseptic effects against a variety of microorganisms. Experiments have also shown that eucalyptus preparations have stimulating expectorant properties.

A combination of eucalyptus and peppermint showed promise as an external application for pain relief in a 1991 study. The researchers concluded that the application "may be beneficial for pain relief and/or useful to athletes."

Eucalyptus is famous for its invigorating scent, characterized by a fresh, camphor-like aroma. This pleasant fragrance has made it a popular choice in perfumes, aromatherapy, and various scented products.

Eucalyptus has been utilized for centuries in traditional medicine for its medicinal properties. Its leaves contain essential oils that possess potent antimicrobial and anti-inflammatory qualities. These properties have led to the use of topical or inhalant eucalyptus-based remedies for treating respiratory conditions, such as coughs, colds, and sinus congestion. Eucalyptus oil is often found in chest rubs, inhalants, and steam therapy to alleviate respiratory discomfort.

Eucalyptus leaves can be used to make herbal teas, which are known to provide relief from respiratory issues when inhaled. The tea's vapors help clear the airways and reduce mucus production, making it beneficial for individuals struggling with asthma and bronchitis.

Eucalyptus oil can be topically applied to soothe sore muscles and joint pain due to its anti-inflammatory and analgesic properties. It is often found in massage oils and ointments designed to relieve muscle tension and promote relaxation.

Eucalyptus is extensively cultivated to produce its essential oil, which is extracted from the leaves through steam distillation. This versatile essential oil is used in aromatherapy, skin care products, and cleaning agents.

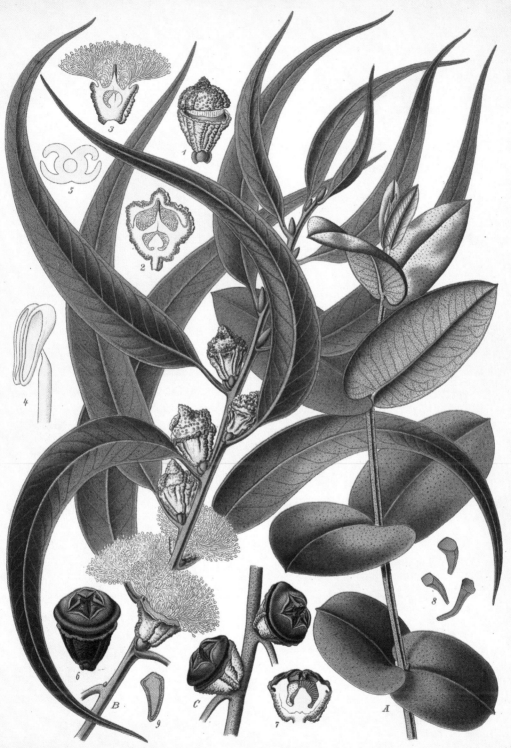

Eucalyptus globulus

EYEBRIGHT
Euphrasia officinalis

Parts used: Herb. *For centuries, this herb has been used as an eye treatment. Various inflammations and irritations were thought to be aided by eyebright.*

TRADITIONAL USAGES

Eyebright is a very old and revered folk medicine for eye troubles. It was first mentioned as a medicinal plant in a 1305 herbal. The powers of eyebright, or euphrasy as it was also commonly called, are even recorded by the poet Milton:

Michael from Adam's eye the film removed,
Which the false fruit, that promised clearer sight,
Had bred; then purged with euphrasy and rue
The visual nerve, for he had much to see.
—*Paradise Lost,* Book XI, lines 412–415

The poet William Shenstone exclaims:

Famed euphrasy may not be left unsung,
That gives dim eyes to wander leagues around.

Euphrasia officinalis

Eyebright had the reputation of being able to restore sight to people over 70 years of age. It was also used to treat cataracts, inflammation, and irritation. In Iceland, the expressed juice of the plant was employed to treat a variety of eye complaints. The Scottish Highlanders mixed the juice with milk and used a feather to apply the lotion to the eyes. The herb also was occasionally employed to treat jaundice, loss of memory, and vertigo (why, we cannot determine).

RECENT SCIENTIFIC FINDINGS

When given internally, eyebright's mechanism of action is not yet known. Externally, compresses relieve conjunctivitis and blepharitis along with other eye inflammations. A mixture of eyebright along with fennel, chamomile, and walnut leaf is a useful application for scrofulous eye conditions in children.

As the name suggests, eyebright is primarily associated with promoting eye health and vision. Herbalists and traditional healers have used this herb to address various eye-related issues, including eyestrain, irritation, and conjunctivitis. It is believed that the compounds in eyebright, such as flavonoids and tannins, have anti-inflammatory and astringent properties that can help soothe and strengthen the eyes.

Eyebright is commonly prepared as eye drops or eyewashes to relieve discomfort and reduce redness and inflammation associated with eye fatigue or minor eye irritations. These preparations are considered a gentle and natural way to refresh and invigorate tired eyes.

Beyond its eye-specific uses, eyebright has been employed in herbal medicine to address respiratory issues. It has been utilized to alleviate symptoms of conditions like colds, sinusitis, and hay fever because of its potential ability to reduce nasal congestion and inflammation.

Eyebright contains compounds known for their anti-inflammatory and antioxidant effects. These properties may extend benefits beyond eye health, potentially supporting overall wellness.

FALSE UNICORN or Helonias Root
Chamaelirium luteum

Parts used: Rhizome. *Also named devil's bit, this was at one time a popular liver remedy.*

TRADITIONAL USAGES
It was sometimes called devil's bit because certain Native American tribes considered this root a cure-all. The name came from the belief that the root's healing properties angered a bad spirit who bit off a portion of the root to prevent its use.

False unicorn was considered a diuretic and emetic, and was used for colic, worms, and fevers. The root was also chewed as a cough remedy. In 19th-century domestic American medicine, it was considered an effective liver remedy.

The rhizome was used in cases of infertility and menstrual irregularities. Thought to relieve symptoms of morning sickness, the root was also promoted to improve low sex drive in some women as well as treating male impotence. We have no definitive proof of any of these claims.

RECENT SCIENTIFIC FINDINGS
Current pharmacology indicates that the steroidal saponins have an adaptogenic effect on ovaries (normalizing function).

FENNEL

Foeniculum vulgare

Parts used: Seeds. *This popular food flavoring agent also soothes gastrointestinal upsets. It is rich in potassium, selenium, phosphate, iron, zinc, manganese, sodium, phosphorus, magnesium, and calcium, as well as vitamin K.*

TRADITIONAL USAGES

The ancient physicians Hippocrates and Dioscorides employed fennel to increase milk secretion in nursing mothers. Recent 2020 research confirms digesting these seeds may also stimulate prolactin to help mothers naturally produce breast milk.

On the basis of the old observation that when they shed their skin, serpents eat fennel to restore their sight, Pliny recommended it for visual problems, including blindness.

The gum resin from the cut stems was applied topically to indolent tumors and chronic swellings. The juice expressed from the root was considered a diuretic and was given for intermittent fever. Externally, fennel was a popular remedy for toothache and earache.

The main applications of the plant were as an aromatic, stimulant, and carminative, especially used to prevent colic in infants. It is often combined with senna or chamomile to make this stronger-tasting medicinal more palatable as well as more tolerable to the upset gastrointestinal tract. An infusion of fennel seeds was administered as an enema to infants to aid expulsion of flatus. Fennel remained an important element of veterinary medicine long after its use in human ailments declined.

The entire plant has a fragrant, aromatic licorice-like odor; it has been widely employed in foods, both for flavoring and as a vegetable, both raw and cooked. Fennel is used to flavor absinthe and other liquors.

RECENT SCIENTIFIC FINDINGS

Oil of fennel is known to contain 50 to 60 percent anethole, and 20 percent fenchose, chavicol, and anisic aldehyde. It is soothing for gastrointestinal upsets as well as being an appetite stimulant. One experiment on adult humans found a kidney stone dissolution effect.

Other studies have observed antimutagenic activity in bacteria as well as antifungal activity against *Aspergillus* and *Trichophyton* in cell culture studies. Antibacterial activity in vitro against several human pathogens has been observed. Fennel exhibited anti-yeast activity against *Candida albicans* and anti-inflammatory activity in humans and rats. The fruit has been shown to be effective as an insect repellent.

In an animal study, a boiled water extract of fennel leaves produced a significant dose-related reduction in arterial blood pressure. Heart and respiratory rates were not affected. Interestingly, a non-boiled extract showed no effect.

Fennel has a long history of medicinal use, particularly in traditional herbal medicine systems. It is believed to possess various potential health benefits, such as aiding digestion, soothing gastrointestinal discomfort, and promoting lactation in nursing mothers. Fennel seeds are often used to make herbal teas or infusions for these purposes.

In addition to its culinary and traditional uses, fennel continues to be valued in modern times. Its seeds are used as a flavoring agent in various cuisines and are a common ingredient in spice blends.

A recent study explored the impact of fennel seed extract on the intestinal epithelium barrier function and the signal transducer and activator of transcription (STAT) pathway, which plays a role in inflammatory bowel disease. The study used monolayers from the T84 colonic cell line challenged with interferon-gamma and monitored with and without fennel seed extract to investigate the protective effects of the extract in vitro. Additionally, the study employed the dextran sodium sulfate–induced murine colitis model to determine if the protective effect of fennel seed extract could be replicated in vivo. Results indicated that fennel seed extract had a positive effect on transepithelial electrical resistance (TEER) in both T84 and murine models and showed an increase in tight junction–associated mRNA in T84 cell monolayers. Both models also displayed a significant decrease in phosphorylated STAT1 (pSTAT1), indicating reduced activation of the STAT pathway. Furthermore, mice treated with fennel seed showed significantly lower ulcer indices than control mice. In conclusion, the study suggests that fennel seed extract improves barrier function of the gastrointestinal tract and may have potential therapeutic applications. Clearly, the simple fennel plant deserves much more research and study!

Foeniculum vulgare

FENUGREEK
Trigonella foenum-graecum

Parts used: Seeds. *Used by the ancient Egyptians and Greeks, the seeds have been found to reduce blood glucose in diabetics. The most popular use was to increase breastmilk production.*

TRADITIONAL USAGES

The ancient Egyptians and Greeks both used fenugreek for respiratory problems. It was also considered a restorative and was given to people recovering from a variety of illnesses.

In traditional Chinese medicine, fenugreek's recorded use dates back a thousand years. The dried seeds are used to treat the kidney meridian. The bitter seeds are dried and given for hernia, beriberi, abdominal pains, and impotence.

Fenugreek has also been utilized as an anti-inflammatory agent and as a mucilaginous poultice. In some societies, it was believed to be an aphrodisiac.

RECENT SCIENTIFIC FINDINGS

Fenugreek is rich in steroid saponins, especially diosgenin. French researchers found that fenugreek reduced blood glucose and plasma cholesterol levels in diabetic dogs.

Human experiments confirmed the animal research. Defatted fenugreek seed powder was added to the diet of diabetic patients and served with both lunch and dinner. This resulted in a 54% reduction in urinary glucose. Blood sugar levels decreased. Cholesterol was also significantly reduced.

Another study with non-insulin dependent diabetics produced similar results. Powdered fenugreek seed soaked in water significantly reduced glucose levels and lowered plasma insulin. These studies indicate that fenugreek may be beneficial in the treatment of diabetes.

Fenugreek has a history of medicinal use, particularly in traditional systems like Ayurveda and traditional Chinese medicine. It is believed to have potential health benefits, including aiding digestion, supporting blood sugar management, and promoting lactation in nursing mothers. Fenugreek seeds are often used to make herbal infusions and supplements for these purposes.

In modern times, fenugreek continues to be a popular ingredient in culinary dishes and dietary supplements. It is used in traditional medicine practices and is also being studied for its potential health effects, such as its impact on blood sugar levels and cholesterol.

FEVERFEW

Tanacetum parthenium, Chrysanthemum parthenium

Parts used: Herb. *This has been in use since the time of the ancient Greeks.*

TRADITIONAL USAGES

Physicians dating back to Dioscorides have considered feverfew to be especially valuable for its action on the uterus. It was employed to stimulate menstruation and in childbirth to aid expulsion of the placenta after birth. Herbalist John Parkinson in 1629 wrote, "It is chiefly used for the diseases of the mother, whether it be the rising of the mother, or the hardness or inflammations of the same."

However, it is a remedy for headaches that feverfew is most noted. This plant's action against fevers earned it its name. Gerard wrote in 1633 that feverfew is "very good for them that are giddie in the head." Echoing that endorsement in 1772, John Hill declared that "in the worst headache this herb exceeds whatever else is known."

Other uses were as an antispasmodic, stomachic, and diuretic, and for rheumatism. A Cuban variety of the plant was used by local practitioners as a febrifuge and antiperiodic to treat intermittent fevers; an American variety was used in the southwest United States as a tonic and antiperiodic.

Feverfew smells, tastes, and looks like Roman chamomile (*Anthemis nobilis*). In France, the two plants were at one time used interchangeably. This perennial herb is sometimes added for its flavor in wine making and certain pastries.

RECENT SCIENTIFIC FINDINGS

At seminars people often ask if feverfew is as effective for treating regular headaches as it is for its accepted use in the treatment of migraine headaches.

A 1988 study may help us to understand why feverfew "works" only for migraine headaches. The researchers reported that crude extracts of the plant both inhibit platelet aggregation and also inhibit secretory activity in platelets, most cells, and PMNs (polymorphonuclear leucocytes). They speculate that such activities are relevant to the plant's medicinal properties.

Feverfew contains the sesquiterpene lactones (parthenolide and parthenolide-like compounds). These compounds bring about the anticlotting effects of extracts. Blood platelets are so affected because the cellular sulfhydryl groups they contain are "neutralized" by this herb. Feverfew extracts also slow the spread of platelets and the formation of clot-like substances on collagen. In a series of novel experiments, the authors demonstrated that extracts of this plant protected the endothelial layer of rabbit aorta from laboratory-induced injury (i.e., perfusion with a salt solution).

As for headaches, it is interesting to note that by inhibiting the secretion of histamines from mast cells, migraine-type pain is controlled or eliminated. In conclusion, Luke Voyno-Yasenetsky and colleagues reconfirmed "feverfew being of value as an antithrombotic agent as well as being of value in migraine and arthritis."

Feverfew to treat migraines came about not by laboratory research but because of a woman in England. For years she had suffered from severe migraines. On the advice of a friend's father, the woman began eating feverfew leaves. Gradually the headaches disappeared. The woman became convinced of feverfew's healing properties and passed on her experience to other migraine sufferers.

Subsequent research by investigators has confirmed feverfew's efficacy in treating migraine. In 1988, a randomized, double-blind, placebo-controlled study with 72 human volunteers was carried out over an eight-month period. The researchers found feverfew significantly reduced migraine attacks.

A double-blind study discovered that a combination of feverfew and ginger may be effective for treating acute migraines. The study showed that 63% of patients taking the herbal preparation experienced pain relief within two hours, while only 39% taking a placebo experienced relief, which was a statistically significant difference. The product used in this study was a proprietary preparation called Lipi-Gesic M (PuraMed BioScience, Inc., Schofield, WI). The liquid from one unit dose applicator was administered sublingually, held under the tongue for 60 seconds, and then swallowed. A second dose was given five minutes later. If pain persisted after one hour, a second treatment of two-unit doses could be given. All treatments mentioned here need to be under the control of a licensed medical practitioner for safety and efficacy.

Chrysanthemum parthenium

FLAX

Linum usitatissimum

Parts used: Seeds. *For centuries, herbalists have recorded that these seeds provide a soothing mucilage.*

TRADITIONAL USAGES

It is estimated that flax has been grown as a fiber crop for weaving into fabric since the 23rd century B.C. Medicinally, the seeds are a valuable demulcent and emollient, with soothing qualities both internally for coughs and externally for skin irritations. The soothing mucilage is obtained by infusing the seeds in water. This infusion is valuable in treating irritations and inflammations of the mucous membranes, particularly of the lungs, intestines, and urinary passages; it has therefore been used for pulmonary catarrhs, dysentery, diarrhea, urinary infections, kidney diseases, and urinary stones. A laxative enema is derived from the decoction.

The meal from the pressed seeds mixed with hot water makes an excellent emollient poultice. Linseed oil, expressed from the seeds, also has emollient properties and is applied externally for burns and scalds, mixed with lime water or oil or turpentine; this treatment is said to reduce the pain considerably and prevent undue blistering.

RECENT SCIENTIFIC FINDINGS

Flax seeds have a thick outer coating of mucilage cells. When water comes in contact with these cells, they swell and give rise to a soothing demulcent and/or emollient protective effect. When the skin or mucous membranes are coated with this mucilage, this effect becomes evident.

The seeds also contain a high concentration of fixed oil, which explains the laxative effect when taken internally.

Flax seeds are renowned for their exceptional nutritional profile. They are an excellent source of dietary fiber, omega-3 fatty acids (alpha-linolenic acid), and lignans, which are compounds with potential antioxidant and hormone-balancing properties. Flax seeds are also rich in vitamins and minerals, making them a valuable addition to a balanced diet.

Flax seeds are used both for culinary and medicinal purposes. They can be ground into flaxseed meal and incorporated into smoothies, yogurt, oatmeal, or baked goods. Flaxseed oil, derived from the seeds, is used as a nutritional supplement and in various recipes. Additionally, flax fibers are used in the textile industry to make linen fabric.

Flax has gained attention for its potential health benefits. The omega-3 fatty acids in flax seeds are associated with heart health and inflammation reduction. The lignans in flax may contribute to hormone regulation and potentially offer protective effects against certain cancers. Some studies also suggest that flax consumption may help improve digestive health and be a critical component to healthy weight loss.

FO-TI or Heshouwu
Polygonum multiflorum

Parts used: Root. *Second only to ginseng in traditional Chinese medicine, this plant has shown positive results in eliminating the symptoms of heart disease.*

TRADITIONAL USAGES

Fo-ti is one of China's main herbal tonics, second only to ginseng in reputed benefits. Its use was first recorded in an herbal written in A.D. 973. It is a key herbal remedy for the elderly. Said to nourish yin, fo-ti is utilized to "replenish sperm," reverse hair graying, and for "pain in the knees and loins." In other words, all the sins that aging flesh is heir to!

The Chinese name, heshouwu, has a colorful history. According to legend, Heshouwu was the grandson of a man who at age 58 had been unable to father a child. A monk advised him to eat the chiao-teng he gathered on the mountain. He then fathered several children. His hair turned from gray to black and his body became more youthful. He lived to the age of 160, still with black hair, while his child lived to be 130. From that time on, fo-ti has been used to strengthen the body and to nourish vital essence.

In Ayurvedic medicine, fo-ti is utilized as a remedy for colic and enteritis, while in Brazil it is employed for gout and hemorrhoids.

RECENT SCIENTIFIC FINDINGS

Chemically, this species of *Polygonum* contains phospholipids, anthraquinones, and bianthraquinonyl glucosides. The principle actions of the major constituents are purgative, cholesterol lowering, anti-inflammatory, cardiotonic, and antiviral. These effects are thought to be due to the plant's leucoanthocyanidins.

In human studies, fo-ti has reduced hypertension, cholesterol levels, and the incidence of heart disease among those prone to the condition. A 1991 study found that emodin, one of fo-ti's active principles, served as an effective immunosuppressive

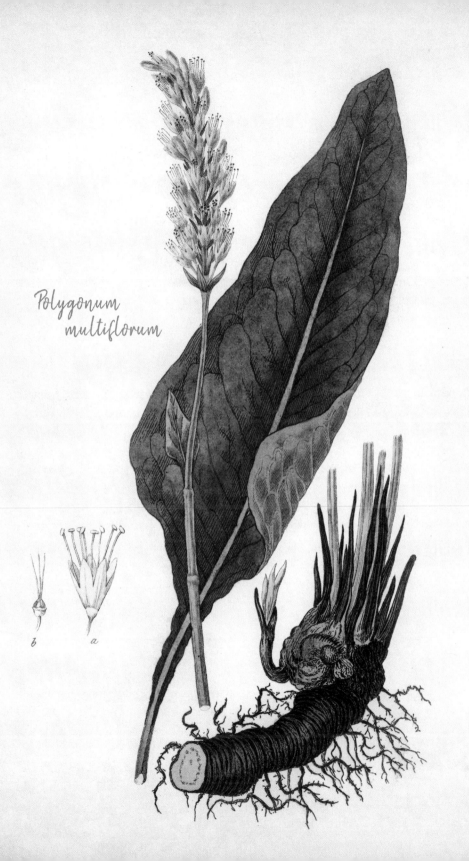

*Polygonum
multiflorum*

Fo-ti is one of China's main herbal tonics,
second only to ginseng in reputed benefits.

agent in human cells. The authors speculate that emodin may be useful against transplantation rejection and autoimmune disease.

In what appears to be an attempt to discredit Chinese herbal remedies, an investigator at the University of California, Berkeley, published an article in 1981 titled "Mutagenic Activity of He Shou Wu (*Polygonum multiflorum*)," which instead exonerated fo-ti. We had to read this brief entry three times to realize that the title held the opposite meaning of the findings. The author subjected this herb to the by now infamous Ames test and discovered "that the herb is not mutagenic," and that "a positive dose-response relationship did not exist." Instead of stating this at the outset, the author saved this for the end, even adding the caveat, "Oxidation and pyrolytic products could be created during the long simmering process. Especially when other herbs are present, molecular recombination and alteration of functional groups may occur." Unable to nail this herb to the cross of scientific bias, he concludes, "Pinpointing herbs with mutagenic potential awaits further investigation." Amen!

Heshouwu has a prominent place in traditional Chinese medicine, where it has been used for centuries. It is often associated with promoting longevity, enhancing vitality, and supporting overall well-being. It is often referred to as the "Elixir of Life" and has been used in traditional Chinese medicine formulations and remedies for a wide range of health concerns, including aging-related issues, hair health, and reproductive health.

Heshouwu is particularly valued for its potential to support the health of the liver and kidneys, which are considered essential organs for longevity and vitality in traditional Chinese medicine.

Scientific studies on heshouwu suggest that it may have antioxidant and anti-inflammatory properties. Additionally, certain compounds in heshouwu, such as stilbenes, have attracted attention for their potential health benefits.

Heshouwu is a culturally significant herb deeply woven into traditional Chinese medicine, with a legacy that spans centuries. Its potential health-promoting properties and historical significance continue to make it a noteworthy herb in the realm of natural remedies.

FOXGLOVE
Digitalis purpurea

Parts used: Leaves. *The leaves of this plant are the source of the well-known heart medicine digitalis.*

TRADITIONAL USAGES

Probably the best example of an herbal remedy that eventually became an indispensable drug to the medical profession are the leaves of foxglove. The point of departure was that foxglove was being used by a Welsh woman as one of several plants in a tea for the treatment of dropsy. (Dropsy is a symptom of a poorly operating heart, with a resulting accumulation of fluid in the body, particularly in the legs and ankles.) English botanist Dr. William Withering observed this use in 1775. Through experimentation he found that the major plant in the mixture responsible for this effect of reducing fluid accumulation was *Digitalis purpurea* leaves. Withering then used an infusion of the leaves of this plant in his medical practice for the treatment of dropsy. For over a decade, Withering recorded his clinical observations and so established guidelines for use of the drug. A remarkable medical pioneer!

Prior to the discovery of its cardiac applications in 1775, foxglove was utilized as an expectorant, in epilepsy, and to reduce glandular swellings. The juice obtained by bruising the leaves was mixed with honey and drunk to purge the gastrointestinal tract in both directions. Famed herbalist Nicholas Culpepper recommended that foxglove be used to treat obstructions of the liver and spleen, as well as externally for scabies. The plant was used externally in Italy to heal wounds and reduce swellings.

Digitalis purpurea

RECENT SCIENTIFIC FINDINGS

Digitalis, the active principle of foxglove, came to be employed as a stimulant in acute circulatory failure, as a diuretic, and as a cardiac tonic in chronic heart disorders.

Both powdered foxglove leaves and digitalis are currently widely used for the treatment of congestive heart failure. A symptom of overdose is vomiting, but when taken in proper amounts, foxglove causes the heart to beat slower and stronger, which then causes fluids to be excreted from the body more efficiently, resulting in a secondary diuretic effect.

The cardiotonic and diuretic effects of digitalis make foxglove very useful in cases of dropsy associated with heart disease. The drug reduces the force and velocity of the circulation and helps to regulate irregular heartbeats.

Foxglove is historically significant for its role in modern medicine. It contains compounds called cardiac glycosides, which have the potential to positively affect heart function. These compounds led to the development of the drug digoxin, which is derived from foxglove and used to treat certain heart conditions, particularly congestive heart failure and atrial fibrillation.

Foxglove-derived medications like digoxin are prescribed by healthcare professionals for specific heart conditions. However, due to its potency and potential toxicity, the use of foxglove as a medicinal herb is strictly regulated and should only be done under medical supervision.

Foxglove is a captivating herb with a dual legacy—celebrated for its ornamental beauty and recognized for its pivotal role in the development of cardiac medications. Its history serves as a reminder of the intricate relationship between plants and human health.

GARLIC

Allium sativum

Parts used: Cloves. *This commonly used plant may help prevent heart disease.*

TRADITIONAL USAGES

The Egyptians employed garlic to give strength and nourishment to the slaves constructing the pyramids. The Romans also gave garlic to their laborers, while Roman soldiers believed that garlic inspired courage and dedicated the plant to Mars, the god of war.

In the Middle Ages, garlic was used to ward off demons and the evil eye. Because of the belief that evil spirits caused diseases, garlic was held to have magical powers.

Garlic also has been utilized for thousands of years as a cancer treatment. Hippocrates wrote about a steam fumigation of garlic to treat cancer of the uterus. Similar usage against various forms of cancer was recorded in ancient Egypt, Greece, Rome, India, Russia, Europe, and China. Pliny wrote that garlic was a useful remedy for a variety of conditions, including ulcers, asthma, and rheumatism.

In Japan, garlic has been a folk medicine for centuries, most commonly for various gastrointestinal ailments.

RECENT SCIENTIFIC FINDINGS

As knowledge about the benefits of garlic continues to spread from folklore into mainstream medicine, numerous claims are being made regarding various garlic products. Before looking at some of these claims, we should summarize the health significance of garlic and garlic constituents.

One of the world's leading authorities on this subject is Dr. Eric Block, a professor of chemistry at the State University of New York at Albany. His review article published in *Scientific American* (Volume 252, pp. 114–119, 1985) remains an important summary of the chemistry of this fascinating plant.

To summarize, here are some of the claimed nutritional and pharmacological properties of garlic:

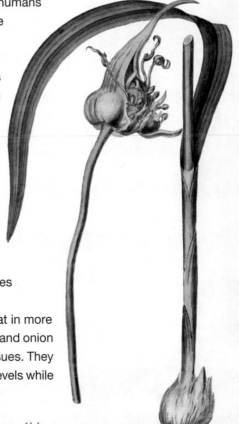

- Lowers serum total and low-density lipoprotein cholesterol in humans
- Raises high density lipoprotein cholesterol in humans
- Reduces the tendency of blood to clot and the aggregation (i.e., clumping) of blood platelets
- Inhibits inflammation by modulating the conversion of arachidonic acid to eicosanoids
- Inhibits cancer cell formation and proliferation by inhibiting nitrosamine formation, modulating the metabolism of polyarene carcinogens, and acting on cell enzymes that control cell division
- Protects the liver from damage induced by synthetic drugs and chemical pollutants
- Kills intestinal parasites and worms, as well as gram-negative bacteria
- Protects against the effects of radiation
- Offers antioxidant protection to cell membranes

Some of these health effects are worth looking at in more detail. Perhaps most significant is the effect of garlic and onion and their extracts on the lipid profile of blood and tissues. They lower cholesterol, triglycerides, and LDL cholesterol levels while also increasing the beneficial cholesterol, HDL.

Allium sativum

In the Middle Ages, garlic was used to ward off demons and the evil eye. Because of the belief that evil spirits caused diseases, garlic was held to have magical powers.

Both garlic and onion oils inhibit the enzymes lipoxygenase and cyclooxygenase. Each of these enzymes is known to act on one of two parallel biochemical pathways (within the arachidonic acid cascade) and only by inhibiting these enzymes can this pathway be arrested. When arrested, the production of prostaglandin is slowed. Since many cancers are prostaglandin dependent, this may explain why these oils have antitumor properties.

Garlic and onion contain over 75 different sulfur-containing compounds. While most of the medical benefits derived from supplementation with extracts of these plants are a result of these sulfurous compounds, recent studies show the additional presence of the bioflavonoids quercetin and cyanidin.

The cellular antioxidant selenium is another constituent found in the *Allium* vegetables and their extracts. The antitumor effects claimed for selenium may be based on its ability to replace the sulphur in the amino acid 1-cystine. Leukemic white blood cells have a rapid turnover of 1-cystine, a similar amino acid, and by substituting selenium for sulphur, leukemia can be suppressed in animals.

Recent research in China demonstrated a significant inverse relationship between the incidence of stomach cancer and the intake of garlic and related *Allium* vegetables. The researchers interviewed 1,131 controls and 564 patients with stomach cancer and found that people with no stomach cancer ate significantly higher amounts of *Allium* vegetables (a mean intake of 19.0 kg/year) than did the cancer patients (a mean intake of 15.5 kg/year). Those people who ate less than 11.5kg/year were more than twice as likely to develop stomach cancer than were people who ate more than 24 kg/year.

Researchers at the Garlic Research Bureau in Suffolk, England, recently found that "even small amounts of garlic, say 3 or 4 grams, will have a pronounced effect on fibrinolytic activity . . . in doses from 25 grams (10 cloves) to 50 grams garlic seems to be highly effective in promoting beneficial changes in blood fat composition and in platelet adhesiveness." To understand which type of garlic—the raw, the cooked, or the preserved—may be most beneficial, we must look at the chemical changes that occur inside a garlic clove. Fresh whole garlic is pharmacologically inactive. When crushed, an internal enzyme acts on allicin, a sulphur-containing amino acid, to produce the reactive compound known as allicin. Left to stand in the air or when cooked, allicin is destroyed.

While there is no final scientific agreement on the therapeutically active component of garlic, there is a consensus that allicin is very important, both as an active component itself or as a precursor of other active components. Because it is unstable, it has been difficult to manufacture a garlic product with significant amounts of allicin. The term "allicin potential" has been created to refer to the established standard of activity found in fresh garlic. Obviously, fresh garlic is highly desirable, for those who can tolerate the strong taste and aroma.

Garlic is a highly aromatic and flavorful herb that has played a prominent role in culinary and medicinal traditions for centuries. Its distinctive taste and scent make it a beloved ingredient in kitchens around the world.

Garlic's reputation extends beyond the kitchen. It has been linked to numerous potential health benefits. Compounds like allicin, responsible for garlic's pungent aroma, are believed to possess antioxidant and anti-inflammatory properties. Garlic consumption has been associated with supporting heart health by potentially lowering cholesterol levels and promoting healthy blood pressure.

Garlic has a rich history in traditional medicine. Ancient civilizations, including the Egyptians and Greeks, valued garlic for its medicinal qualities. Today, research continues to explore its potential role in immune system support, antimicrobial properties, and even the possible contribution to reducing the risk of certain chronic diseases.

Garlic has often been regarded as a symbol of strength and protection. Throughout history, it has been used to ward off evil spirits and illnesses. Its cultural significance extends to various cuisines, where it serves as a foundation for iconic dishes.

GINGER
Zingiber officinale

Parts used: Rhizome. *For centuries, this popular condiment has been an effective medicinal remedy for upset stomach and nausea, and its properties continue to be confirmed in clinical research.*

TRADITIONAL USAGES
There are more than 80 species of ginger spread throughout tropical Asia, east to Australia, and north to Japan. To encounter *Zingiber zerumbet,* or wild ginger, in full bloom

in a Hawaiian rainforest and to drink the sweet juice from the stems of flower heads after a long hike, as did the ancient Hawaiians, is the stuff that dreams are made of.

This widely used condiment has a recorded history of medicinal usage in China dating from the fourth century B.C. Today, the condiment is commonly found in many Chinese food preparations, indicating well established culinary as well as medicinal uses.

Ginger is mainly employed in gastrointestinal upsets. As a stimulant and carminative (removing gas from the gastrointestinal tract), it is used to treat indigestion and flatulence. Because of these properties, as well as its aromatic qualities, it is often combined with bitters to make them more palatable; ginger adds an agreeable, warming feeling.

In Ayurveda, the traditional Indian system, ginger is employed to treat arthritis, pain, fever, and blood clumping—all related to the metabolism of arachidonic acid as it affects various eicosanoids.

RECENT SCIENTIFIC FINDINGS

Currently, ginger has received new attention as an aid to prevent nausea from motion sickness. Ginger tea has long been an American herbal remedy for coughs and asthma related to allergy or inflammation; the creation of the soft drink ginger ale sprang from the common folkloric usage of this herb and still today remains a popular beverage for the relief of stomach upset. Externally, ginger is a rubefacient and has been credited in this connection with relieving headache and toothache.

The mechanism by which ginger produces anti-inflammatory activity is that of the typical NSAID (nonsteroidal anti-inflammatory drug). This common spice is a more biologically active prostaglandin inhibitor (via cyclooxygenase inhibition) than onion and garlic.

By slowing associated biochemical pathways, an inflammatory reaction is curtailed. In one study, Danish women between the ages of 25 and 65 years consumed either 70 grams of raw onion or 5 grams of raw ginger daily for a period of one week. The author measured thromboxane production and discovered that ginger, more clearly than onion, reduced thromboxane production by almost 600 percent. This confirms the Ayurvedic "prescription" for this common spice and its anti-aggregatory effects.

By reducing blood platelet "clumping," ginger, onion, and garlic may reduce our risk of heart attack or stroke. In a series of experiments with rats, scientists from Japan discovered that extracts of ginger inhibited gastric lesions by up to 97%. The authors concluded that the folkloric usage of ginger in stomachic preparations were

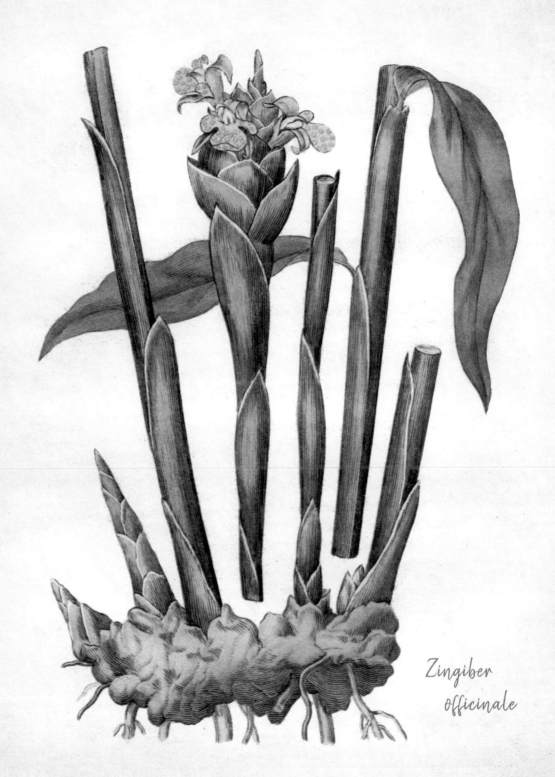

Zingiber
officinale

> *This widely used condiment has a recorded history of medicinal usage in China dating from the fourth century B.C.*

effective owing to the constituents zingiberene, the main terpenoid and 6-gingerol, the pungent principle.

In an earlier look at how some of the active components of ginger (and onion) act inside our cells, it was found that the oils of these herbs inhibit the fatty acid oxygenases from platelets, thus decreasing the clumping of these blood cell components.

A 1991 double-blind, randomized cross-over trial involved 30 women suffering from hyperemesis gravidarum. Ginger was alternated with a placebo. Seventy percent of the women confirmed they subjectively preferred the period in which they took the ginger. More objective assessment verified the subjective reactions, as significantly greater relief was found after the use of the ginger.

Ginger has a rich history of medicinal use alongside its culinary appeal. Its bioactive compounds, which include gingerol, have been associated with various health benefits. Ginger is widely used to alleviate digestive discomfort, motion sickness, and nausea. Additionally, it is currently being studied for its potential to support immune health and reduce inflammation, while addressing pain.

Ginger is known to possess anti-inflammatory and antioxidative effects, making it a popular herbal supplement for treating inflammatory diseases. According to a study led by Michigan Medicine and published in *JCI Insight*, the main bioactive compound in ginger root, 6-gingerol, has therapeutic effects in combating the mechanism that fuels certain autoimmune diseases in mice. Specifically, researchers examined lupus, a disease that attacks the body's immune system, and its associated condition antiphospholipid syndrome, which causes blood clots. Both conditions cause extensive inflammation and damage organs over time.

Ginger's healing properties have been valued for centuries, with use in ancient healing practices like Ayurveda and traditional Chinese medicine. In contemporary times, ginger's reputation as a natural remedy is on the rise, leading to a wide range of ginger-based products and supplements.

GINKGO

Ginkgo biloba

Parts used: Leaves. *For thousands of years, the leaves of this ancient tree have been recognized for their benefits as a geriatric drug. It is hard to understate the many purported benefits of ginkgo, which range from heart health improvement to brain function health, and many other critical anti-inflammatory and antioxidant properties.*

TRADITIONAL USAGES

Ginkgo, also known as maidenhair, is the oldest living tree, dating to the age of the dinosaurs. A common tree, it can live a thousand years! It has been recognized in Chinese medical practice for nearly 3,000 years. In Japan, it has been planted in temple gardens since antiquity. In 1730, the tree was introduced to Europe.

In traditional Chinese medicine, ginkgo was used for a variety of respiratory ailments, including asthma. It was also employed for urinary problems.

RECENT SCIENTIFIC FINDINGS

Ginkgo research has proceeded in many different areas. The most interesting and important relate to vascular diseases, brain function, impotency, dopamine synthesis, inflammation, and asthma.

An extract from ginkgo leaves is marketed as Tebonin. Clinical research has shown that Tebonin achieves vasodilation and improved blood flow, especially in deeper-seated medium and small arteries. The flow rate in capillary vessels and arteries is increased. In elderly subjects, Tebonin alleviated dizziness and loss of memory. Ginkgo has proven to be a particularly valuable geriatric drug.

Mild memory loss continues to be one of humankind's tragedies and one of medicine's greatest challenges. Interestingly, ginkgolides and a bilobalide possess a structure that is unique in the vegetable kingdom. A double-blind, placebo-controlled study shows yet another powerful benefit from this ancient Chinese herbal medicine.

Thirty-one patients showing mild to moderate memory impairment were followed for six months while taking a standardized extract of *Ginkgo biloba* (GBE). (All were over the age of 50.) The extract contained 24% flavonoid glycosides and 6% terpenes. The results show that GBE "has a beneficial effect on mental efficiency in elderly patients showing mild to moderate memory impairment of organic origin."

Ginkgo, also known as maidenhair, is the oldest living tree, dating to the age of the dinosaurs.

Sixty patients suffering from arterial erectile dysfunction received a daily treatment with 60 mg of an extract of *Ginkgo biloba*. After six months, 50 percent of the subjects once again were able to achieve penile erections. Upward of 45% of the remaining subjects showed some improvement.

Another study found that *Ginkgo biloba* extract (GBE) might prevent radical mediated human kidney and liver damage caused by cyclosporin A, an immunosuppressive drug used in transplants. This herbal product was found to be as effective as vitamin E and glutathione in protecting against such damage, adding to our understanding of the value of incorporating nutritional and herbal supplements in modern medicine. The protective effects of GBE were diminished in the presence of iron, owing to the limits imposed by this powerful oxidant.

Ginkgo's effect as an anti-allergic, antiasthmatic agent has also been demonstrated. The platelet activating factor (PAF) has been implicated in pathophysiological states including allergic inflammation, anaphylactic shock, and asthma. One study concluded that ginkgolide B is the most active PAF antagonist found in this class of ginkgolides. It appears that ginkgo relieves bronchoconstriction due to its PAF antagonist activity. A randomized, double-blind, placebo-controlled crossover study in eight atopic asthmatic patients showed that ginkgo achieved significant inhibition of the bronchial allergen challenge compared to placebo.

The leaves of the ginkgo tree contain flavonoids and terpenoids, which are bioactive compounds that may have potential health benefits. Ginkgo extract is commonly utilized to enhance cognitive function and memory, promote circulation, and improve overall well-being. In traditional herbal medicine, particularly in Chinese medicine, Ginkgo has been a staple.

Ginkgo supplements, which are derived from the leaves, are widely available and often used to support cognitive health and circulation. While research is ongoing, Ginkgo's potential benefits have garnered attention in the areas of natural medicine and health.

In Europe, Ginkgo is widely used to treat dementia. Initially, it was believed to improve blood flow to the brain, but research now suggests that it may protect damaged nerve cells in Alzheimer's disease. Numerous studies have demonstrated that Ginkgo has a positive impact on memory and thinking in individuals with Alzheimer's or vascular dementia.

Because Ginkgo improves blood flow, it has been studied in people with intermittent claudication, a condition characterized by pain in the legs due to reduced blood flow. An analysis of eight studies revealed that those taking ginkgo tended to walk about 34 meters farther than those taking a placebo. However, regular exercise is more effective than ginkgo in improving walking distance. One feels that ginkgo supplements in collaboration with a well-planned walking regime might be the best course of action for those suffering from leg pains, as the research is not overwhelmingly conclusive that ginkgo alone is helpful. Clearly, more research is required.

One preliminary study discovered that a specific extract of ginkgo called EGB 761 may help reduce anxiety. Individuals with generalized anxiety disorder and adjustment disorder who took this extract experienced fewer anxiety symptoms than those who took a placebo.

Another small study found that individuals with glaucoma who took 120 mg of ginkgo daily for eight weeks experienced improvements in their vision.

Ginkgo is widely regarded as a "brain herb." Certain studies have shown that it helps improve memory in individuals with dementia. However, it is unclear whether ginkgo aids memory in healthy individuals with normal, age-related memory loss. Some studies have shown slight benefits, while others have shown no effect. Ginkgo has been shown to enhance memory and thinking in healthy young and middle-aged individuals in some studies. Preliminary studies suggest that it may be beneficial in treating attention-deficit/hyperactivity disorder (ADHD). Ginkgo is frequently added to nutrition bars, soft drinks, and other products, yet the jury is still out. This is an herb that continues to garner international queries and will continue to have new science reports. We look forward to the new works!

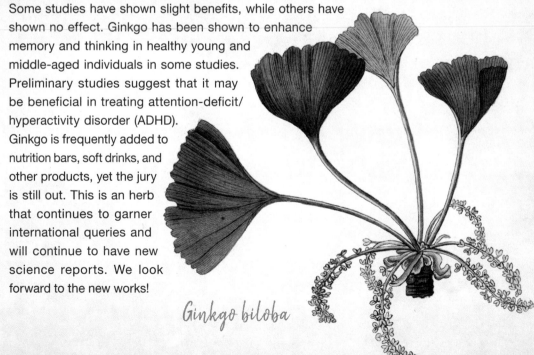

Ginkgo biloba

GINSENG (American)

Panax quinquefolius

Parts used: Root, leaves. *Preliminary studies indicate that this North American species is quite similar in its effects to the more widely known Asian variety of this famous herb.*

TRADITIONAL USAGES

A number of North American Indian tribes used ginseng as an ingredient in love potions, reinforcing its international reputation as an aphrodisiac. The Meskwakis prepared a love potion consisting of ginseng root, mica, gelatin, and snake meat. In the words of one Meskwaki, it is "a bagging agent women . . . use when they get a husband." The Pawnee made a powerful love charm by combining ginseng with three other plants (wild columbine, cardinal flower, and carrot-leaved parsley). According to anthropologist M. R. Gilmore, when the suitor added hairs "obtained by stealth through the friendly offices of an amiably disposed third person from the head of the woman who was desired, she was unable to resist the attraction and soon yielded to the one who possessed the charm."

Many tribes used ginseng as a normal remedy, not ascribing it the magical powers believed inherent in the plant by the Chinese, French, and English. Some Chinese viewed the plant as a panacea. The root's shape was especially important; one small piece resembling a man might bring a higher price than an entire bale. The ginseng trade was especially brisk during the 16th century; sometimes entire Indian villages engaged in foraging for the root. In the 1790s, the root sold for as high as one dollar a pound. By 1900, the commercial price was five dollars a pound. Before World War I, ginseng was one of the chief money-making crops in America; exports in 1906 amounted to 160,949 pounds, which was then valued at $1,175,844.

A second species found is red American ginseng (*Rumex hymenosepalus,* family Polygonaceae). It is native to the southwestern United States but has been introduced in other parts of the country. Indeed, it has also been used as an adulterant for ginseng. Originally utilized by the Hopi and Tohono O'odham Indians to treat colds and sore throats, the plant soon found its way into early American medicine, primarily in Texas. It was employed as an astringent for colds, loose teeth, and sore throats, and to heal sores.

RECENT SCIENTIFIC FINDINGS

There are two species of *Panax* normally found growing in North America, only one of which is found in relative abundance, *Panax quinquefolius*. Until recently, 90–95 percent of all *Panax quinquefolius* collected from wild-growing plants, or cultivated in the United States and Canada, was exported to the Orient. Undoubtedly, "American ginseng" sold in the Orient was simply sold as "ginseng," resulting in a great deal of confusion. Much of the scientific research in support of certain effects of ginseng was carried out in the Orient. The evidence needed to substantiate which species was used in these experiments was never given in the scientific reports. Hence, prior to about 1965, we really cannot say whether "ginseng" scientific studies were conducted with extracts of *Panax ginseng* (see section on Korean ginseng) or *Panax quinquefolius.*

As the situation exists today, there is not a single definite report existing in the scientific literature concerning the pharmacologic testing of authentic *Panax quinquefolius.* Only preliminary studies have been carried out to identify American ginseng's chemical constituents, yet they seem to be quite similar to those in *Panax ginseng.* Several of the ginsenosides are common to both species. Thus, at this point, and until further studies are reported, we can only presume that the biological effect of *Panax quinquefolius* is similar to that of *Panax ginseng.*

Recent purveyors of red American ginseng allege effects similar to those of *Panax ginseng,* especially its supposed aphrodisiac properties. Needless to say, there is no evidence for any ginseng-like activity for red American ginseng. The roots contain anthraquinone derivatives that would predictably result in a laxative effect if ingested. If you purchase a ginseng product and the use results in loose bowel movements, it can be suspected that the product did not contain ginseng, but rather *Rumex hymenosepalus.*

American ginseng is celebrated for its adaptogenic qualities, which means it may help the body cope with stress and maintain balance. It is believed to support the adrenal glands, helping to regulate the body's response to stressors and promoting overall resilience.

This herb has also gained attention for its potential cognitive benefits. Some studies suggest that American ginseng may help improve cognitive functions

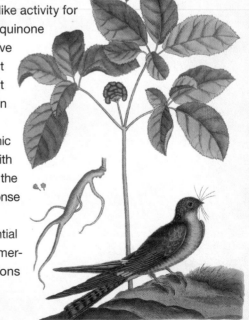

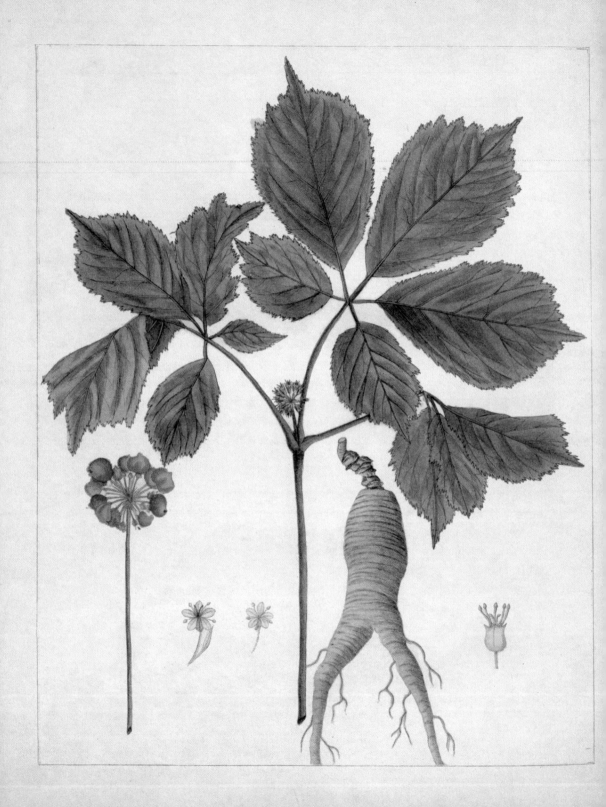

such as memory, focus, and mental clarity. It is thought to have a positive impact on neurotransmitter activity and cerebral circulation.

American ginseng has been traditionally used to enhance physical endurance and vitality. It is believed to support energy levels by improving the body's capacity to utilize oxygen efficiently, thus contributing to enhanced stamina and overall vitality.

Rich in antioxidants, American ginseng is thought to provide immune system support by helping to protect cells from oxidative stress. Some research suggests that its immune-modulating properties may contribute to maintaining a healthy immune response.

Traditional herbalists have used American ginseng to help regulate blood sugar levels, making it potentially useful for individuals seeking natural support in managing their glucose levels.

GINSENG (Korean)
Panax ginseng

Parts used: Root. *Long considered one of our most effective tonics or adaptogens, this popular herb is now also receiving a great deal of attention as a means to enhance endurance.*

TRADITIONAL USAGES
The genus name, *Panax,* is derived from the Greek goddess who "heals all," Panacea. In the Orient, ginseng has been long revered as a tonic. It was first mentioned as a superior herb in an ancient Chinese herbal dating from A.D. 25. Chinese herb practitioners use tonics to increase overall physical strength and promote the proper functioning of the body organs. Along with being prescribed for general energy deficiency, ginseng is used for specific ailments such as hypertension and diabetes. Ginseng is viewed as an herb that heals the spirit as well as the body.

RECENT SCIENTIFIC FINDINGS
Currently, there are three major types of ginseng available in North America. Since the names of these are often confusing, the situation needs to be clarified. Confusion results when manufacturers of ginseng products do not clearly indicate on the label the exact Latin name for the product being sold. The name ginseng on a bottle tells us very little about the content. One often finds labels such as Manchurian ginseng, Swiss ginseng, Korean ginseng, Oriental ginseng, and the like, with no further elaboration. Indeed, we have examined a large number of these products and find that they

contain neither *Eleutherococcus senticosus* (see section on Siberian ginseng) nor any of the common *Panax* species. According to a test of ginseng products selected at random, the West German government's State Product Test Institution reported that 25% of all ginseng products contained little or no active ingredients.

One should presume any mention of ginseng prior to about 1965, relative to human use, means *Panax ginseng* (family Araliaceae). This species is primarily found in the Orient, and it does not grow naturally in North America. Thus, Korean ginseng is *Panax ginseng,* Chinese ginseng is *Panax ginseng,* and so on.

The biological effects of *Panax ginseng* root extracts are fairly well defined, as are the chemical constituents responsible for most of these effects. Ginseng's main active principles are complex glycosides known as ginsenosides. These are classified as triterpene saponins and consist of about 20 identified structures. Ginsenosides of the Rb grouping are "slightly sedative," while those of the Rg grouping are more stimulating. Both types of ginsenosides show some anti-fatigue activity.

All of the ginsengs are used primarily as adaptogens, or substances that produce nonspecific resistance in the body. By definition, an adaptogen usually exerts no specific biological effects, but it tends to normalize adverse conditions of the body; at least this is the claim of Russian scientists, who have contributed immensely to this field of research. Thus, a person with mild high blood pressure, after taking an adaptogen, will usually have normal blood pressure. Conversely, a person with low blood pressure will also have normal blood pressure.

A great deal of evidence from animal studies, as well as data from dozens of human experiments, verifies the adaptogenic effects of *Panax ginseng.* However, the major use for *Panax ginseng* seems to be as a preventive medicine against various forms of stress, the common cold, and similar conditions. A popular belief is that *Panax ginseng* has aphrodisiac properties, but there is no evidence, in animals or humans, to verify such an action.

This herb, which has long been utilized for tonic or adaptogenic effects, is now also receiving attention for its capacity to act as an enhancer of performance and endurance. While not strictly a stimulant in the sense of being a primary central nervous system activator (such as caffeine and ephedrine-containing plants), the various ginsengs do show some central nervous system stimulant activity. Ginseng is utilized for its reputed anti-fatigue effects, improved performance, and stamina, as well as to improve concentration and reaction times in the elderly.

There are no reports in the scientific literature (and there have been more than 1,400 scientific papers published on this subject) that indicate any adverse effects for *Panax ginseng*. However, there are indications that regular use of this plant may cause mild insomnia in some people. Thus, it should not be taken in the early evening or at bedtime.

Buying a concentrated extract of ginseng offers the consumer a far more reliable assurance that the active constituents are present at precise levels as stated on labels.

Korean ginseng is a highly regarded herb deeply rooted in traditional Asian medicine. Renowned for its potential health benefits, this herb has earned a reputation as a natural tonic for various bodily systems.

Korean ginseng is celebrated as a powerful adaptogen, aiding the body in adapting to stressors and promoting overall balance. It is believed to support the adrenal glands, helping to regulate the body's response to stress and potentially mitigating its adverse effects.

Among its many qualities, Korean ginseng is renowned for its potential to enhance energy levels and physical stamina. Traditional use suggests that it may improve endurance, making it a favorite among individuals seeking a natural boost in vitality.

Some studies propose that Korean ginseng may support cognitive function by promoting mental clarity, focus, and memory. Its potential influence on brain health and neurotransmitter activity has piqued scientific interest.

Packed with antioxidants, Korean ginseng is believed to fortify the immune system by helping to counter oxidative stress. Its potential immune-modulating effects could contribute to maintaining a robust immune response.

GINSENG (Siberian)
Eleutherococcus senticosus

Parts used: Root. *This has long been studied in Russia, and recent research indicates that an extract stimulates cellular immunity.*

TRADITIONAL USAGES

During the past decade, a new ginseng has appeared in the marketplace in North America; indeed, it is being widely used throughout Europe also. This is the so-called Siberian ginseng, or *Eleutherococcus senticosus,* sometimes erroneously named *Acanthopanax senticosus*. Since the family Araliaceae is known popularly as the ginseng family, many different species of this family are referred to as ginseng. Since the habitat for *Eleutherococcus senticosus* is primarily in Siberia, the vernacular name Siberian ginseng was given to this plant. Indeed, because of the amazing similarity of pharmacologic effects of the *Panax* species, with comparison to *Eleutherococcus senticosus,* it seems that the name Siberian ginseng is appropriate.

It has been used for centuries in Russian folkloric medicine as an immune-enhancing agent. It is also employed as an anti-inflammatory; in cardiovascular disease; to restore concentration, memory, and cognition; and as a remedy for stress, depression, fatigue, or complete nervous breakdown.

RECENT SCIENTIFIC FINDINGS

Traditionally touted for its aphrodisiac effect, many people are under the impression that ginseng is only a "male" herb. In actuality, Siberian ginseng is highly valued by both sexes for its adaptogenic abilities. An adaptogen is a substance that "normalizes" adverse conditions of the body.

Ginseng has always been perceived as a stimulant. In Russia, a great deal of publicity comes from its use by cosmonauts and Olympic athletes to provide energy and negate stress effects.

Most remarkably, victims of the Chernobyl nuclear disaster were given courses of *Eleutherococcus* to aid them with an anti-radiation effect. Russians prescribe Siberian ginseng for patients undergoing chemotherapy and radiotherapy.

While the chemical constituents, eleutherosides, differ from those of *Panax* species, the pharmacological effects of Siberian ginseng are quite similar to those of *Panax ginseng.* This plant has been studied more rigorously by the Russians than *Panax ginseng.* Extracts of Siberian ginseng have been shown to relieve stress, lower the toxicity of some common drugs that tend to produce side effects in humans, increase mental alertness, improve resistance to colds and mild infections, and be beneficial in cases where a person is continuously in contact with environmental stresses.

A 1987 first-rate double-blind study demonstrated that a Siberian ginseng extract stimulated cellular immunity. Thirty-six healthy volunteers received 10 milliliters of an alcohol extract of Siberian ginseng three times daily for four weeks. A placebo of plain ethanol was used. A "drastic increase in the absolute number of [immune] cells," especially T lymphocytes, was shown using flow cytometry. The T helper/inducer cells, as well as cytotoxic and natural killer cells, were increased in number, which is a clear demonstration that the human immune system can be augmented with this herb. As expected, no side effects were observed during the experiment or afterward, a period of six months.

Flow cytometry is a highly advanced means for observing cells that permits an analysis of individual living cells. Using this method to study human immune reactions,

Traditionally touted for its aphrodisiac effect, many people are under the impression that ginseng is only a "male" herb. In actuality, Siberian ginseng is highly valued by both sexes for its adaptogenic abilities.

German researchers proved that an extract of Siberian ginseng stimulated T cell production, especially helper cells. This proof that such an adaptogen truly works pushes herbal science into mainstream medicine with wide application in numerous immune-related disorders.

The German scientists stated Siberian ginseng "could be considered a nonspecific immunostimulant." This may help explain why it has been said to be of benefit or cited in "protective effects against viral infections, retardation of neoplastic growth and metastasis, or better tolerance of chemotherapy and radiation." They further speculated about a "positive effect of *Eleutherococcus* in very early stages of HIV (AIDS) infection by preventing or retarding the spread of the virus, mediated by a synergistic action of elevated numbers of both helper and cytotoxic T cells."

It is not likely that any of the eleutherosides or ginsenosides will ever be used as adaptogens by themselves, since they are only present in their respective plants in small amounts. Similarly, they are too complex to expect a commercially feasible synthesis. Professor I. I. Brekhman, who has conducted numerous animal and human experiments with both *Panax ginseng* and *Eleutherococcus senticosus,* claims that the adaptogenic effect requires the total mixture of eleutherosides, in the case of Siberian ginseng at least, and that the full effects cannot be obtained with any one of the pure eleutherosides.

Unlike *Panax ginseng, Eleutherococcus senticosus* does not seem to cause insomnia, and like *Panax ginseng,* there do not appear to be any adverse effects in humans from the use of Siberian ginseng. In recent years, a flood of products claiming to contain Siberian ginseng have appeared on the market. We have found that most of these contain no *Eleutherococcus senticosus* root. The substitute products most frequently are offered for sale in capsule form. Unlike authentic Siberian ginseng, we have found that most of the substitute products have an intense bitter taste and a characteristic "vanilla-like" odor, but it is not the typical pleasant odor of vanillin.

Siberian ginseng is a remarkable herb deeply rooted in traditional herbal practices. Hailing from the rugged Siberian terrain, this herb is celebrated for its potential to enhance resilience and support overall well-being.

Siberian ginseng shines as an adaptogen, assisting the body in adapting to stressors and promoting a balanced response. It is believed to bolster the adrenal glands, helping the body better cope with stress and potentially reducing its negative impact.

This herb is renowned for its ability to boost energy levels and physical endurance. Traditional wisdom suggests that Siberian ginseng may enhance stamina, making it a go-to choice for those seeking natural support for an active lifestyle.

Enriched with antioxidants, Siberian ginseng is thought to strengthen the immune system by combating oxidative stress. Its potential to support immune function can contribute to overall wellness.

Some studies propose that Siberian ginseng might have cognitive benefits, potentially improving mental focus, clarity, and alertness. Its effects on neurotransmitter activity have intrigued researchers.

Siberian ginseng is often consumed as a tonic to support general well-being. It is available in various forms, including extracts, capsules, teas, and dried root preparations.

GOLDENSEAL
Hydrastis canadensis

Parts used: Rhizome and root. *This was widely used by Native American healers for skin diseases, and recent research has discovered potent hypotensive properties.*

TRADITIONAL USAGES

Here is another native American plant with wide usage by Native American healers. An infusion of the roots was made into an eyewash for sore eyes. It was also used for inflammation of the mucous membranes. The Cherokees pounded the rootstock together with bear fat and smeared it on their bodies as an insect repellent. The root was boiled in water and the resulting liquid applied as a wash for skin diseases by Native Americans and later in domestic American medicine. From 1831 to 1842, the dried rootstock was official in the *U.S. Pharmacopoeia*; it was readmitted in 1863 and remained until 1936.

Three components of the plant were at one time official drugs; hydrastine was official in the *U.S. Pharmacopoeia* from 1905 to 1926, and hydrastinine hydrochloride was in the *U.S. Pharmacopoeia* from 1916 to 1926 and the *National Formulary* from 1926 to 1950. All were classified as internal hemostatics. Goldenseal enjoys a tremendous reputation for its medicinal virtuosity. It has been recommended in the treatment of dozens of ailments.

RECENT SCIENTIFIC FINDINGS

Recent research has corroborated goldenseal's biological activities. The dried rhizome possesses cytotoxic activity, indicating it is useful against viruses. Since 1950, its antibacterial properties have been well-established, especially against *E. coli* and *Staphylococcus aureus.* Not to be overlooked is goldenseal's potent hypotensive activity. In one experiment in rabbits, an extract of the root brought about a severe drop in blood pressure.

Goldenseal owes its effect primarily to the alkaloids hydrastine and hydrastinine, in addition to berberine.

Three components of the plant also produce a strong astringent effect on mucous membranes, reduce inflammation, and have antiseptic effects.

Goldenseal can be used as an external application to the arms and legs in the treatment of disorders of the blood vessels and lymphatics. Berberine was found to have an anticonvulsive effect against the bacterial *Staphylococcus aureus*.

As a treatment for uterine complaints, it was given to arrest uterine hemorrhage, as well as to check excessive menstrual evacuation. In very small dosage, it was advocated to cure morning sickness; however, it is critical to note that in large doses goldenseal may produce abortion, and in fact has been used deliberately as an abortifacient.

Moreover, taken in too large a dose, goldenseal can dangerously overstimulate the nervous system. It is inadvisable to continue even limited usage for extended periods of time since the alkaloids are eliminated quite slowly from the body.

This is a potent plant that must be utilized with care. One of its constituent alkaloids, L-canadine, reportedly paralyzes the central nervous system and causes severe peristalsis.

Hydrastis canadensis

Goldenseal has a rich history of use among Indigenous communities for its potential health benefits. It has been valued for its purported antimicrobial, anti-inflammatory, and immune-supporting properties.

This herb is believed to have immune-modulating effects due to its alkaloids, which may aid in supporting the body's natural defense mechanisms against infections and illnesses.

Goldenseal is thought to support digestive health by promoting a healthy gut environment. Its potential to soothe mucous membranes may contribute to digestive comfort.

The roots of goldenseal have been used topically for skin concerns. Its potential antimicrobial and anti-inflammatory properties might make it a valuable addition to natural skin care routines.

GOTU KOLA
or Chi-Hsing or Pai Kuo
Centella asiatica

Parts used: Whole plant. *Long known to Fijian healers, this herb awaits discovery and possible wide adoption by the medical establishment.*

TRADITIONAL USAGES

Gotu kola is used primarily as a sedative, diuretic, and tonic, and to accelerate healing of wounds. It is claimed to strengthen and energize the brain. In large doses, it is said to act as a narcotic, causing stupor, headache, and sometimes coma.

It has been employed to alleviate bowel complaints and to treat syphilis and tubercular inflammation of the cervical lymph nodes. Its ability to aid in these and urinary tract disorders has been attributed to its demulcent properties.

Fijian healers have long known of the values of this plant; it is the most frequently utilized medicinal plant in their pharmacopoeia. It has long been known in India, and its use was probably brought to Fiji by Indian settlers.

RECENT SCIENTIFIC FINDINGS

Recent pharmacological studies have shown that extracts of gotu kola exhibit a sedative activity. The mode of action appears to be mainly on the cholinergic mechanism in the central nervous system. The major active principle in this plant is most probably the triterpene glycoside asiaticoside. Asiaticoside is well tolerated when given by mouth

> *This small, green herb is often referred to as the "herb of longevity" due to its potential to support various aspects of well-being.*

to mice and rabbits at a single dose of 1.0 gram. This would imply that it is a relatively safe substance. When asiaticoside is implanted under the skin, or injected subcutaneously in mice, rats, guinea pigs, or rabbits, improved blood supply of connective tissue occurs. A rapid thickening of the skin is also noted in the treated animals, as well as an accelerated growth of hair and nails.

There is some evidence that in humans, because of the sum total of these effects, that asiaticoside, and hence extracts of *Centella asiatica,* accelerates healing of wounds. There are indications that asiaticoside is useful for infectious diseases such as tuberculosis and leprosy. The microbes that cause both of these diseases are well known to have a waxy coating that most other disease-producing organisms lack. This waxy coating prevents the body's own defense mechanisms from killing the organisms, hence it is difficult to cure both of these diseases. It is thought that asiaticoside acts to dissolve the waxy covering on the organisms, which then allows the normal defense mechanisms of the body to destroy the causative organisms of leprosy and/or tuberculosis.

It must be pointed out that the foregoing is indicated only as a reasonable explanation for part of the useful action of *C. asiatica* preparations. Further work must be carried out to determine whether or not this is the case.

An extract, CATTF, has been found to be effective in promoting wound healing in vivo. Following up on this research, a 1991 study involving patients with post-phlebitic syndrome (PPS) confirmed that gotu kola has a regulatory effect on vascular tissue. Another study of patients with varicose veins also substantiated this effect.

Two other extracts, TTFCA and TECA, have also proven effective in treating venous hypertension. In one study involving 62 patients, after four weeks of treatment, those receiving TTFCA showed significant improvement while the placebo group showed no change. In another study, 94 patients suffering from edema in the lower limbs were given two different doses of TECA or a placebo. The patients given the TECA exhibited a significant difference in comparison to the placebo group.

It has also been shown that asiaticoside-pretreated rats (12.5 mg/kg/day for 3 days, subcutaneously), who were subjected to cold conditions, did not develop gastric ulcers. Control animals in the experiment did develop gastric ulcers under these conditions.

Recent pharmacological studies have shown that extracts of gotu kola exhibit a sedative activity similar to that of meprobamate and chlorpromazine.

Because of the pronounced effect of asiaticoside on skin, a study was carried out to determine if repeated applications would produce cancer. A 0.10% solution of asiaticoside was applied to the back of hairless mice twice weekly for the lifetime of the animals (about 18 months). It was found that sarcomas (cancers) were produced on the skin of 2.5% of the treated mice. These findings probably have little significance, since the test is not specific, and is recognized as invalid for weak carcinogens. The results of this experiment would indicate that in that test, asiaticoside would be classified as a weak carcinogen. Despite these minor pharmacological problems, gotu kola awaits discovery and possible wide adoption by the medical establishment.

Caution: Overdose may cause narcotic stupor.

This small, green herb is often referred to as the "herb of longevity" due to its potential to support various aspects of well-being. Gotu kola is renowned for its adaptogenic properties, which means it helps the body cope with stress and adapt

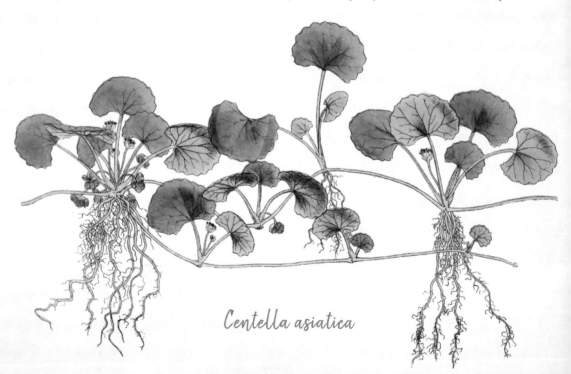

Centella asiatica

to changes. Traditionally used to improve memory and cognitive function, the herb's name is linked to its role in enhancing mental clarity and cognitive vitality.

Beyond its cognitive benefits, gotu kola has gained a reputation for promoting skin health. Rich in triterpenoids and antioxidants, it is believed to support the production of collagen, aiding in skin elasticity and wound healing. It has also been used to address conditions like varicose veins and cellulite due to its potential to improve blood circulation and strengthen blood vessels.

The soothing and calming effects of gotu kola have led to its association with tranquility and relaxation. In certain cultures, it is considered a nervine tonic, often used to alleviate anxiety and promote a sense of calmness. This reputation has earned it the nickname the "herb of tranquility."

GREEN TEA
Various species

Parts used: Leaves.

TRADITIONAL USAGES
For centuries, tea has been the most commonly consumed beverage in the world, except for water. Since antiquity, green tea has been thought to provide various pharmacological benefits, such as combating mental fatigue as well as colds and flu. Many 19th-century chemists and medical scientists believed that tea produced healthful effects on the digestive and nervous systems, facilitated cardiovascular function, and decreased blood pressure.

RECENT SCIENTIFIC FINDINGS
Modern scientists are discovering new healthful benefits from the consumption of green tea. According to Hirota Fujiki, a chemist at the National Cancer Center Research Institute in Tokyo, "Green tea cannot prevent every cancer, but it's the cheapest and most practical method for cancer prevention available to the general public."

The majority of teas produced worldwide can be classified into two types: black tea, which is most common in Western nations, and green tea, which predominates in the Far East, especially China and Japan. When consumed, green tea provides more healthful advantages than black tea because it contains larger amounts of such important substances as vitamins, including twice as much vitamin C as black tea. Green tea contains more than twice the catechins of black tea; tea's "tannins" consist mostly of these catechins. Though the content of vitamin P in other foods is very low, tea catechins have been found to have high vitamin P activity. In fact, the regular consumption of catechin-rich tea may meet the human requirements for vitamin P, according to some researchers.

While tea's favorable effect was once attributed to its caffeine content, biochemical studies have shown that tea's catechins may play an even greater role. It has been demonstrated that peculiar features of the chemical composition of tea are responsible for its important pharmacological and physiological properties. Tea's beneficial effects that were first discovered empirically over many generations have been corroborated by present-day scientific investigations.

The catechins in tea are formed by polyphenic compounds. Many researchers have found that phenolic compounds, including tea catechins, delay the development of arteriosclerosis. Clinical investigations ascertained that consumption of green tea had a therapeutic effect on infectious diseases, particularly dysentery. Incorporating green tea in the treatment of rheumatism had a favorable effect on both the general condition and capillary resistance of patients. The researchers concluded that green tea exerts a favorable regulatory effect on every vital component of human metabolism.

Green tea polyphols, which comprise from 17 to 30% of the dry weight of green tea leaves, are now known to explain the panacea-like properties of the world's most popular beverage. Found recently to account for the antiviral, antioxidant effects in green tea, these unique polyphenols also enhance immunity and destroy bacteria. Epidemiological surveys suggest that green tea consumption is associated with a reduced incidence of pancreatic and stomach cancers.

In recent years, there has been a growing interest in identifying the antimutagenic and anticarcinogenic constituents of the human diet. Here again, researchers are discovering that green tea provides healthful benefits. From a series of mouse experiments, Wang and his colleagues concluded, "These results, in conjunction with our prior publications, suggest that consumption of green tea may reduce the risk of some forms of human cancer induced by both physical and chemical environmental carcinogens."

At the Fourth Chemical Congress of North America, Japanese and U.S. researchers reported that green tea helps shield mice against tumors of the liver, lung, skin, and digestive tract and may do the same for humans. In 1987, scientists identified epigallocatechin gallate (EGCG) as the key protective compound in green tea. EGCG is the most potent among the various polyphenols found in green tea, constituting over 50% of its total polyphenol content. Researchers believe that this antioxidant

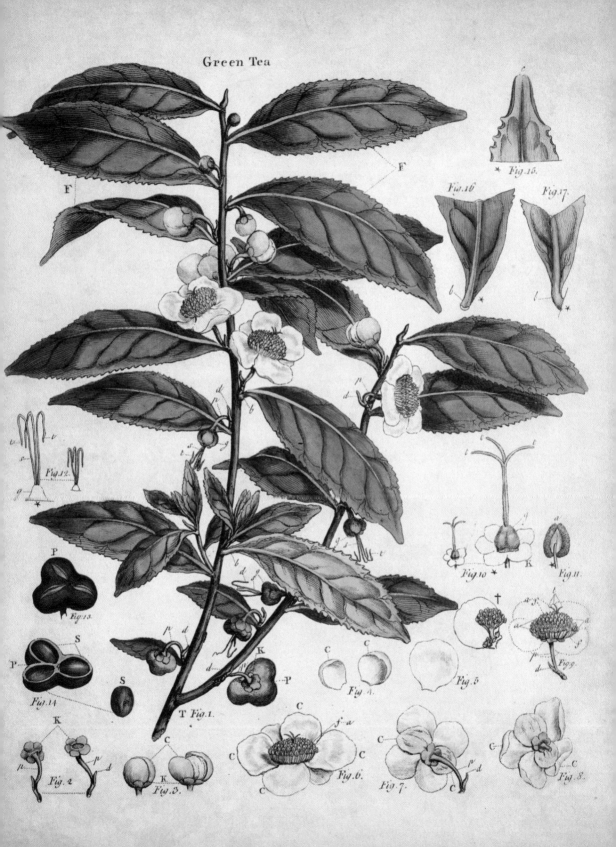

Green Tea

Green tea polyphols, which comprise from 17 to 30% of the dry weight of green tea leaves, are now known to explain the panacea-like properties of the world's most popular beverage.

might safeguard against tumor formation by neutralizing harmful free radicals—highly reactive molecules that can damage DNA and interfere with normal cellular functions. In a study involving mice exposed to a carcinogenic substance affecting the digestive system, only 20% of the mice treated with EGCG developed intestinal cancer, compared to 63% of those not receiving EGCG.

At the same time, EGCG may prevent the activation of certain carcinogens so that free radicals never form. Researchers at Rutgers University reported similar findings regarding skin cancer. The incidence of skin cancer is steadily increasing, and the disease represents a major health and economic problem in the modern industrialized world. Mice that drank green tea instead of plain water for 10 days before and during exposure to ultraviolet light proved less susceptible to skin damage. "These broad effects of the green tea are quite interesting. There aren't that many things that have as broad a spectrum," mused study director Allan H. Conney. Much research remains to be done in this area, however. "The results are encouraging, but I think it would be premature to extrapolate these studies to humans," said Conney. It is not yet known how well the mouse data may apply to humans.

Currently, the speculation of green tea's cancer inhibiting effects in humans is based on demographic extrapolations. It has been surmised that green tea may explain why Japanese cigarette smokers have a lower rate of lung cancer than smokers in the United States. People residing in Shizuoka, Japan's tea-growing region, use tea leaves only once instead of using the same leaves several times, as in other areas of Japan. Therefore, the people of Shizuoka consume greater quantities of the tea's chemicals. In Shizuoka, the death rate from cancer, especially stomach cancer, is markedly lower than in the rest of Japan. Significant differences for habitual green tea consumption between Nakakawane City and Osuka City were observed. In Osuka, people drink less tea and have a high mortality rate due to stomach cancer. In Nakakawane, people drink more tea and have a low rate of stomach cancer.

Green tea also stabilizes blood lipids and may therefore be of value in an overall cardiac-care regimen. According to a 1991 study on mice, green tea extract prevented an increase in serum cholesterol even when the animals were fed an atherogenic (i.e., artery-damaging) diet. Serum lipid peroxides were also diminished, while the destruction of lecithin was reduced.

An antioxidant fraction of green tea extract has been shown to efficiently scavenge the prooxidants hydrogen peroxide and superoxide anion radical, and to protect against the cytotoxicity of paraquat, a biocide that exhibits cellular toxicity via a prooxidant intermediate. Studies evaluating the ability of various polyphenols and condensed tannins (procyanidins linked to gallic acid) to scavenge the various pro-oxidants revealed that EGCG was the most potent; EGCG was also most effective at inhibiting lipid peroxidation in brain tissues from animals, exhibiting over 200 times greater activity than vitamin E (alpha-tocopherol). These investigators postulated that the galloyl groups may lend themselves to increasing antioxidant effectiveness.

EGCG and epicatechin gallate have recently been shown to selectively inhibit reverse transcriptase in human immunodeficiency virus (HIV-RT), whereas the constituent building blocks of these compounds had no inhibitory activity. The most attractive feature of these results rests upon the observation that inhibition of HIV-RT was observed at gallocatechin concentrations over five times less than that which inhibited "normal" cellular DNA polymerases. This is a promising finding in that the side effects of many currently employed antiretrovirals are due to inhibition of host cellular DNA polymerases. This means that green tea polyphenols inhibit viral replication at low concentrations, low enough to avoid destroying normal cells, which suggests that side effects from EGCG would be minimal.

As can be seen, green tea possesses unique and broad effects. While much research must yet be done to see if all these conclusions will apply to humans, we can safely assume that the wisdom of the ages is not to be ignored. In the future, having a cup of tea might mean more than just enjoying a pleasant beverage.

GRINDELIA
Grindelia spp.

Parts used: Leaves and flowering tops. *Also known as gum plant, this has a long history of use as an expectorant.*

TRADITIONAL USAGES
The principal use of grindelia (or gum plant) in traditional medicine was for the treatment of bronchial catarrh, or inflammation of the bronchial mucous membranes,

particularly in cases of asthma. Grindelia was thought to act as a stimulating expectorant and antispasmodic.

When combined with stramonium, grindelia was used in "asthma powders," which were also given for whooping cough and hay fever.

RECENT SCIENTIFIC FINDINGS

The herb contains an essential oil, over 20% resin, grindelol, saponin, tannin, and robustic acid. In one study, a fluid extract of the aerial parts of *Grindelia squarrosa* (curlycup gumweed) was tested in guinea pigs, rabbits, and cats for expectorant activity. The fluid extract was administered orally. Expectorant effects were shown in the cat experiments, but not in the rabbit and guinea pig experiments. Species variation in drug testing is not uncommon, and so the results are inconclusive but promising in verifying grindelia's expectorant properties.

In the form of topical poultices and solutions, grindelia has been reported to be useful in treating burns, vaginitis, and genitourinary membrane infections and inflammation. *G. squarrosa* has been found to be beneficial in the treatment of poison ivy and other skin irritations and rashes.

Grindelia, also known as gumweed or resinweed, is a remarkable botanical treasure celebrated for its therapeutic properties in supporting respiratory health. Native to North America, this herb has been cherished for centuries by Indigenous communities for its potential to alleviate respiratory discomfort. Grindelia is renowned for its high resin content, which contains compounds that can have a soothing effect on the respiratory system. Whether in the form of teas, tinctures, or herbal remedies, this herb has traditionally been used to ease coughs, clear congestion, and promote easier breathing.

The herb's potential lies in its ability to help relax bronchial passages and promote the expulsion of mucus, making it a valuable ally during seasons when respiratory challenges are prevalent. Its gentle yet effective nature has led to its incorporation into various natural remedies and herbal blends designed to provide relief for those seeking a holistic approach to respiratory wellness.

As interest in herbal remedies continues to grow, grindelia shines as a reminder of the wisdom passed down

Grindelia spp.

through generations. It serves as a bridge between traditional knowledge and modern wellness, offering a natural option to those seeking respiratory comfort and a deeper connection to the healing power of plants.

GROUNDSEL
Senecio vulgaris

Parts used: Herb. *Both European and Native American practitioners used this in place of ergot.*

TRADITIONAL USAGES

Groundsel was used to stimulate menstruation and to ease painful menstruation, both by European and American domestic practitioners. Native Americans used the plant to speed childbirth. All these functions recall the applications of ergot, and groundsel was employed at various times as a substitute for that fungus, such as in controlling pulmonary hemorrhage. In general, the plant has been utilized as a diaphoretic, diuretic, and tonic. In dentistry, the herb is employed for bleeding gums.

Groundsel, scientifically known as *Senecio vulgaris*, is an herbaceous plant that has a history deeply intertwined with human traditions and herbal medicine. This unassuming herb, often found in fields, gardens, and disturbed areas, possesses a rich cultural and botanical significance.

While groundsel may seem modest with its small yellow flowers and jagged leaves, it has been recognized for its potential medicinal properties for centuries. In folk medicine practices across various cultures, different parts of the groundsel plant have been utilized for their alleged benefits, including promoting digestion, soothing skin irritations, and addressing respiratory discomfort. However, it's important to note that the plant also contains potentially toxic compounds, which have led to concerns about its safety for consumption.

Historically, groundsel has been both revered and reviled. Some ancient societies held the herb in high regard, using it cautiously for its potential therapeutic effects. Others saw it as a pest, as it can quickly establish itself in disturbed areas, competing with crops and other desirable plants.

In the realm of modern botanical exploration, groundsel remains a subject of interest and study. Researchers

Senecio vulgaris

seek to unravel the complexities of its chemical composition and its potential benefits and risks. This pursuit underscores the delicate balance between the historical uses of plants and the scientific scrutiny required to fully understand their properties.

GUARANA
Paullinia cupana

Parts used: Seeds. *This traditional Brazilian beverage alleviates migraine headaches.*

TRADITIONAL USAGES

A traditional beverage of the Brazilian Indians, guarana is prepared from the dried seeds, which are powdered, sometimes mixed with cassava flour, then kneaded into dough and formed into cylindrical or globular masses. It may also be mixed with chocolate. Besides having refreshing and nutritive value, guarana has been used medicinally by Indigenous communities in Brazil for bowel complaints, both as a curative and as a preventive.

The plant was introduced into France by a physician who had been working in Brazil. It came to be employed in the treatment of migraine and nervous headaches, neuralgia, paralysis, urinary tract irritation, and other ailments, as well as continuing to be administered for chronic diarrhea.

RECENT SCIENTIFIC FINDINGS

The medicinal virtues of the plant are probably largely due to its caffeine content, which is higher than in any other plant source and two and a half times that of coffee. The caffeine explains the efficacy of guarana in alleviating the pain of migraine headaches. The tannins undoubtedly act as an astringent to alleviate diarrhea.

Aqueous extracts of guarana have shown positive results in a study of platelet aggregation. In both humans and rabbits, the guarana extracts inhibited platelet aggregation following either oral or intravenous administration. Guarana has also exhibited central nervous system stimulant activity in adult humans.

Guarana is a climbing plant native to the Amazon rainforest that has captured the attention of both traditional healers and modern enthusiasts for its potential to invigorate and stimulate. This herb has a rich history and a range of uses that make it a unique addition to the world of botanical remedies.

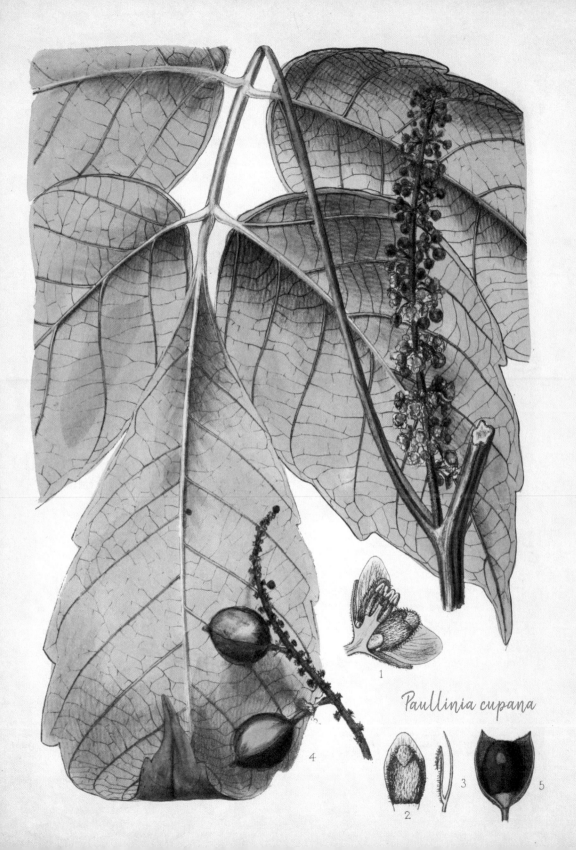

Paullinia cupana

1

2   3   4   5

The seeds of the guarana plant are particularly renowned for their high caffeine content. Traditionally, Indigenous communities in the Amazon basin have utilized guarana as a natural stimulant, incorporating it into beverages and rituals to boost energy, enhance focus, and combat fatigue. These seeds are often ground into a powder and incorporated into various formulations, including teas, energy drinks, and dietary supplements.

What sets guarana apart is its gradual caffeine release. Unlike the abrupt jolt often associated with coffee, guarana provides a sustained release of energy due to the presence of tannins that slow down the caffeine absorption process. This unique attribute has made guarana a popular choice for those seeking a more balanced and prolonged energy boost.

Beyond its stimulating effects, guarana contains antioxidants and other bioactive compounds that contribute to its potential health benefits. Research suggests that it may have cognitive-enhancing properties and could play a role in supporting weight management and digestive health.

GUAR GUM
Cyamopsis tetragonoloba

Parts used: Ground endosperm of seeds. *At one time a popular laxative in southern Asia, preparations have decreased serum cholesterol.*

TRADITIONAL USAGES

Guar gum is the ground endosperm of the seeds of *Cyamopsis tetragonoloba,* a plant native to India and Pakistan. When mixed with water, it rapidly forms high viscous colloidal solutions.

Traditionally, guar gum was most commonly used as a bulk laxative. It was also employed as an appetite suppressant and as a treatment for diabetes.

RECENT SCIENTIFIC FINDINGS

Along with psyllium, guar gum preparations have been found to decrease serum cholesterol, especially LDL cholesterol. Researchers have discovered that patients given guar gum preparations exhibit anywhere from a 5% to a 17% reduction of serum cholesterol.

Guar gum stabilizes the blood sugar level by delaying action on the absorption of carbohydrates in the gut. In both rabbit and human models, guar gum exhibited an anti-hyperglycemic effect. Anti-hyperlipemic activity has been observed in animal modals.

Guar gum is a versatile and widely used herbal extract with a range of applications in various industries. This natural thickening and stabilizing agent has earned a place as a valuable ingredient in food, pharmaceuticals, cosmetics, and other commercial products.

One of the primary attributes of guar gum is its exceptional ability to create viscosity in liquid solutions. When mixed with water, guar gum forms a gel-like substance that lends a smooth and consistent texture to foods, beverages, and various products. This quality has made guar gum a popular additive in items such as ice cream, sauces, dressings, and gluten-free baked goods.

Beyond its role in the culinary world, guar gum has found applications in pharmaceuticals and cosmetics due to its binding and emulsifying properties. In the pharmaceutical sector, it's utilized as a binder in tablets and a thickening agent in syrups. In cosmetics, it can enhance the texture and stability of lotions, creams, and other personal care products.

Guar gum's significance extends to the oil and gas industry, where it is used as a natural thickener in hydraulic fracturing fluids. This application highlights the diverse uses of this herbal extract and its ability to adapt to specific industrial needs.

While guar gum has numerous benefits, it's important to use it judiciously. Excessive consumption of guar gum in food products can sometimes lead to digestive discomfort for some individuals. As with any ingredient, moderation is key.

GUGGAL

Commiphora mukul

Parts used: Gum resin. *A doctoral student's curiosity led to the discovery of this gum resin's cholesterol-lowering properties.*

TRADITIONAL USAGES

The 2,500-year-old Ayurveda treatise *Sushruta Samhita* recommends gum guggal as a treatment for obesity as well as "coating and obstruction of channels." Guggal is derived from the resin of *Commiphora mukul,* a small, thorny tree four to six feet tall that grows in the semi-arid regions of Rajasthan, Gujarat, and Karnataka in India. The tree exudes a yellowish gum resin with a balsamic odor. When tapped during winter, the average tree yields 700–900 grams of resin. Guggal oleoresin contains a complex mixture of diterpenes, esters, and higher alcohols. The active components for lowering cholesterol are believed to be two steroids, guggalsterones Z and E.

RECENT SCIENTIFIC FINDINGS

In the mid-1960s, doctoral student G. Satyavati's curiosity was piqued by the *Sushruta Samhita*'s description of guggal's uses with the ancient concept of *medoroga* (obesity) and contemporary knowledge of atherosclerosis (believed to be the principal cause of coronary heart disease). Might this mean, mused the student, that guggal lowers cholesterol and excess fat? Satyavati's initial findings, published in 1966, supported her conjecture. Since this pioneering doctoral work, more than 20 clinical studies have been published on the lipid-lowering effects of guggal. The results clearly show that guggal can lower blood cholesterol, lower blood triglycerides, lower blood LDL (the "bad" cholesterol fraction), and raise blood HDL (the "good" cholesterol fraction).

While there currently does not appear to be support in scientific literature for the anti-inflammatory properties described in ancient Ayurvedic texts, guggal demonstrates a cholesterol-lowering ability rivaling any natural substance—total blood cholesterol reduction of over 20% has been achieved by the use of guggal alone without dietary modifications.

The connection between cholesterol and heart disease has been well documented both in medical journals and the popular press. Cholesterol is manufactured to provide building materials for the body, including hormones and cell membranes. However, an excessive level of cholesterol in blood vessels leads to hyperlipidemia, that is, excess lipids in the bloodstream. Lipids are fatlike materials consisting of phospholipids and cholesterol and may be the prime cause of atherosclerosis, or narrowing of the arteries, and therefore, heart disease. The American Heart Association estimates that at least 60% of Americans have cholesterol levels that place them in the high-risk category for heart disease. If guggal lowers cholesterol, then this gum resin may significantly reduce that risk.

Detailed pharmacological studies on guggal have been conducted on animals and humans. Several animal studies showed a lowering of serum cholesterol by 34 to 40% and a lowering of serum triglycerides by 26 to 30%. In human clinical studies, reductions in cholesterol and triglyceride levels of 15 to 21.5% have been achieved. The lipid-lowering effect has no correlation to age, sex, or body weight, and no side effects were found. The authors of one study stated, "From these studies we conclude

Commiphora mukul

The resin contains active compounds known as guggalsterones, which are thought to influence lipid metabolism and contribute to cardiovascular well-being.

that gugulipid is a safe and effective lipid-lowering agent comparable in its efficacy to clofibrate but with better compliance and fewer side effects."

Clofibrate is a standard lipid-lowering drug. Comparison studies showed that guggal was equal to or better than clofibrate regarding normalizing blood lipid profile. Other preliminary studies have demonstrated that guggal decreases platelet adhesiveness and increases the blood's fibrinolytic (fibrin-breaking) activity. Both of these actions are extremely beneficial in protecting against thrombosis (heart attack and stroke). If further research confirms these findings, this would be an important breakthrough because few nutrients both normalize blood lipids and protect against thrombosis.

Twenty years after her initial doctoral research, Satyavati wrote, "In conclusion, the saga of gum guggal serves as a highly fascinating and inspiring account of how an 'ancient insight' can lead to a significant 'modern discovery,' provided modern scientists with an open mind (i.e., those without any prejudice against the traditional systems of medicine) care to undertake a serious study of ancient Ayurvedic texts and then carry out carefully planned scientific studies to test some of the rich fundamental concepts and hypotheses available in time-honored ancient systems of medicine."

Guggal has a long-standing tradition of use in Ayurveda, where it is believed to possess a range of health benefits. One of its primary traditional uses is related to promoting healthy cholesterol levels already within the normal range. The resin contains active compounds known as guggalsterones, which are thought to influence lipid metabolism and contribute to cardiovascular well-being.

Beyond cardiovascular health, guggal is also recognized for its anti-inflammatory properties. It has been employed to address joint discomfort and support musculoskeletal health, aligning with Ayurveda's holistic approach to overall vitality.

In contemporary times, guggal has gained attention as a natural remedy for various wellness goals. It is often included in dietary supplements and herbal formulations aimed at cardiovascular support, joint comfort, and overall wellness.

HAWTHORN

Crataegus oxyacantha

Parts used: Flowers, leaves, and berries. *In Europe, this is often prescribed as a substitute for digitalis.*

TRADITIONAL USAGES

Hawthorn is a versatile and widely used herbal remedy with a rich history of medicinal applications. This deciduous shrub or small tree is native to Europe, Asia, and North America and is characterized by its thorny branches and clusters of vibrant red berries. The hawthorn plant's leaves, flowers, and berries are all valued for their therapeutic properties. Hawthorn leaves and berries were used for digestive and urinary ailments. Parkinson recommended the berries or seeds as a remedy for kidney stones and dropsy.

Hawthorn has a history of use for various heart conditions dating from the 17th century. However, its use as a heart medicine was not widespread until the late 19th century, when an Irish doctor became well known for his secret remedy for heart disease. After his death in 1894, the doctor's daughter disclosed that the remedy was a hawthorn berry tincture. Hawthorn then became a popular remedy for heart and cardiovascular ailments. It was believed to strengthen the heart muscle and, taken over a long period of time, to lower blood pressure.

Other uses for hawthorn include as a diuretic and astringent. A tea was drunk as a nerve tonic.

Hawthorn has a long history of use in traditional Chinese medicine. It was given as a treatment for dyspepsia as well as to improve digestion of both children and adults.

RECENT SCIENTIFIC FINDINGS

Since the turn of the century, hawthorn has been a widely used heart remedy. Hawthorn exhibits vasodilatory action and lowers peripheral resistance to blood flow. The mode of action and active principles are still being investigated, though it is known that hawthorn is not a digitalis-like substance. Hawthorn is rich in flavonoids, which in general are known to have cardiotonic attributes. Because the flowers and leaves contain different amounts of flavonoids, preparations commonly combine the parts.

In Europe, where hawthorn is more widely prescribed than in the United States, it is often given in conjunction with digitalis or in place of digitalis when the latter's side effects need to be avoided. In hawthorn's nearly 100 years of clinical use, there has

Crataegus oxyacantha

yet to be a reported case of a toxic reaction. In animal studies where even high doses of hawthorn were administered, there weren't any toxic reactions.

Hawthorn has been traditionally employed to support cardiovascular health. It is believed to enhance blood circulation, regulate blood pressure, and strengthen the heart muscle. Its potent anti-oxidant compounds, including flavonoids and proanthocyanidins, help protect the heart from oxidative stress and inflammation, potentially reducing the risk of heart disease.

The specific cardiac symptoms for which hawthorn is most commonly prescribed include myocardism, geriatric or stressed heart, hyperten-sion, and dysrhythmia. In combination with digitalis, hawthorn is given for cardiac disturbances such as palpitations, angina complaints, and tachycardia (rapid heart action). It is recommended that treat-ment be long-term, at least several months.

A 1981 double-blind placebo study was conducted with 120 patients suffering from loss of cardiac output. The researchers found that in compar-ison to the placebo group, the hawthorn group exhibited improvement both in subjective symptoms, especially palpitations and shortness of breath, and in cardiac function.

A 1990 experiment found that a mixture of hawthorn and motherwort might prove an effective preventive and/or treatment for atherosclerosis. Also, dried hawthorn flowers were tested pharmacologically and found to have a positive inotropic effect.

This herb is also used to alleviate symptoms of anxiety, particularly those asso-ciated with mild forms of heart-related conditions. Hawthorn may promote a sense of calm and relaxation, which can be beneficial for individuals experiencing nervous-ness or tension.

In addition to its cardiovascular and calming effects, hawthorn is recognized for its potential to aid in digestion. It may soothe digestive discomfort and promote healthy gastrointestinal function.

HENNA

Lawsonia alba

Parts used: Leaves and fruit. *Since antiquity, henna leaves have been used as a hair dye.*

TRADITIONAL USAGES

Henna leaves were used by the people of ancient civilizations to dye the manes and tails of their horses. The Arabs have employed the leaves for centuries to dye their beards, nails, palms, and soles. Henna imparts a reddish tint to the hair. Mixed with indigo, it imparts a fine blue-black gloss to beard and hair.

Interestingly, the mummies of ancient Egypt were found wrapped in henna-dyed cloth. In Africa, the flowers are used to give a fine scent to pomades and oils.

The fruit has been thought to stimulate the menstrual function. In powdered form, the leaves have been utilized both internally and externally to treat various skin diseases, including leprosy. In Arabic medicine, the powder was employed in the treatment of jaundice, most likely on the basis of coloration (as implied by the doctrine of signatures); it is unlikely that henna benefitted patients at all and perhaps it only turned them more yellow. In India, the leaves were made into an astringent gargle.

RECENT SCIENTIFIC FINDINGS

Extracts of henna leaves have been shown to act in a manner similar to ergot with respect to inducing uterine contractions. It is therefore quite possible that extracts of this plant could induce menstruation and be effective emmenagogues. In test-tube experiments, extracts of the leaves of henna have shown good antibacterial activity, although not specifically against the leprosy bacillus, which is not possible to test against since it does not grow in non-living tissues. The active principle for these effects most likely is the coloring principle, lawsone.

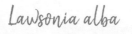

Lawsonia alba

The topical application of two chemical components of this shrub, lawsone and dihydroxyacetone, has been reported useful as a protective filter against ultraviolet light for people with chlorpromazine-induced light sensitivity. Experimentally, a water extract of the leaves inhibited gram-positive and gram-negative bacteria. Antitumor activity in experiments with mice tends to support folkloric uses of henna as an anticancer agent.

Henna is a natural herb with a history of traditional use in various cultures. This small flowering shrub is primarily cultivated in regions of North Africa, the Middle East, and South Asia. Its leaves are the primary source of a vibrant red-orange dye, which has been utilized for centuries in body art and hair coloring.

Henna has experienced a renewed popularity as a hair dye. Henna's dyeing properties come from the lawsone molecule found in its leaves. When mixed with a mildly acidic liquid, such as lemon juice or tea, the crushed henna leaves create a paste that can be applied to the skin or hair. This paste leaves behind temporary color when used for body art, commonly referred to as mehndi, and imparts auburn or reddish hues to the hair.

Beyond its cosmetic applications, henna has been recognized for its potential therapeutic benefits. In some traditional systems of medicine, it is believed to possess cooling and anti-inflammatory properties, making it useful for soothing minor skin irritations, sunburn, or as a natural hair conditioner.

Henna is a natural alternative to synthetic hair dyes and temporary skin adornments, offering a safe and eco-friendly option for those seeking to experiment with color or intricate designs without long-term commitment.

HOLLY

Ilex aquifolium (European Holly), *Ilex opaca* (American Holly)

Parts used: Leaves and berries. *Both the European and American varieties were at one time employed for a variety of uses.*

TRADITIONAL USAGES

The leaves of European holly were employed medicinally for their ability to increase perspiration. In infusions, they were also utilized to treat inflammations of the mucous membranes, pleurisy, gout, and smallpox.

The leaves also enjoyed a brief reputation in France as a cure for intermittent fevers. The berries were said to have purgative, emetic, and diuretic properties, and the juice of the berries has been used in the treatment of jaundice.

American holly was used for essentially the same purposes. Two species growing in the southern United States, *I. vomitoria* and *I. dahoon,* were utilized by North Carolina tribes in ritual as well as medicine.

A decoction made from the toasted leaves, known as black drink or yaupon, had emetic properties.

RECENT SCIENTIFIC FINDINGS

Holly leaves are known to contain theobromine, which explains the diaphoretic and febrifuge effects attributed to herbal teas prepared from them. No studies have been reported on the berries of this plant.

This plant has a rich history of symbolism and traditional significance, often associated with various cultural and religious practices.

Beyond its symbolic significance, holly has had limited use in herbal medicine. Some herbalists have explored its potential as a remedy for certain ailments, such as coughs and colds, although it is not a widely recognized or extensively studied herbal remedy.

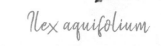

Ilex aquifolium

The holly herb's enduring presence in cultural traditions, folklore, and seasonal celebrations underscores its enduring importance in human history, providing a sense of connection to nature and a reminder of the enduring cycle of life and renewal.

HOLY THISTLE

Cnicus benedictus

Parts used: Leaves and flowering tops. *Used as a medicinal for 2,000 years, the leaves contain cnicin, which stimulates gastric juices.*

TRADITIONAL USAGES

Holy thistle has been recorded as a medicinal since the first century A.D. Credited with the medical virtues of a diuretic, diaphoretic, febrifuge, and cholagogue, it has been used to treat a variety of ailments. A bitter tonic and a good appetite stimulant, it is still used today to treat indigestion. At one time this herb was ascribed the nearly supernatural qualities of a "cure all," but current knowledge yields no evidence to support such a belief.

RECENT SCIENTIFIC FINDINGS

While there is no direct experimental evidence that preparations of holy thistle leaves will give the emetic effect claimed by some writers, if given in large enough quantity, most any plant would produce emesis due to the presence of low concentrations of irritant principles.

On the other hand, the use of leaf decoctions as a bitter tonic is well founded. The bitter principle in this plant is known to be cnicin, and human experiments have shown that extracts of holy thistle stimulate the production of gastric juices.

Although widely used as an herbal tea for the treatment of amenorrhea (absence of menses), there is no experimental evidence that holy thistle seeds have this effect.

Holy thistle, or blessed thistle, is an herb with a history of medicinal use dating back centuries. This annual plant, native to the Mediterranean region but now found in various parts of the world, is characterized by its spiky leaves and vibrant yellow flowers.

Holy thistle has earned its name from its traditional association with healing and protection. It was believed to have sacred and beneficial properties, often used in herbal remedies for a wide range of ailments. In traditional herbal medicine, it was used to stimulate digestion and alleviate indigestion and gas, and as a general tonic to improve overall health. It was also considered an herbal remedy for fevers, infections, and respiratory conditions.

Holy thistle is sometimes confused with milk thistle, another herb known for its potential liver-protective properties. While they share similar names, they are distinct plants with different uses.

HONEYSUCKLE (Japanese)
Lonicera japonica

Parts used: Flowers, leaves, and stems. *Japanese honeysuckle, known for its sweetly scented, tubular white and yellow flowers, has a variety of anti-inflammatory and skin-healing properties.*

TRADITIONAL USAGES

Japanese honeysuckle has been a cherished plant in various cultures for its therapeutic properties. Traditionally, its flowers, leaves, and stems have been utilized for a range of medicinal purposes.

Infusions made from the flowers and leaves of Japanese honeysuckle have been employed as a traditional remedy for soothing respiratory issues such as coughs,

> *In traditional herbal medicine, this herb has also been recognized for its potential to support the immune system and offer relief from symptoms associated with colds and flu.*

bronchitis, and asthma. The plant's natural compounds are believed to possess anti-inflammatory and antimicrobial properties, making it a valuable choice for treating respiratory discomfort.

Japanese honeysuckle has also been used externally for its potential skin-healing properties. Poultices and topical preparations made from its stems and leaves have been applied to minor skin irritations, burns, and insect bites to alleviate discomfort and promote healing.

In traditional herbal medicine, this herb has also been recognized for its potential to support the immune system and offer relief from symptoms associated with colds and flu.

RECENT SCIENTIFIC FINDINGS

Modern scientific research has begun to uncover the bioactive compounds within Japanese honeysuckle that contribute to its traditional uses. The plant contains various phytochemicals, including flavonoids, saponins, and essential oils, which may explain its anti-inflammatory and antimicrobial effects.

Studies have also identified potential antioxidant properties in Japanese honeysuckle, which could contribute to its ability to protect cells from oxidative stress and support overall health.

In recent years, Japanese honeysuckle has gained attention for its potential as a natural ingredient in cosmetics and skin care products, thanks to its skin-soothing and healing properties.

Lonicera japonica

HOPS

Humulus lupulus

Parts used: Strobiles. *This well-known ingredient in beer contains a complex mixture of substances with proven sedative action.*

TRADITIONAL USAGES

Best known as a flavoring and preservative ingredient in the brewing of beer, the hops plant has also been utilized traditionally in the treatment of hysteria, restlessness, and insomnia. In 1633's *The Herbal*, John Gerard wrote, "The buds or first sprouts which come forth in the spring are used to be eaten in sallads; yet are they, as Pliny saith, more toothsome than nourishing, for they yield but very small nourishment." Only the young shoots are tasty; the older ones being so bitter and tough that they are softened by bleaching with sulphuric oxide. King Henry VIII feared that he would be poisoned by this violent bleaching agent; he passed an edict that forbade the addition of hops to ale brewed in his household. In 1787, when King George III was seriously ill, the court physicians filled his pillow with hops instead of opiates to calm his nerves and to promote sleep.

The ancient Hebrews relied on hops to ward off the plague. Hops contain effective antibacterial principles and were in fact valuable against the infectious agent *Yersinia pestis,* the plague bacillus.

In North America, Native Americans discovered hops' value independent of Europeans. The Mohegans prepared a sedative medicine from the conelike strobiles and sometimes heated these blossoms and applied them for toothache. One Meskwaki practitioner cured insomnia with hops. The Dakotas prepared a tea of the steeped strobiles to relieve digestive pains.

At the end of the 19th century, hops were widely used in American medicine for their tonic, diuretic, and sedative properties. Hops were believed to exert calming effects on the heart and nervous system. The side effects described were colic and constipation.

RECENT SCIENTIFIC FINDINGS

The dried strobiles of hops contain a complex mixture of substances known as "hop acids" (although not all of them are acids), which are all very bitter substances. Some of these hop acids are very effective sedatives, as determined from animal experiments. However, it is most likely that an essential oil in hops also contributes to the sedative effects, although the active principle(s) in the oil has not yet been identified.

Best known as a flavoring and preservative ingredient in the brewing of beer, the hops plant has also been utilized traditionally in the treatment of hysteria, restlessness, and insomnia.

Pillows stuffed with hops have been used to produce sleep in nervous disorders. To prevent rustling of the contents, it is advisable to moisten them with water and glycerin or spirits before placing them under the head of the patient.

A 1966 experiment validated hops' sedative action. One recent study showed that hops was truly a sedative and not merely a muscle relaxant. Other experiments have found antihyperglycemic activity in human adult models and antibacterial activity in vitro against *Staphylococcus aureus*.

The hops plant is a flowering vine, primarily used in the brewing of beer. Native to Europe, Asia, and North America, hops are recognized for their distinctive cone-like flowers, or strobiles, which contain compounds essential for imparting bitterness, flavor, and aroma to beer.

Hops have been an integral ingredient in the brewing process for centuries. They not only contribute to the characteristic taste and aroma of beer but also serve as a natural preservative. The bitter compounds in hops, particularly alpha acids, balance the sweetness of malted barley and help to prevent spoilage, allowing beer to mature and develop its complex flavors over time.

In addition to their role in brewing, hops have been explored for their potential therapeutic properties. They are believed to have mild sedative and anxiolytic (anxiety-reducing) effects, making them a popular ingredient in herbal remedies for promoting relaxation

Humulus lupulus

and aiding sleep. Hops are often used in conjunction with other calming herbs such as valerian or chamomile.

Hops are also valued for their phytonutrients, including antioxidants and essential oils, which may offer health benefits. These compounds have been studied for their potential anti-inflammatory and anticancer properties, although research in these areas is ongoing.

Overall, the hops plant is a versatile plant with a strong cultural and economic impact, notably in the world of brewing. Its contributions to beer production and its potential role in herbal medicine make it a noteworthy herb with both traditional and contemporary relevance.

HOREHOUND
Marrubium vulgare

Parts used: Leaves and flowering tops. *This popular folk remedy for respiratory problems contains high concentrations of mucilage.*

TRADITIONAL USAGES

A very popular folk remedy, horehound is mainly tonic and laxative in its action, but it has also been considered valuable for removing obstructions in the system. It was used to treat chronic hepatitis and a wide range of ill health due to malignancies, advanced pulmonary tuberculosis, leukemia, malaria, and hysteria.

In domestic use, however, it is more often employed in respiratory complaints, such as in the treatment of sore throats, to promote the expectoration of phlegm in bronchitis, for asthma, for pulmonary consumption, and for obstinate cough.

RECENT SCIENTIFIC FINDINGS

White horehound has a high concentration of mucilage, which would be expected to ease the irritation accompanying sore throats.

This perennial plant is characterized by its woolly, gray-green leaves and clusters of small, white flowers. Native to Europe, it has become naturalized in various regions across the world.

In traditional herbal medicine, horehound has been highly regarded for its potential therapeutic properties. It is commonly used to alleviate respiratory ailments such as coughs, colds, and bronchitis. The herb contains compounds that help to soothe

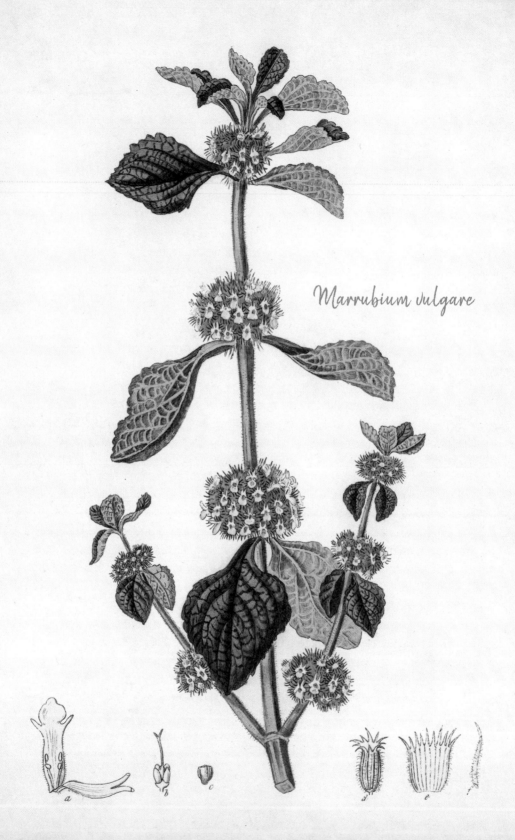

Marrubium vulgare

irritated throats and promote the release of mucus, making it valuable in cough syrups and lozenges.

Horehound's bitter taste has also earned it a place in traditional digestive remedies, where it is believed to stimulate digestion and ease indigestion. Its use extends beyond respiratory and digestive support; horehound has been studied for its potential as an antimicrobial and anti-inflammatory agent, although further research is needed in these areas.

Culturally, horehound has found its way into various culinary applications. It has been used as a flavoring agent in candies and liqueurs, notably in the production of horehound candy, which combines its slightly sweet and bitter taste.

Horehound remains a respected herb in herbal medicine and enjoys a unique role in both traditional remedies and culinary delights, continuing to offer its valuable contributions to wellness and taste.

HORSE CHESTNUT
Aesculus hippocastanum

Parts used: Bark, leaves, and nut (kernel and oil). *The seeds of this beautiful tree contain escin, a widely used anti-inflammatory agent.*

TRADITIONAL USAGES

This easily recognized, stately tree migrated originally from the north of Asia about the middle of the 16th century. It is not known in what year, but Matthiolus is the first botanist to mention horse chestnut. Parkinson states in his *Paradisus* that he cultivated it in his orchard as a fruit tree, esteeming the nuts superior to the ordinary sort.

The powdered kernel of the nut causes sneezing, and the oil extracted with ether from the kernels has been used in France as a topical remedy for rheumatism. A decoction of the leaves was formerly employed in the United States as a treatment for whooping cough, while the seed oil has been considered useful against sunburn. Native American tribes in California combined bear fat with the nut kernel as a paste for hemorrhoids. Dr. Charles Millspaugh described the nuts of the horse chestnut as narcotic and stated that "10 grains are equal to 3 grams of opium."

RECENT SCIENTIFIC FINDINGS

The active principle of horse chestnut seeds is the complex triterpene glycoside escin. Escin is not absorbed in the stomach when taken in its natural form. However, when converted to an amorphous form, a derivative (which is sold as Reparil) can be taken orally. Escin is widely utilized in Europe as an anti-inflammatory agent for a variety of conditions, in addition to being used for vascular problems. There is ample evidence supporting the folkloric usage of horse chestnut to treat varicose veins and inflammatory disorders of the legs. Ointments and gels are applied externally in conjunction with the internal preparation.

Many animal experiments have repeatedly confirmed the anti-inflammatory and anti-edema actions of escin. One group of researchers studied the process of inflammation in detail and learned that escin inhibits the movement of inflammatory cells, especially macrophages, without lessening their activity or phagocytic properties.

This remarkable glycoside also has potent powers to reduce edema. It achieves this by normalizing the permeability of blood vessel walls. In human therapy, Italian researchers found this compound to be "well tolerated throughout treatments lasting 50 consecutive days."

The leaves of *A. glabra,* the Ohio buckeye, were felt to be quite efficacious in the treatment of chest congestion. Buckeye seeds contain constituents similar to those in *A. hippocastanum* seeds and thus would be expected to have beneficial effect in the treatment of portal congestion.

When next you gaze at these thickly armored fruits, consider the sweet healing balm contained therein.

Horse chestnut seeds contain a compound called escin, which is believed to have anti-inflammatory and vasoconstrictive properties. In herbal medicine, horse chestnut extracts are used topically in creams and ointments to alleviate the symptoms of chronic venous insufficiency (CVI), a condition that can lead to varicose veins, swollen legs, and discomfort. Escin is thought to reduce swelling and improve blood circulation.

The tree's bark and leaves, however, contain a toxic compound called esculin and are not used in herbal remedies. Proper preparation to remove the toxic components is essential when using horse chestnut seeds for medicinal purposes.

Aesculus hippocastanum

Although horse chestnut has demonstrated efficacy in managing CVI-related symptoms, it should be used under the guidance of a healthcare professional, as it may interact with certain medications and is not suitable for everyone. In the realm of herbal medicine, horse chestnut serves as a reminder of the importance of harnessing nature's resources while respecting their potential risks and benefits.

HORSETAIL or Shavegrass
Equisetum arvense, E. hyemale

Parts used: Whole plant. *Used by Native Americans to help wounds to heal, this plant's high silica content makes it ideal for sitz baths.*

TRADITIONAL USAGES

Also known as shavegrass, horsetail was used by Native Americans as a poultice to promote wound healing. The Thompson tribe in British Columbia applied the ashes of horsetail fern stems to burns. A mild diuretic, horsetail was administered to promote urination in dropsical complaints and kidney dysfunctions. Because the diuretic action of horsetail is quite weak, it is likely to have been utilized in cases of very sensitive or weakened patients, or for pregnant women, as there were no deleterious side effects.

The cuticle of the stems contains abrasives that made the plant useful in scouring metal culinary articles; it was widely used by artisans for polishing wood, ivory, brass, and objects of similar materials.

RECENT SCIENTIFIC FINDINGS

Although diuretic effects are attributed to extracts of *Equisetum hyemale* very frequently in literature, very few experiments have been carried out to verify this effect. At best, the experiments show a low level of diuretic activity, which is almost entirely attributable to the irritant action of silica that is present in the plant in high concentrations. It is highly questionable whether diuresis should be induced on the basis of a purely irritant effect on the kidneys, in that long-term ramifications of this continuous irritation could be detrimental.

Horsetail's silica content makes it useful in sitz baths, which aid in treating peripheral vascular disorders, chilblains, and post-thrombotic swelling, as well as treating ligaments and tendons after ankle sprains and fractures. The silica horsetail contains is highly absorbable and is utilized to promote bone growth and collagen formation, two very important functions for menopausal women. Horsetail has a high content of minerals in general, such as calcium, which promote the rebuilding of body tissue.

Current pharmacology indicates a reduction of edema in some cases of arthritis and swelling of legs, and tuberculostatic activity. A horsetail tea has been recommended for stomach ulcers.

Caution: Long-term use could be detrimental to kidney function.

This ancient herb is characterized by its distinctive hollow jointed stems and feathery branches, resembling the tail of a horse.

In traditional herbal medicine, horsetail has been valued for its high silica content, which lends it potential benefits for hair, skin, and nail health. Silica is believed to promote the formation of collagen, a crucial component of healthy connective tissues.

Horsetail has also been used as a natural diuretic, aiding in the elimination of excess fluids from the body and potentially supporting kidney and urinary tract health. It is sometimes included in herbal remedies for conditions like urinary tract infections and edema.

Additionally, horsetail's astringent and anti-inflammatory properties have made it a candidate for external use, such as in poultices and ointments for wound healing and minor skin irritations.

IPECAC

Cephaelis ipecacuanha, Euphorbia ipecacuanha

Parts used: Root. *The Aborigines of Brazil first discovered the properties of this popular emetic.*

TRADITIONAL USAGES

The name *ipecacuanha,* from the language of the Brazilian Aborigines, has been applied to various emetic roots of South America. The Portuguese learned of this remedy for bowel problems when they settled Brazil, and the root was introduced to Europe around 1672 as a remedy for dysentery.

Originally sold in Paris as a secret cure, the plant showed such value in bowel affections that no less a personage than Louis XIV eventually bestowed a large sum of money and public honors on the physician who popularized its use, on the condition that he make it public.

Like many other similar drugs, ipecac is emetic only in large doses. In intermediate doses, it is a nauseant, diaphoretic, and expectorant; in small doses, it is a mild stomach stimulant, increasing the appetite and aiding digestion. Very small doses have also been used to treat the vomiting of pregnancy. When used as a nauseant, ipecac was also observed to exert a sedative effect on the vascular system; hence it came to be employed for hemorrhages, particularly of the uterus.

RECENT SCIENTIFIC FINDINGS

After it was introduced in Europe, ipecac appeared to work extremely well in some cases of dysentery while it did nothing in others. Later evidence showed that the drug has no value against bacteria. Since there are two types of dysentery, one due to a specific amoeba and one due to a bacillus, ipecac is useless against the bacillary form, while its amebecidal properties account for its being considered probably the most efficacious remedy available against the amoebic type of dysentery. The major active constituents of ipecac root are the alkaloids emetine and cephaeline. These potent drugs can cause adverse effects on the heart, but in proper dosage, they are not appreciably absorbed from the stomach or intestinal tract, and thus the bad effects are rarely encountered.

Perhaps the major use for ipecac is in the form of syrup of ipecac, which is widely publicized as a useful vomitive (emetic) to administer when people (especially children) have accidentally swallowed a poisonous substance and it is desired to remove the

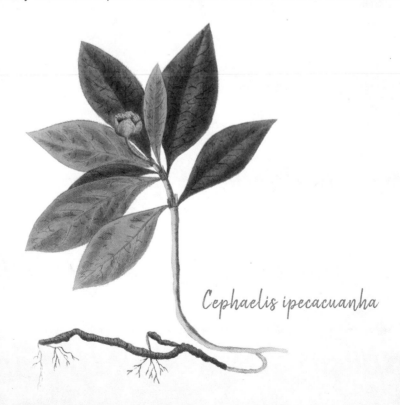

Cephaelis ipecacuanha

poison by using an emetic agent. If the proper amount is administered, emesis will take place within 15–20 minutes, and no adverse effects are noted.

Unfortunately, there have been a large number of cases in which fluid extract of ipecac has been erroneously used for this purpose, and several deaths have been recorded due to such mistakes. Fluid extract of ipecac is about 20 times more potent than syrup of Ipecac. When utilized as an expectorant, very small doses of ipecac are required.

Recently, physicians have been recommending and research supports the use of activated charcoal instead of ipecac in pediatric medicine.

JUNIPER BERRY
Juniperus communis

Parts used: Berries. *Long used as a gentle diuretic, preliminary studies indicate this may also be a valuable arthritis treatment.*

TRADITIONAL USAGES
Juniper berries act as a gentle stimulant and diuretic, imparting an odor of violets to the urine. Taken in large quantities, they occasionally produce irritation of the urinary passages. Their principal use was as an adjuvant to more powerful diuretics in problems of fluid retention. The berries were also used as carminatives, stomachics, antiseptics, and stimulants. The volatile oil distilled from the berries was used as a carminative to aid the expulsion of intestinal flatulence and also as a diuretic. For a period of time, the *U.S. Pharmacopoeia* recommended them to promote menstruation. The aromatic berries have been employed in folk medicine to lower serum cholesterol and as an anticancer remedy.

Juniper berries make an excellent survival food because they are edible and available through part of the winter. The tree's inner bark is also edible and was eaten by many Native Americans to fight off starvation. Some tribes dried the berries and baked the ground fruits into cakes or mush. Roasted juniper berries were ground and substituted for coffee. In British Columbia, the stems and leaves were boiled to make an astringent tea. Juniper berries are also the primary source of flavoring for gin.

RECENT SCIENTIFIC FINDINGS
Though the USFDA considers this plant an "unsafe herb," there is no known data to substantiate this conclusion. Experimentally, antitumor activity has been shown in

animals, along with strong cytotoxic activity in cell culture against HELA cancer cells. Studies have also found antiviral activity in cell culture against influenza virus A2 and herpes simplex virus I and II, as well as antibacterial activity in vitro against several human pathogens.

The primary use, however, has been as a diuretic, and this effect has been substantiated in animal studies. The active diuretic principle has been shown to be a simple terpene, terpinen-4-ol.

Although there is no direct experimental evidence that juniper berries would be effective in the treatment of gout, studies have been conducted in humans that indicate a value in treating arthritis. Both gout and arthritis are acute inflammatory conditions, and drugs effective for one of these conditions are usually found useful for the other.

The mildly stimulant effect attributed to juniper berries is due to the action of constituents in the essential oil.

Caution: May irritate kidneys. Do not use more than six consecutive weeks. Juniper may stimulate uterine contractions and cause abortion.

Juniper berries are a widely recognized herb used for various culinary and medicinal purposes. These small, aromatic, blue-black berries have a long history of use, particularly in traditional European cuisine and herbal medicine.

In culinary applications, juniper berries are prized for their piney and slightly citrusy flavor. They are a key ingredient in many dishes, most notably in the preparation of gin, where they impart a distinctive and complex flavor. In traditional European cuisine, juniper berries have been used to season game meats, sauerkraut, and other dishes, adding a unique earthy aroma and taste.

Medicinally, juniper berries have been used for their potential diuretic and digestive properties. They were historically used to aid digestion, alleviate stomach discomfort, and promote urinary health. The essential oil derived from juniper berries contains compounds that are believed to have antimicrobial and anti-inflammatory effects.

Juniperus communis

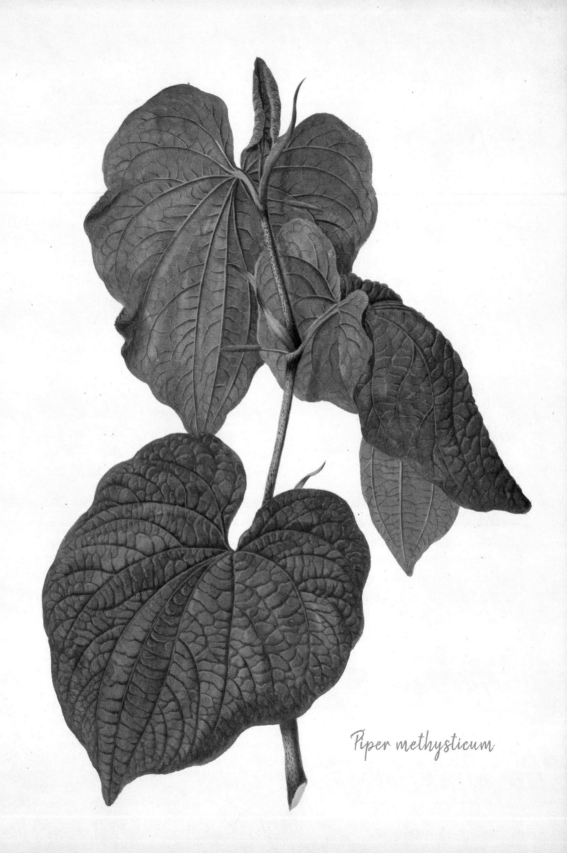

Piper methysticum

KAVA KAVA

Piper methysticum

Parts used: Root. *This drink has been a part of Polynesian religious and social life since antiquity.*

TRADITIONAL USAGES

Kava is native to the Pacific Islands. In early times, it was distributed eastward through tropical islands by migrating people, who valued the root both as a drink and medicine. In Hawaii, more than 15 varieties were known. In many islands of the Pacific, kava has long played an important part in the life of the people, being used in ceremonies and festivals and as a sign of goodwill.

The root is used to prepare the ceremonial drink of many inhabitants of Melanesia and Polynesia. This drink is reputedly a sedative, aphrodisiac, tonic, stimulant, diuretic, and diaphoretic. While both men and women drink kava nowadays, in former times tribal custom forbade women to partake. Young virgins would masticate the root to prepare the beverage for the men's ceremonial purposes. The root has a faint but characteristic odor, an aromatic, bitter, pungent taste, with a slight local anesthesia resulting.

RECENT SCIENTIFIC FINDINGS

A number of compounds referred to as "kava pyrones" (for example, kawain, dihydro-kawain, methysticin, and dihydromethysticin) are claimed to have mild sedative and tranquilizing effects. Kawain is marketed in Europe as a mild sedative for the elderly. Extracts of kava, and most of the kava pyrones have been shown to have antiseptic properties in test-tube experiments.

Animal studies clearly point out a marked ability of extracts of kava to calm enraged animals. Anticonvulsant activity has been observed in adult human and animal models. The principle responsible for this effect has not yet been discovered. Regular and prolonged use of kava extracts results in the production of a skin rash, which is pigmented yellow. This condition, among kava users in the South Pacific, is known as "kawaism." The condition subsides following restriction of the kava beverage, with no ill effects. It is important to remember that this plant has been utilized for its calming effects in Oceania since antiquity. While the introduction of alcohol has created many social problems, those groups still using this plant in its traditional way enjoy a mild insulation from life's vicissitudes.

It is renowned for its traditional use in the preparation of a ceremonial beverage with sedative and anxiety-reducing properties. The roots of the kava plant are processed to create a beverage that is consumed in social and cultural gatherings.

Kava has been used for centuries by Pacific Island communities as a means of relaxation and stress relief. It contains compounds known as kavalactones, which are believed to have calming effects on the central nervous system. This has made kava popular for its potential to reduce anxiety, ease muscle tension, and induce a state of mild euphoria.

The cultural significance of kava as a social and ceremonial drink, along with its potential as a natural relaxant, showcases the rich diversity of traditional herbal remedies from around the world.

KINO
Pterocarpus marsupium, P. indicus, P. echinatus

Parts used: Exudate (juice from incisions in trunk of tree). *Kino is a powerful astringent.*

TRADITIONAL USAGES

Kino is the name given to the juice that exudes from incisions in the trunk of the tree *Pterocarpus marsupium.* It was deemed a powerful astringent and as such was used externally to check discharges from wounds, scrapes, and skin ulcers. In combination with opium or chalk mixtures, it was administered to treat noninflammatory diarrheas. Kino was never given in the presence of fever.

It has also been used to treat diabetes and passive hemorrhages of the intestines and uterus, and as a gargle to relax the throat. Aromatic substances were often added to the kino to make it more palatable.

A related species, from Africa, *P. angolensis* (bloodwood), used as substitute for Indian teak, is famed as an aphrodisiac. The roots were employed for this activity in the Congo, Angola, Tanzania, Mozambique, and the Transvaal.

RECENT SCIENTIFIC FINDINGS

Kino's astringent action is primarily due to the presence of a tannin-like substance, kino-tannic acid, which also gives it application in the treatment of leucorrhea by injection.

Kino, also known as gum kino, is a natural resin extracted from various species of trees belonging to the *Pterocarpus* genus. This herbal resin has a long history of

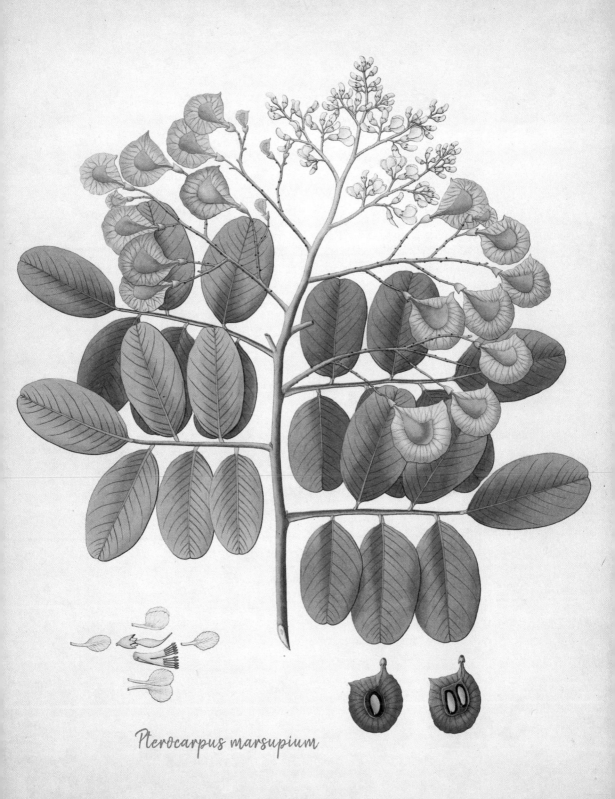

Pterocarpus marsupium

traditional use for its astringent and wound-healing properties. It has been valued for its ability to stop bleeding, making it a valuable remedy for minor cuts, abrasions, and other skin injuries.

Kino has a dark reddish-brown appearance and was used in traditional medicine as a topical application to help control bleeding and promote the healing of wounds. It contains tannins and other compounds that have astringent qualities, which enable it to constrict blood vessels and reduce bleeding.

Although the use of kino has decreased in modern medicine due to the availability of more advanced wound care products, it remains an example of nature's contributions to early healthcare practices. Its historical use as a natural remedy for managing bleeding underscores the resourcefulness of traditional herbal medicine.

LADY SLIPPER (Domesticated)
Cypripedium parviflorum

Parts used: Root. *This beautiful flower deserves further research as a mild nerve medicine.*

TRADITIONAL USAGES

Several North American tribes used lady slipper as a nerve medicine. It later became an accepted cure for insomnia in domestic American medicine. A medical botanist of the first half of the 19th century, Constantine Rafinesque, introduced lady slipper to medical circles.

"Of this beautiful genus, all the species are equally medical; they have been long known to the Indians . . . They produce beneficial effects in all nervous diseases and hysterical affections, by allaying pain, quieting the nerves and promoting sleep."

The roots were official in the *U.S. Pharmacopoeia* from 1863 to 1916. They were primarily used as an antispasmodic and a nerve medicine. Dr. Charles Millspaugh wrote, "This is one of our drugs that has not been sufficiently thought of by provers. It merits a full proving."

And it still does!

Cypripedium parviflorum

RECENT SCIENTIFIC FINDINGS

Lady slipper is another drug plant that was once popularly prescribed but has been superseded by synthetic agents. Lady slipper may act similarly to valerian, in milder form, to lessen anxiety and restlessness.

Lady slipper is a captivating herbaceous plant known for its distinctive and enchanting slipper-shaped blossoms. This unique and rare orchid species can be found in various regions across the Northern Hemisphere, where it graces woodlands and damp, shaded areas with its elegance.

Beyond its aesthetic appeal, lady slipper has historical significance in traditional medicine. Indigenous peoples and early settlers recognized the plant's therapeutic potential and utilized it to address a range of health concerns. The herb's root was believed to possess medicinal properties and was often employed to alleviate nervous conditions and anxiety.

Today, due to its limited availability and protected status in many areas, the use of lady slipper in herbal remedies has become rare. Its conservation is prioritized to ensure the continued existence of this exceptional species.

LAVENDER

Lavandula officinalis (*L. vera* and *L. spica*)

Parts used: Flowers (and oil). *The aromatic oil of the flower is often used in combination with other herbs and pharmaceuticals.*

TRADITIONAL USAGES

The flowers, as well as the oil, are employed chiefly in perfumery, but their fragrance also led to their use to disguise nasty-smelling herbal and other pharmaceutical preparations. Bunches of the dried flowers are used to make sachets and for imparting a gentle scent to linen.

Oil distilled from lavender flowers is utilized medicinally as an aromatic stimulant, mild carminative, and tonic, and to treat nervous languor and headache. Interestingly, the oil (known as "oil of aspic") is also used in varnishes to dilute delicate colors on painted china.

Lavandula officinalis

RECENT SCIENTIFIC FINDINGS

Chemically, the plant contains 1-linalyl acetate, geraniol, and linalool. Lavender flowers contain large amounts of a highly aromatic oil and have definite spasmolytic, antiseptic, and carminative properties. These activities are all attributed to the essential oil and its aromatic principles.

Lavender is a fragrant and versatile herb widely recognized for its aromatic qualities and diverse applications. This herb, native to the Mediterranean region, is characterized by its vibrant purple flowers and soothing, sweet scent. Lavender has been cherished for centuries for its calming and therapeutic properties. Its essential oil, derived from the flowers, is known for its ability to reduce stress and anxiety, promote relaxation, and improve sleep quality. Lavender oil is often used in aromatherapy, massage oils, and bath products for its soothing effects.

Medicinally, lavender has a history of use in herbal remedies for conditions such as headaches, digestive discomfort, and skin irritations. It contains compounds with anti-inflammatory and antimicrobial properties, which contribute to its healing qualities.

LEMONGRASS
Cymbopogon citratus

Parts used: Oil. *This tasty tea has long been a mild sedative due to myrcene, an analgesic that may also reduce cholesterol.*

TRADITIONAL USAGES

Lemongrass tea has long been used as a before bed drink to promote sleep. In traditional Brazilian medicine, lemongrass has been widely used as an analgesic and as a sedative.

Lemongrass oil is a common food flavoring and ingredient in cosmetics and perfumes. The oil is a source of ionone, which is made into a synthetic violet.

RECENT SCIENTIFIC FINDINGS

Lemongrass's essential oil contains the monoterpene myrcene, an analgesic, thus confirming lemongrass tea's traditional use as a mild sedative. One team of researchers concluded, "Terpenes such as myrcene may constitute a lead for the development of new peripheral analgesics with a profile of action different from that of the aspirin-like drugs."

> *Lemongrass tea has long been used as a before bed drink to promote sleep. In traditional Brazilian medicine, lemongrass has been widely used as an analgesic and as a sedative.*

Myrcene was also found to reduce the toxic and mutagenic effect of cyclophosphamide in in vitro experiments. In other words, myrcene may possess antimutagenic properties.

Lemongrass oil has also been reported to possess strong antibacterial activity in vitro against several human pathogens. For instance, a 1988 study found an appreciable increase in activity against *Escherichia coli* and *Staphylococcus aureus*.

Lemongrass oil is also rich in geraniol and citral, both of which may contribute to lowering serum cholesterol levels. In one study involving 22 hypercholesterolemic patients, cholesterol levels were lowered.

However, to date there is no laboratory evidence to support lemongrass's reputed folkloric ability to relieve anxiety.

Lemongrass is a fragrant and versatile herb appreciated for its fresh, lemony aroma and various culinary and medicinal applications.

Culinary use of lemongrass is prevalent in Southeast Asian cuisine, where it imparts a distinctive citrusy flavor to dishes. The tender inner portion of the stalks is typically used in cooking, adding a zesty, aromatic essence to soups, curries, and stir-fries.

Beyond its culinary contributions, lemongrass has been valued for its potential health benefits. It contains essential oils, notably citral, which give it a lemony scent and offer various therapeutic properties. Lemongrass has been traditionally used to aid digestion, alleviate muscle pain, and reduce fever.

Moreover, lemongrass is a popular choice for herbal teas, often consumed for its relaxing and calming effects. The tea is believed to help reduce stress and anxiety, making it a soothing beverage choice.

Lemongrass's versatility in the kitchen and its potential for wellness highlight its significance as a beloved herb. Its delightful aroma and ability to enhance the flavor of dishes and offer therapeutic qualities make it a cherished addition to many cultures and cuisines.

LETTUCE (Wild)

Lactuca elongata

Parts used: Latex. *Since ancient times, the milk latex has been an effective, mild sedative.*

TRADITIONAL USAGES

Wild lettuce has been used as a painkiller and relaxant since ancient times. It is mentioned by Dioscorides, Galen, and Theophrastus, among others.

In North America, Meskwaki women imbibed a lettuce leaf tea to promote the secretion of milk after childbirth, as did the Flambeau Ojibwas. The Menominees applied the milky juice to poison ivy rash.

The medicinal effects depend upon the milky juice that exudes when the stem or the flower stalks are lacerated. In color, taste, and odor, this juice strongly resembles opium. The medicinal preparation consists of the juice in hardened, evaporated form and is known as lactucarium. As a sedative and diuretic, it was official in the *U.S. Pharmacopoeia* from 1820 to 1926. More recently, it has been revived to some extent among the drug culture in the form of a commercial preparation known as "lettuce opium."

RECENT SCIENTIFIC FINDINGS

Lactucarium, found in this and other species of lettuce, is obtained by wounding the plants in the flowering season when their vessels are filled with juice and so irritable that they often spontaneously burst or are ruptured by very slight accidental injuries.

This fresh milky latex contains a sedative principle known as lactucopicrin. The best way to collect this juice is by placing successive small pieces of cotton on the cut stem and throwing them into a little water. Once a certain amount has been gathered, the water containing the dissolved contents of the cotton pieces is evaporated, resulting in the extraction of the desired substance. An easier way to collect the latex is by macerating the stems

Lactuca elongata

and leaves in water, just after the seeds have matured and before the plant decays. The maceration is to be continued for 24 hours, then the liquid is boiled for 2 hours, and finally evaporated in shallow basins.

Lactucarium has very mild pain allaying and calmative effects, somewhat like a weak dose of opium. It may best be employed as a mild sedative. It was also used as a draught in constipation, for intestinal disorders such as engorgements, and for other gastric upsets.

Lactuca elongata, commonly known as wild lettuce or tall lettuce, is an herbaceous plant that grows in various regions, including North America. Unlike its cultivated relative used in salads, this wild variety is recognized for its potential medicinal properties.

The leaves of *Lactuca elongata* contain lactucarium, which has mild sedative and analgesic effects. This has led to its historical use in traditional herbal medicine for addressing conditions such as pain, anxiety, and sleep disturbances. The herb is sometimes referred to as the "poor man's opium" due to its subtle sedative qualities, although it is not as potent or addictive as opium.

LICORICE
Glycyrrhiza glabra

Parts used: Root. *The roots contain glycyrrhizin, which is about 50 times sweeter than sugar and exhibits a powerful cortisone-like effect.*

TRADITIONAL USAGES

Among the ancient Greeks, licorice root had a reputation for quenching thirst and was used in this connection to treat dropsy. It is an excellent demulcent and is soothing to the mucous membrane, hence it was given to treat irritated urinary, bowel, and respiratory passages. It was often given in combination with senega and mezereon when these drugs were used on people with irritated or inflamed eliminatory organs. The root also reportedly had expectorant and laxative properties.

The Blackfoot steeped the leaves in water and used this liquid for earaches. The edible roots of American licorice were boiled, and the tea drunk by the early white settlers, who either learned of this remedy from Native Americans or adapted a European remedy.

In China, licorice root became a major tonic to combat fevers and as a remedy for infections. For centuries, it has been one of the most commonly employed herbs in Chinese medicine; most prescriptions include licorice as a component.

Children suck on licorice sticks both as a candy and as a remedy for coughs. Licorice is a valuable flavoring adjunct to medicines with unpleasant tastes. The powdered root was utilized in the preparation of pills, both to give them more substance and to coat the surfaces to prevent their sticking together.

In the 1940s, Dutch physicians tested licorice's reputation as an aid for indigestion. Their research resulted in the drug carbenoxolone, which was used to aid peptic ulcer patients. Though the drug proved effective, it also resulted in the adverse side effect of excessive swelling of the limbs and face.

RECENT SCIENTIFIC FINDINGS

The multitude of pharmacological effects of licorice rhizomes and roots are practically all attributed to the presence of a triterpene saponin called glycyrrhizin, which is about 50 times sweeter than sugar and has a powerful cortisone-like effect. Several cases have been reported in medical literature in which humans ingesting 6–8 ounces (a very large amount) of licorice candy daily for a period of several weeks are "poisoned" due to the cortisone-like effects of licorice extract in the candy. Proper treatment restores patients to normal. This amount of this compound is very large compared with the relatively small amount found in supplements.

In addition, licorice rhizomes and roots have a high mucilage content. When mixed with water, the resulting preparation has a very pleasant odor and taste and acts as an effective demulcent on irritated mucous membranes, such as those that accompany a sore throat. One study found that glycyrrhizin was as effective a cough suppressant as codeine. A 1991 experiment with mice found that glycyrrhizin protected against skin cancer. The authors speculated that it might prove useful in protecting against some forms of human cancer as well.

It is not surprising that licorice and glycyrrhizin have such wide applications. It should be noted that this chemical constitutes only 7 to 10% of the total root (on a dry weight basis). Glycyrrhetic acid (G.A.) is obtained when acid hydrolysis is applied to the main component of

Glycyrrhiza glabra

licorice. This compound is extensively used in Europe for its anti-inflammatory properties, especially in Addison's disease and for peptic ulcers. Some European researchers concluded that G.A. may be preferred to cortisone because it is safer, especially when prolonged treatment is required.

A recent study (1990) demonstrated that G.A. exerts its activity not as a direct effect but by reducing the conversion of cortisol to cortisone, its biologically inactive product. The authors concluded that hydrocortisone, a "weak anti-inflammatory agent," can be greatly potentiated (i.e., made more powerful) by the addition of 2% G.A. To lessen the toxic effects of corticosteroids, the authors suggested that patients use hydrocortisone together with G.A. Here is another example of the growing marriage between prescription pharmaceuticals and herbal preparations.

Glycyrrhizin has also exhibited antiviral activity. A 1979 study demonstrated that glycyrrhizin inhibited Epstein-Barr virus (EBV), cytomegalovirus (CMV), and hepatitis B virus. In Japan, glycyrrhizin has long been successfully used to treat chronic hepatitis B. This has led to speculation that glycyrrhizin holds promise in the treatment of HIV.

Caution: Side effects from the ingestion of large amounts of licorice have been reported. Glycyrrhizin in very large amounts can promote hypokalemia and hypertension. For these reasons, people with heart problems and high blood pressure are advised to avoid consuming large quantities of licorice or its components.

Licorice is a versatile herb with a long history of use in various cultural and medicinal traditions. In traditional herbal medicine, licorice has been utilized for its demulcent and expectorant qualities. It is often employed to soothe respiratory discomfort, such as coughs and sore throats. Its natural sweetness makes it a favored ingredient in herbal cough syrups and teas.

Licorice root contains glycyrrhizin, a compound responsible for its sweet taste and believed to have anti-inflammatory and antiviral properties. This has led to its use in addressing various health concerns, including digestive problems and immune support.

Moreover, licorice has been used in traditional Chinese medicine and Ayurveda for its adaptogenic properties, which are believed to help the body adapt to stress and maintain balance.

Despite its potential benefits, it's important to use licorice with care, as excessive consumption can lead to adverse effects. In particular, glycyrrhizin can affect blood pressure and potassium levels. It is advisable to seek guidance from a healthcare professional before using licorice for medicinal purposes, especially for those with preexisting health conditions or who are taking medications.

LILY-OF-THE-VALLEY

Convallaria majalis

Parts used: Root, fruit, and flowers. *This lovely flower contains glycosides that make a powerful cardiotonic that is currently popular in Europe.*

TRADITIONAL USAGES

The major traditional use for lily-of-the-valley seems to be as a cardiotonic. It has long been used as a popular remedy for dropsy. It was also employed to expel worms from the intestinal tract.

The flowers were believed to stimulate the secretions of the mucous membranes of the nose. They also were employed in the treatment of apoplexy, epilepsy, coma, and vertigo. Spirits distilled from the flowers were applied externally on sprains and to treat rheumatism.

The root was employed for the same maladies as the flowers. Also, an extract of the root was used for its gentle stimulant and laxative properties.

RECENT SCIENTIFIC FINDINGS

Lily-of-the-valley's effective use as a cardiotonic is explained on the basis of the presence of cardiac glycosides similar in structure and effect to the digitalis glycosides. The major cardiac glycoside in lily-of-the-valley is convallatoxin.

Since there are no advantages of *Convallaria* as a cardiotonic over the effect of *Digitalis purpurea* (foxglove), it is not commonly used in the United States. However, it is employed extensively in Europe. Lily-of-the-valley is a small and enchanting herbaceous plant celebrated for its elegance and delicate, bell-shaped white flowers. This herb carries a sweet, intoxicating fragrance that has made it a symbol of spring and romance.

While lily-of-the-valley is cherished for its aesthetic qualities and scent, it has a limited role in traditional herbal medicine due to its toxic nature. The plant contains compounds called

Convallaria majalis

cardiac glycosides, which can have severe effects on the heart if ingested. Historically, it was used cautiously and under professional guidance to address certain heart-related conditions, although its use has declined in modern herbal practices due to safety concerns.

LINDEN
Tilia cordata, T. europaea

Parts used: Flowers and leaves. *This was a popular home remedy in Europe and North America, but little recent research has been conducted to confirm or deny folkloric claims.*

TRADITIONAL USAGES
The flowers of many of the different species of this tree were used in both Europe and North America as a home remedy for colds, sore throats, coughs, and flu. The leaves were also sometimes used in North America for the same afflictions. The flowers were also an antispasmodic and nervine.

The inner bark's mucilage was applied for various skin conditions, such as sores, burns, and wounds. The burned wood was also used as a wound application.

RECENT SCIENTIFIC FINDINGS
Linden contains flavonoids. This herbaceous tree, native to North America, Europe, and Asia, is characterized by its heart-shaped leaves and clusters of small, pale-yellow flowers.

Linden flowers have a long history of use in herbal remedies, primarily for their calming and soothing effects. They are known for their ability to promote relaxation, alleviate anxiety, and aid in sleep. The herbal infusion made from linden blossoms is often enjoyed as a comforting tea, especially in the evening, due to its mild sedative qualities.

In addition to its calming attributes, linden has been used in traditional herbal medicine to address various ailments, including respiratory conditions and digestive discomfort. Its pleasant taste and gentle nature make it a popular choice for herbal infusions and syrups.

Linden's aromatic charm and potential health benefits highlight its role in traditional and modern herbal practices. Its fragrant blossoms and therapeutic qualities offer a bridge between the world of natural remedies and the pursuit of well-being and relaxation.

LOBELIA

Lobelia inflata

Parts used: Leaves and seeds. *This controversial herb was at the center of the Thomsonian system of herbal medicine. Current evidence suggests that lobelia may help smokers to quit.*

TRADITIONAL USAGES

Sometimes called Indian tobacco, this species of *Lobelia* is a very common weed and grows throughout the United States. The Meskwaki tribe finely ground the roots of red and blue lobelias and secretly put it into the food eaten by a quarreling couple. This tribe felt this preparation "averts divorce and makes the pair love each other again." The Iroquois used a root decoction of lobelia to treat syphilis. In the early 1800s, English physicians adapted this cure. Dr. Charles Millspaugh theorizes why the plant failed to effect a cure when employed in Europe:

"The natives of North America are said to have held this plant a secret in the cure of syphilis, until it was purchased from them . . . and introduced . . . as a drug of great repute in that disease. European physicians, however, failed to cure with it, and finally cast it aside, though Linnaeus, thinking it justified its Indian reputation, gave the species its distinctive name, *syphilitica.* The cause of failure may be the fact that the aborigines did not trust to the plant alone, but always used it in combination with May-apple roots (*Podophyllum peltatum*), the bark of the Wild Cherry (*Prunus virginiana*) and dusted the ulcers with the powdered bark of New Jersey tea (*Ceanothus americanus*). Another chance of failure lay in the volatility of its active principle, as the dried herb was used."

This controversial herb was the mainstay of the system of herbal medicine introduced by Samuel Thomson, who wrote in the third edition of his *Botanic Family Physician* (Boston, 1831): "In consequence of their [accredited doctors] thus forming an erroneous opinion of this herb, which they had no knowledge of, they undertook to represent it as a deadly poison; and in order to destroy my practice, they raised a hue and cry about my killing my patients by administering it to them." Thomson's book largely contained passionate protestations toward the medical establishment, which he felt was persecuting him.

Lobelia was reported useful in treating bronchitis, laryngitis, asthma, and convulsive and inflammatory disorders such as epilepsy, tetanus, diphtheria, and tonsillitis.

As a muscle relaxant, lobelia was employed in midwifery to alleviate rigidity of the pelvic musculature during childbirth, according to the recommendations of one of

Thomson's followers. Used externally in a poultice with slippery elm and a little soap, lobelia was helpful in bringing abscesses and boils to a head.

RECENT SCIENTIFIC FINDINGS

The precautions about the poisonous potential of the plant are always mentioned by herbalists other than those practicing the Thomsonian system. Lobelia, along with 26 other plants, has been declared an "unsafe herb" by the U.S. Food and Drug Administration, which describes it as "a poisonous plant which contains the alkaloid lobelia, plus a number of other pyridine alkaloids. Overdoses of the plant or extracts of the leaves or fruits produce vomiting, sweating, pain, paralysis, depressed temperatures, rapid but feeble pulse, collapse, coma and death in the human being." The effects of excessive doses, classified by herbalists as "aeronarcotic," are similar to those of tobacco; hence its popular name, Indian tobacco.

Lobelia leaves and flowering tops do contain the alkaloid lobeline, which is known to relax smooth muscle and thus would give rise to an antispasmodic effect. Extracts of the leaves have been shown experimentally to have expectorant properties, most likely due to the lobeline content.

Lobeline is used to stimulate respiration in newborn infants. It is a popular smoking deterrent when taken orally in small doses. Human experimental evidence attests to its value in aiding smokers to drop the habit, contradicting the possibly excessive cautions of the USFDA.

Lobelia's active compounds, particularly lobeline, have been traditionally utilized for their potential therapeutic effects. The herb is best known for its ability to support respiratory health and has been used to help alleviate conditions such as asthma, bronchitis, and coughs. Its bronchodilatory properties may help to relax and open airways, aiding in easier breathing.

In addition to its respiratory benefits, lobelia has been employed as a natural remedy for digestive discomfort and as an agent to promote relaxation and stress reduction.

It's essential to use lobelia with care, as excessive consumption can lead to adverse side effects.

Lobelia inflata

MAGNOLIA

Magnolia glauca and other *Magnolia* species

Parts used: Bark and root bark. *The bark of this beautiful tree mitigates malaria, and future research may confirm preliminary antitumor findings.*

TRADITIONAL USAGES

Various Native American tribes employed magnolia as a remedy for rheumatism, to expel worms, and for cramps. Colonial settlers employed the bark by putting it into brandy or boiling it with any other liquor. They used it to ease pectoral diseases, as well as internal pains, fever, and dysentery.

Owing to their diaphoretic properties, the barks of various magnolias were taken to mitigate the ravages of malarial as well as other intermittent fevers. Used in place of cinchona (quinine), magnolia could be administered for longer periods of time with no side effects.

There is some record of magnolia bark's usefulness as a substitute for tobacco and as an aid for breaking the habit of chewing tobacco. Official in the *U.S. Pharmacopoeia* from 1820 to 1894, the dried bark of three magnolia species (*M. virginiana, M. acuminata,* and *M. tripetala)* was recommended in doses of 2.0 to 3.9 grams.

M. officinalis is prized in Chinese herbalism as a tonic and is considered aphrodisiac. In Mexico, *M. schiedeana* in a flower decoction applied topically is used to treat scorpion stings. Perhaps most interesting of all medicinal properties of magnolias is reported of a species found in Brazil (*M. pubescent).* The stems, leaves, and seeds contain saponins capable of stupefying fish and are employed for this purpose by fishermen wanting an easier catch.

RECENT SCIENTIFIC FINDINGS

Only recently have the various magnolias begun to be subjected to the scrutiny of the laboratory. One team of researchers isolated three neolignans from

Magnolia glauca

magnolia bark. They found that these extracts exhibited "remarkable inhibitory effects" on tumors in mice and in vivo.

One of these three extracts, magnolol, possessed the qualities of an antiplatelet agent in a preliminary study.

Magnolia, scientifically known as *Magnolia grandiflora*, is a captivating and aromatic herb appreciated for its graceful evergreen foliage and large, fragrant flowers.

In traditional herbal medicine, various parts of the magnolia tree have been employed for their potential therapeutic properties. The bark, in particular, is used to create magnolia bark extract, which has been explored for its anti-inflammatory and antianxiety effects. The extract contains compounds such as magnolol and honokiol, which are believed to offer calming and relaxation benefits, making it a notable option in traditional and alternative medicine for stress and anxiety management.

Additionally, magnolia flowers are renowned for their enchanting fragrance and are sometimes used in perfumery and aromatherapy to promote a sense of tranquility.

MARIGOLD
Calendula officinalis

Parts used: Flowers. *This is considered a natural antiseptic, and an Austrian patent was issued for the flowers as an emollient.*

TRADITIONAL USAGES
Applied locally as a tincture, oil, or lotion, marigold is considered a "natural antiseptic" by homeopaths. The crushed petals may be combined with olive oil to form an ointment for external application to cuts, bruises, sores, and burns.

The infusion was used to soothe watery, irritated eyes and for relief of bronchial complaints. Marigold was frequently used as a home remedy in liver disorders. It was also thought to induce perspiration in fever.

RECENT SCIENTIFIC FINDINGS
The flowers contain an essential oil, an amorphous bitter compound, and calendulin. Experimentally, marigold flower extracts have been shown to lower blood pressure and to have sedative effects in several animal species, and it thus seems that the use of marigold tea would have a beneficial effect on these conditions as well. Marigold is a common adulterant to saffron.

An Austrian patent was issued in 1955 for the use of extracts of marigold flowers as an emollient in the treatment of burns in humans.

Marigold, scientifically known as *Calendula officinalis*, is a cheerful and versatile herb admired for its vibrant golden and orange flowers. Native to the Mediterranean region, marigold has a long history of cultural and medicinal significance.

In traditional herbal medicine, marigold blossoms are prized for their anti-inflammatory, antimicrobial, and wound-healing properties. The flowers are often used to create topical salves, creams, and ointments for treating skin irritations, minor wounds, and insect bites. Marigold's soothing qualities make it a popular choice for alleviating skin discomfort.

Marigold is also known for its mild astringent properties, which are useful for skin toning and maintaining skin health. Its bright blossoms are sometimes used to create herbal teas and infusions.

MARIJUANA
Cannabis sativa

Parts used: Flowering tops. *This weed has proven to be an effective treatment for glaucoma and an aid for cancer patients undergoing chemotherapy.*

TRADITIONAL USAGES

Marijuana has enjoyed a long and respectable history as a medicinal agent. As early as 2737 B.C., the plant was included in the pharmacopoeia of the Chinese emperor Shen Nung. The ancient Scythians used it in their funeral rites, and seeds have been found in funerary urns dating back to the fifth century B.C.

Marijuana was formerly utilized in medicine to treat insomnia, allay pain, and soothe restlessness. The herbalist Culpepper recommended it in the treatment of colic, bloody noses, and jaundice. Marijuana has been given in the treatment of neuralgias and spasmodic coughs, as in pertussis and asthma, as well as in tetanus and hydrophobia and other painful spasmodic diseases.

Inhalation of marijuana smoke produces great exhilaration and can cause muscle fatigue to temporarily disappear. These psychic effects of the drug have made it useful as a nervine and stimulant for raising the spirits. Held to be narcotic and antispasmodic, it was recognized in the 1918 *Dispensatory of the United States* as a general nerve sedative for use in hysteria, mental depression, and neurasthenia.

Besides its medicinal applications, hemp is an important fiber crop; it has been observed that plants grown in colder climates yield better fiber while those from warmer climates have more pronounced intoxicant and medicinal properties, owing to a higher content of the resin that contains the active principles.

The fruits, known as hemp seeds, are a popular ingredient in birdseed. At one time they were employed medicinally in the treatment of mucous membrane inflammations.

RECENT SCIENTIFIC FINDINGS

Currently, it is estimated that one in seven Americans twelve years of age or older has used marijuana, and its number seems to have stabilized over the past few years. Although many refer to marijuana as a "narcotic" or "hallucinogen," in a strict scientific sense neither term is applicable. Marijuana is not addicting, nor does it produce true hallucinations, except in extremely high doses. Its anodyne and soporific action resembles that of opium, but without the undesirable aftereffects of constipation and appetite loss.

Pharmacologists have been unable to place marijuana into a neat "category" for purposes of explaining its effects; it is a drug in a class by itself. However, it is safe to say that currently the most popular use for marijuana is as a recreational euphoriant.

The major active euphoric principle in marijuana is a substance known as delta-9-tetrahydrocannabinol (THC). It is an extremely unstable substance in its pure form, but in the living or dead plant it is quite stable. It is amazing to learn that there is only one plant, *Cannabis sativa*, known to contain THC, or compounds related to this principle. Although some botanists, with reasonable arguments, claim three major species of marijuana exist—*Cannabis sativa* (most common), *Cannabis indica,* and *Cannabis ruderalis*—most chemical and pharmacological evidence seems to support the existence of only one species (i.e., *Cannabis sativa*).

Recent clinical experience demonstrates that marijuana has a wide range of useful applications in medicine. Certain types of glaucoma that are resistant to conventional types of treatment can be controlled by smoking marijuana. Administration of THC to cancer patients who experience nausea and vomiting as a common side effect of chemotherapy produces relief of these symptoms. Marijuana or its constituents, however, do not have anticancer properties.

Based on results of human studies, other remarkable effects of THC are to relieve pain, control seizures of epilepsy, relieve symptoms of asthma, and act as a sedative. Newly available evidence supports earlier findings that the use of cannabidiol products probably reduces the frequency of seizures among children with drug-resistant epilepsy. It is now well established that the use of marijuana in the treatment of pain, to induce sleep, and for other maladies has been fully justified on the basis of solid scientific evidence.

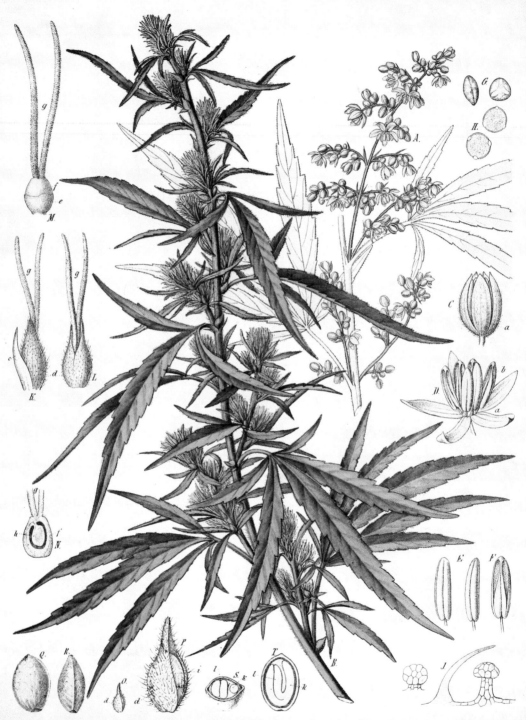

Cannabis sativa

In recent years, other types of marijuana-based products claiming to contain only cannabidiol—more commonly known as CBD—have become popular. Unlike THC, cannabidiol is nonintoxicating, meaning it does not produce the euphoric feeling that is traditionally associated with marijuana products. Products containing CBD include oils, edibles, and topical creams. They have been shown to relieve pain, anxiety, and some sleep disorders.

However, these products should be regarded with caution. Today's CBD products—many of which are being marketed and sold as candy or gummies—are not regulated by the FDA. Many CBD products contain trace amounts of THC. Manufacturers are not regulated by any THC content standards. There are too many variables to guarantee a standard product. Just because the product is packaged nicely does not guarantee its content. Caution therefore must be observed as the incidence of ER admissions by people—particularly youth—attributing mental problems due to CBD intake has surged.

In general, young people should exercise extreme caution when consuming marijuana. A study published in 2021 in *Jama Psychiatry* found that marijuana use negatively altered the development of the cerebral cortex, the portion of the brain responsible for reasoning and executive function. Other studies have shown increased risks of anxiety and depression in marijuana users between the ages of 13 and 25.

Recent studies have also revealed other significant risks for people of all ages. Beyond the immediate psychoactive effects of THC, which can impair cognitive and motor functions, chronic or heavy use of marijuana has been linked to an increased risk of mental health issues, including anxiety and depression, and an elevated risk of psychosis, particularly among individuals with a predisposition to these conditions. Respiratory problems are also a concern, especially when marijuana is smoked, as it can lead to bronchitis and, in the long term, may affect lung health similarly to tobacco. There is also evidence of potential cardiovascular risks, such as increased heart rate, which can lead to a higher risk of heart attacks, especially in older populations or those with preexisting heart conditions. A study published in the journal *Addiction* in 2023 reported that "adults who overuse cannabis are 60 percent more likely to experience heart failure, strokes, or heart attacks compared to adults of the same age and sex without cannabis use disorder."

As of June 2024, there is pending U.S. DEA legislation that will reclassify the status of medical marijuana from Schedule I to Schedule III, acknowledging its medical benefits while maintaining its prohibition for recreational use. This change, initiated by a directive from the Department of Health and Human Services, aims to ease research restrictions, adjust regulatory controls, and reflect the evolving public and scientific perspective on cannabis.

MARSHMALLOW
Althaea officinalis

Parts used: Root, leaves, and flowers. *Considered a cure-all by the ancient Greeks, the roots' mucilage content makes this plant an excellent emollient.*

TRADITIONAL USAGES

The ancient Greeks praised the virtues of marshmallow and seemed to consider it a medicinal that would help cure any ailment. Hippocrates especially felt it was an immense aid in the treatment of wounds.

During the Renaissance, herbalists used marshmallow to treat sore throats, stomach problems, gonorrhea, leucorrhea, toothaches, and mouth infections.

Marshmallow root is an excellent demulcent and emollient. The decoction is taken internally to relieve irritation and inflammation of the mucous membranes. The crushed leaves and flowers are boiled and applied externally in poultice form as a soothing dressing for scrapes, chafing, and other irritated skin conditions.

RECENT SCIENTIFIC FINDINGS

Marshmallow root is well known to have a very high mucilage content. When the mucilage comes into contact with water, it swells and forms a very soft, soothing, and protective gel. Thus, the external application of water extracts of this plant will have a demulcent and emollient effect on mucous membranes or on the skin, or will have a lubricant effect. If a water extract of marshmallow was applied to a burn or

Althaea officinalis

skin abrasion, its emollient effect would reduce the amount of pain from the burn or abrasion, and in this context, it would have pain-relieving properties.

Marshmallow, scientifically known as *Althaea officinalis*, is a versatile and soothing herb with a long history of medicinal use. This perennial plant, native to Europe and parts of Asia, is celebrated for its gentle, mucilaginous properties.

In traditional herbal medicine, marshmallow has been prized for its ability to ease respiratory and digestive discomfort. The root and leaves of the plant contain a slippery, gel-like substance that can provide relief for irritated mucous membranes and help alleviate issues like coughs, sore throats, and digestive irritation. This mucilaginous quality has made marshmallow a valued ingredient in cough syrups.

MATE
Ilex paraguariensis

Parts used: Leaves. *Due to its high caffeine content, this is used in South America to make a popular drink.*

TRADITIONAL USAGES
Just as millions of people drink coffee and tea in other parts of the world, millions in South America enjoy mate. The characteristic aromatic flavor and the stimulant caffeine are extracted by pouring water, either hot or cold, over dried leaves. As with tea, the most expensive grade of mate is composed of the youngest leaves, while cheaper grades contain twigs, stems, and older leaves. Botanically, mate is a species of holly. It is cultivated and is also found growing wild.

RECENT SCIENTIFIC FINDINGS
Mate is a rich source of caffeine. At the Sixth International Caffeine Workshop in Hong Kong, researchers concluded that the consumption of "normal levels" of caffeine posed "no significant health hazards."

The recurring concern of the putative link between cancer and caffeine was specifically dispelled, there being no association for esophageal, stomach, or liver cancer; a slight relationship for pancreatic cancer; and a protective effect against colorectal cancer.

Pregnant women who consumed the substance were studied over a seven-year period with no effect seen on newborns, infants, or four- to seven-year-old children.

Coffee and tea drinkers no longer need be overly fearful of their "daily cup" so long as they follow a "moderate" intake (2–3 cups per day). What remains to be studied, in the editor's opinion, is the relationship between Styrofoam containers and cancer of the pancreas as well as the health effects of highly sweetened caffeinated beverages.

It will not surprise inveterate coffee drinkers to learn that caffeine promotes the burning of fat. A series of studies, most notably that of Astrup and colleagues, confirms what coffee and tea "addicts" have long known, that these beverages promote slimming in humans.

It has been discovered that caffeine stimulates the expenditure of energy and the burning of fats.

Astrup's was a placebo-controlled, double-blind, dose-response study. (In other words, it met all the requirements of mainstream science.) Caffeine was tested in dosages of 100, 200, and 400 mg and compared against three different doses of ephedrine and two placebos.

Six healthy subjects were recruited from the University of Copenhagen Medical School. Excluded were people habituated to caffeine from other sources—coffee, tea, colas, chocolate, and cocoa. The test subjects were put on a weight-controlling diet consisting of about 250 grams of carbohydrate and a fixed amount of sodium. Their body fat content was measured before and after taking the placebo (lactose) or caffeine (100, 200, or 400 mg) in gelatin capsules. Through a series of wonderful experimental analyses, the authors discovered that caffeine has a thermogenic effect (i.e., raises body heat) when taken in moderate doses on a daily basis. "A significant thermogenic effect was found even after the lowest dose of caffeine (100 mg)." Interestingly, even this relatively small intake of caffeine was found to produce a lasting effect on energy expenditure. When caffeine was taken together with physical activity, the thermogenic effect was enhanced.

The mechanism by which caffeine exerts this fat-burning effect is thought to be associated with the thermogenic Cori cycle. This is where glycogen and glucose are converted to lactate in fat and muscle tissue. Lactate then triggers thermogenic processes in the liver.

Mate is prized for its leaves, which are used to prepare a stimulating and invigorating beverage known as mate or yerba mate.

Ilex paraguariensis

Mate has a long-standing tradition in South American countries, particularly in Argentina, Paraguay, Uruguay, and parts of Brazil, where it is considered a national drink. The preparation of mate involves steeping dried leaves in hot water, usually within a hollowed gourd or a special cup, and it is usually sipped through a metal straw called a bombilla.

This herbal infusion contains caffeine and theobromine, providing an energy boost and mental alertness similar to that of coffee and tea. However, mate is also celebrated for its potential health benefits. It is rich in antioxidants and nutrients, which are believed to contribute to its capacity to improve mental focus, aid digestion, and boost the immune system.

MATHAKE or Tropical Almond
Terminalia catappa

Parts used: Leaves and bark. *Commonly used in the South Pacific, tropical almond is one of the most effective antifungal plants.*

TRADITIONAL USAGES
This species, widely distributed in the tropics, is one of the most effective antifungal plants, yet it is not widely known.

RECENT SCIENTIFIC FINDINGS
In 1984, I introduced tropical almond to several physicians who reported strong activity against *Candida albicans* in trials with patients. My decision to bring this plant into Western medicine was based on firsthand observations of its powerful antifungal activity when used in Fijian folk medicine.

Subsequent literature analysis indicated that a decoction of the leaves (mixed with other plants) is used to induce abortion in New Guinea. However, mathake by itself is perfectly safe; it is used as a tonic in Mexico, and the nuts have been eaten by children since antiquity. The compounds found within the leaves kill *staphylococci,* which may explain its folkloric use as a tonic.

A related species, *T. arjuna,* has been shown to reduce total cholesterol and triglycerides while raising HDLs in experiments with rabbits. This study was based on an Ayurvedic prescription for the treatment of cardiovascular disorders.

At this time, we do not know if mathake acts directly to kill yeast or if any of its compounds enhances the immune system. Owing to its clinical effectiveness in initial

Castor oil, derived from the seeds, is the most well-known product associated with mathake.

trials and its long history of usage, this plant is worth utilizing as part of an overall immune-enhancing program.

The following was written about mathake by Richard W. Noble, MD, a physician familiar with herbal medicine.

"It would be difficult to overstate the usefulness of the medicinal herb mathake in my medical practice. I am particularly grateful for your effort to make this material available for use in this country...I was looking for alternatives to oral nystatin, particularly in children with candidiasis. In the intervening years, mathake has become the first treatment of choice for patients with chronic candidiasis-related illness. The wide variety of agents, both prescription and nonprescription, that are available to treat yeast infections is well known. As a medical doctor experienced in the use of botanical medicine, I have used through the years a variety of these agents, including garlic, pau d'arco, grapefruit seed extract, and caprylic acid.

All of these materials may be helpful in certain cases but none of them provide the ease of use, the economy, and the low side effects I have experienced in patients using mathake. It will be readily verified by any physician who has attempted to treat this puzzling problem that continued therapy measured in months, not days or weeks is the usual case. It is for this reason prolonged use of prescription medications are not advised . . .

Mathake can be used for up to three months at a time. It has the advantage of being an easily prepared medication. All that is necessary is boiling water to produce a pleasant tasting cup of tea. Children, particularly, accept this method. Adults find the ease of use and the low toxicity very appealing. Thank you again for your efforts in bringing this valuable herb to the continent. Please keep me advised of your research with mathake."

Mathake is a remarkable herb recognized for its versatile uses and unique characteristics.

Mathake has a history of traditional uses, with various parts of the plant being employed for different purposes. Castor oil, derived from the seeds, is the most well-known product associated with mathake. Castor oil has been used for its potential laxative effects and as a soothing agent for skin and hair.

MEZEREON
Daphne mezereum

Parts used: Bark and berries. *The bark of this plant contains mezerein, a substance that could be a cocarcinogen.*

TRADITIONAL USAGES
Caution: While the berries and bark of mezereon have reportedly been useful in European folk medicine (to cure paralysis of the mouth), the plant is a strong internal poison. However, an ointment made of the berries gained a folkloric reputation in northern Europe as a treatment for cancer, canker sores, and ulcerous lesions.

Linnaeus stated that the Swedes applied the bark to parts bitten by poisonous reptiles and rabid animals.

RECENT SCIENTIFIC FINDINGS
Mezereon contains an extremely irritant substance, known as mezerein, that is toxic to cells. In animal experiments, mezerein, as well as extracts of mezereon, inhibit experimental tumors. These properties explain most of the effects claimed for this plant.

It must be pointed out that mezerein is a chemical substance closely related to other substances classified as cocarcinogens. This means that by itself the substance cannot cause cancer. However, it will increase the cancer-causing effects of other chemical substances when they are put together. Thus, it is possible that the use of mezereon by a tobacco user will increase the risk of cancer, due to this additive effect. Other environmental cancer-causing agents, which we are all exposed to continuously, could possibly react with mezerein and enhance the production of cancer cells in humans who are exposed to both types of agents.

For these reasons, one must understand the risk potential in using mezereon for any purpose.

Daphne mezereum

MILK THISTLE
Silybum marianum

Parts used: Seeds. *The seeds contain silymarin, a flavonoid that is effective for liver disorders.*

TRADITIONAL USAGES

For centuries, milk thistle has been used in folkloric medicine. The seeds were believed to act most directly to protect the liver.

RECENT SCIENTIFIC FINDINGS

One active component extracted from milk thistle seeds, silymarin, is a flavonoid long recognized for its ability to benefit people with liver disorders and as a protective compound against liver-damaging agents as diverse as mushroom toxins, carbon tetrachloride, and other chemicals. This flavonoid demonstrates good antioxidant properties, both in vivo and in vitro.

Chilean scientists found that silymarin also increases the content of liver glutathione (GSH), an effect not known with other closely related flavonoids such as (+)-cyanidanol-3 (catechin). These experiments also showed an increase of glutathione content and antioxidant activity in the intestine and stomach. The effects selectively occur only in the digestive tract, and not in the kidney, lungs, and spleen.

A double-blind, prospective, randomized study performed on 170 patients with cirrhosis of the liver supported the fact that silymarin protects the liver. All patients received the same treatment with a mean observation period of 41 months. The four-year survival rate was significantly higher in silymarin-treated patients than those in the placebo group. No side effects of drug treatment were observed.

Another study found that milk thistle may offer us some protection against the toxic side effects of the common pain-relieving drug acetaminophen, which is

Silybum marianum

a widely used analgesic and fever medication. In overdosage, severe hepatotoxicity may result, characterized by glutathione (GSH) depletion, suppression of GSH biosynthesis, and liver damage. GSH is considered the most important biomolecule against chemically induced cytotoxicity.

Silybin, a soluble form of silymarin, is thought to exert a membrane-stabilizing action that inhibits or prevents lipid peroxidation. Silybin and silymarin may be useful in protecting the liver in many cases besides acetaminophen overdosage. Alcohol also depletes GSH, and these flavonoids offer protection for those who continue to drink. Interestingly, silybin dihemisuccinate remains medicine's most important antidote to poisoning by the mushroom toxins alpha-amanitin and phalloidin.

Milk thistle is a remarkable herb with distinctive, spiky leaves and striking purple flowers. This herb has a rich history in herbal medicine, primarily known for its potential liver-protective properties. The active compound in milk thistle, silymarin, is believed to have strong antioxidant and anti-inflammatory effects, which make it invaluable in liver health support. It is often used to help with liver conditions, such as cirrhosis, hepatitis, and fatty liver disease. Milk thistle serves as a testament to nature's capacity to provide remedies for the well-being of vital organs.

MORNING GLORY

Ipomoea purpurea and other *Ipomoea* species

Parts used: Seeds. *Of the more than 175 varieties of this flower, only seven have been found to contain hallucinogenic components.*

TRADITIONAL USAGES

A great deal of confusion revolves around the use of morning glory as an herbal remedy. This is due to more than one plant species being widely used. A great deal of difference in effect occurs, depending on whether the seeds or the roots are used.

The most common cultivated ornamental morning glory is *Ipomoea purpurea.* No part of this species is capable of producing hallucinogenic effects. However, the roots contain a complex mixture of fatty acid–like substances that produce a rather harsh purgative effect.

In recent years, the seeds of *Ipomoea violacea (Ipomoea tricolor)* have been widely employed as a hallucinogen in North America. Ironically, this use was known in Mexico for centuries for a plant known as badoh negro, and it was only about two decades ago that badoh negro was botanically authenticated as *Ipomoea violacea.*

RECENT SCIENTIFIC FINDINGS

The hallucinogenic effect of this plant is due to chemical substances very closely related to lysergic acid diethylamide (LSD). The active compounds are found in trace amounts in all parts of the plant, the highest concentrations being found in the seeds. More than 175 horticultural variants of *Ipomoea violacea* are known, but the lysergic acid–like substances have only been found in seven of these.

Early controversy arose as to whether or not morning glory seeds were, in fact, hallucinogenic. Some people taking the seeds claimed this effect while others failed to experience the effect. This variance in experience is explained by the fact that the seeds are very hard, and if boiled in water, the active constituents will probably not be extracted. Similarly, when the whole seeds have been taken by mouth, most people who have used them have found that the seeds were not digested and thus little or no effect was experienced. It has been estimated that about 350 seeds are required to produce hallucinations in most humans.

Morning glory encompasses a wide range of flowering plants, some of which are cultivated for their attractive, trumpet-shaped blooms. However, there are certain species of morning glory that contain psychoactive compounds, including lysergic acid derivatives. In some Indigenous cultures, these hallucinogenic morning glory varieties have been used in shamanic rituals and spiritual practices. Their psychoactive properties have drawn the interest of those exploring altered states of consciousness.

MOTHERWORT

Leonurus cardiaca

Parts used: Tops and leaves. *For centuries, this herb was given for menstrual problems, and modern research reveals it may also aid the heart.*

TRADITIONAL USAGES

In Chinese legend, motherwort prolonged life. The herb's name comes from the fact that the fruit, stem, and leaf are always thick and abundant. Motherwort was commonly prescribed for menstrual disorders, during childbirth to aid the placenta, and for general abdominal pains. In Western medicine, motherwort was recommended as a treatment for vaginitis when employed as a douche. The plant has been utilized to provoke menstruation and to aid the continuation of the flow of the lochia following childbirth.

Reportedly, it was used to calm epileptics during the 17th century, and more recently, it has been employed as a nerve tonic and sedative, especially for administration after childbirth.

RECENT SCIENTIFIC FINDINGS

While most uses of this aromatic perennial herb, as evidenced by the common name, have been directed toward the female anatomy, recent evidence has confirmed its utility in heart problems. Experimentally, motherwort extracts have been reported to have cardiotonic effects based on experiments involving application of extracts of the plant on isolated animal hearts. The action was confirmed in whole animals. Hot water extracts also show sedative and anti-epileptic effects in animals. These experiments tend to confirm the accuracy of the species epithet (*cardiaca*).

A 1990 experiment found that a mixture of hawthorn and motherwort might prove an effective preventive and/or treatment for atherosclerosis. Animal experiments have produced interesting results that warrant further investigation in regard to motherwort's effect on breast cancer. A methanol extract of motherwort was added to the drinking water of mice. The extract stimulated the excretion of carcinogenic factors and suppressed the development of one type of mammary cancer. Yet, it also enhanced the development of a different type of mammary cancer.

After flowering, the herb is richest in its components, consisting of various glycosides, resins, tannins, saponins, and organic acids.

Motherwort is an herb that derives its name from its traditional use as a tonic for women. It is characterized by its deeply lobed leaves and small, pink or white flowers. Motherwort has been esteemed for its calming properties, often used to ease nervousness, anxiety, and stress. Additionally, it has a historical association with women's health, particularly in addressing menstrual discomfort and menopausal symptoms. The herb's Latin name, *cardiaca*, alludes to its traditional role in heart-related remedies, emphasizing its multifaceted significance in herbal medicine.

Leonurus cardiaca

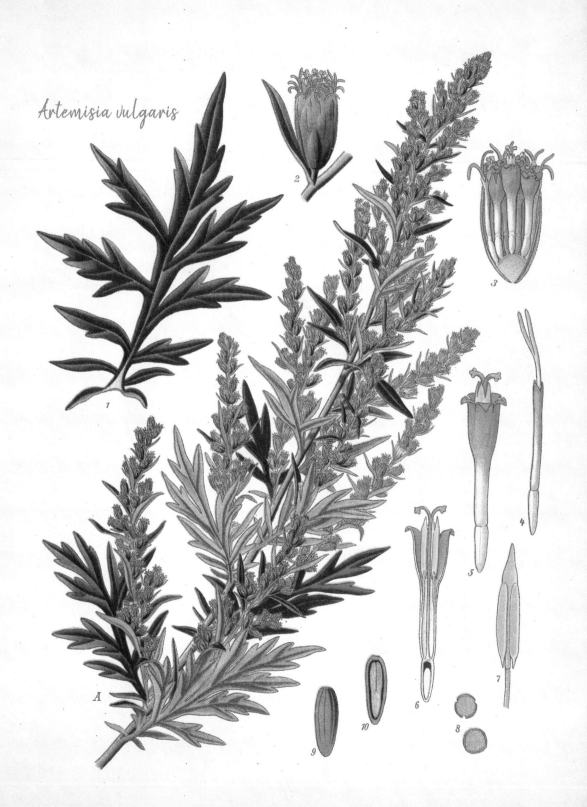

Artemisia vulgaris

MUGWORT

Artemisia vulgaris

Parts used: Leaves and flowering tops. *This plant has been used by cultures throughout the world to assist and promote menstruation.*

TRADITIONAL USAGES

The leaves of the common mugwort were used to make "moxas." The term "moxa" designates a small mass of combustible matter, which by being burnt slowly in contact with the skin, produces an eschar, a slough or scab produced from cauterization. As a treatment for disease, cauterization by fire has been commonly practiced from the earliest periods of history both by primitive tribes and advanced civilizations. The ancient Egyptians and Greeks were acquainted with the use of moxa, as were the ancients in China, Japan, and other Asian countries.

The early Portuguese navigators brought the practice from Asia to Europe. In the 1830s, moxas were a popular remedy in France for amaurosis, loss of taste, deafness, paralytic affections of the muscles, asthma, chronic catarrh and pleurisy, phthisis, chronic engorgement of the liver and spleen, rachitis, diseased spine, coxalgia, and other forms of scrofulous and rheumatic inflammation of the joints. The *British Flora Medica* has this to say:

"The dried leaves, bruised in mortar, and rubbed between the hands until the downy part is separated from the woody fiber, and rolled into little cones, is a good substitute for Chinese moxa. The part is first moistened and then a cone of the moxa is applied, which is set on fire at the apex and gradually burns down to the skin, producing a dark-colored spot; by repeating this painful process an eschar is formed, and this on separation leaves an ulcer which may be kept open or healed as circumstances may require."

Hippocrates recommended mugwort taken internally to aid in the delivery of the placenta; Dioscorides utilized it to expedite labor and delivery. It has been used as a tonic and as a cure for intermittent fever.

RECENT SCIENTIFIC FINDINGS

Mugwort is one of the most commonly employed herbal preparations for the treatment of amenorrhea, i.e., used to assist and promote menstruation. We have records showing that it is used in the Philippines, Vietnam, India, Korea, China, Europe, and the United States for this purpose. There is evidence that water extracts of mugwort will cause a stimulation of uterine muscle in the test tube; thus, on a theoretical basis, it could act as an emmenagogue in humans. There is no really effective means to establish whether or not a substance has an emmenagogue effect in animals or in humans, and thus it is difficult to use evidence such as this in support of this effect. However, when a plant is used for the same purpose in as many geographically separated areas as is mugwort, this adds credibility to the alleged effect.

Certain of its extracts injected into laboratory animals give rise to a sedative effect. Thus, it is possible that this sedative effect could be beneficial in a person with epilepsy, an illness in which mugwort has been employed.

Mugwort is a versatile herb with a long history in traditional medicine. Its deeply lobed leaves and silvery undersides make it easy to identify. Mugwort has been used for its potential digestive benefits, such as alleviating indigestion and supporting healthy digestion. Additionally, it has been employed as an antiparasitic agent in some traditional remedies. Mugwort holds cultural and spiritual significance in various societies and has played a role in rituals and practices aimed at enhancing awareness and intuition.

MULLEIN
Verbascum thapsus

Parts used: Leaves and flowers. *This plant has long been used as a treatment for respiratory problems.*

TRADITIONAL USAGES

Mullein was introduced from Europe into North America. In all probability, Native Americans learned from early settlers to treat respiratory problems with mullein. The Menominees smoked the pulverized, dried root for respiratory complaints. The Potawatomis, Mohegans, and Penobscots smoked the dried leaves to relieve asthma. The Mohegans steeped the leaves in molasses to make "an excellent cough remedy." Catawbas prepared a sweetened syrup from the boiled root as a cough medicine for their children.

During the Civil War, the Confederate Army used mullein to treat respiratory problems. Dr. Charles Millspaugh noted that mullein was principally employed around 1887 to relieve painful, phlegmy coughs. He also described a "cure" for hemorrhoids consisting of a fatty oil that resulted after the bottled flowers were allowed to sit in the sun.

Verbascum thapsus

By 1913, mullein had become extremely popular in America as a treatment for coughs and inflamed mucous membranes lining the throat. The corolla of the golden yellow flowers brought a wholesale price of 70 to 80 cents a pound. The steam was often inhaled to relieve cold symptoms such as nasal congestion and throat irritation.

RECENT SCIENTIFIC FINDINGS

Mullein leaves have high concentrations of mucilage, which is responsible for the emollient and demulcent effects of water extracts of this plant. In its application as an external emollient, a fomentation of mullein leaves in hot vinegar and water makes an agreeable application to hemorrhoids and itching complaints. Boiled with lard, it makes an ointment for dressing wounds. Fomentations or poultices of the leaves or flowers beaten up with linseed meal have been applied to burns, scalds, and boils.

Internally demulcent, mullein soothes the throat and lungs. It is also a diuretic, allays pain, and is antispasmodic. It does not have a very pleasant taste, so the addition of an aromatic, together with boiling the herb in milk, is advised.

This herb has had a consistent presence in herbal remedies, particularly for addressing respiratory conditions. It is valued for its soothing and expectorant properties, making it a popular choice for herbal teas, tinctures, and herbal remedies aimed at relieving coughs, bronchitis, and other respiratory discomforts. Mullein's tall, stately appearance reflects its historical and contemporary role in respiratory health support.

MUSTARD

Sinapis alba, S. nigra

Parts used: Seeds. *Mustard plasters continue to be a common remedy.*

TRADITIONAL USAGES

Powdered mustard seeds are a common condiment; they promote the appetite and stimulate the gastric mucous membrane, with some effect on pancreatic secretions, thereby aiding digestion. By virtue of these effects, they can sometimes relieve obstinate hiccups.

Mustard is also a valuable emetic, when it is desired to empty the stomach without accompanying depression of the system, as in cases of narcotic poisoning. Taken whole, the seeds have a laxative effect and can aid in upset stomach due to acid indigestion.

An important use of mustard has been externally, as a rubefacient (reddening the skin, producing local congestion, the vessels becoming dilated and the supply of blood increased); with longer applications, vesication, or blister formation, occurs, drawing deeper fluids to the surface. Mustard poultices may be mixed with alcohol, almond oil, or olive oil. The poultice should be carefully attended, as too long an application can result in pain and tissue damage.

RECENT SCIENTIFIC FINDINGS

Black and white mustard seeds both contain highly irritating so-called "mustard-oil" glycosides, typified by mustard oil, or allyl isothiocyanate. The irritant effect is mild in water extracts, but in concentrated extracts, the irritation can actually induce blistering. A combination of mild irritation due to the mustard-oil glycosides, in addition to a high fat content, causes the laxative effect of mustard seeds. In larger doses, the irritant action of the mustard-oil glycosides causes emesis.

Mustard plasters are still widely used, and their effective utility requires special handling. The mustard plaster is simply a thin layer of deflated mustard seeds applied to a piece of paper with a suitable glue. Prior to use, the mustard plaster is dipped into lukewarm (never hot) water. This contact with water sets off a chemical reaction in which the end product is mustard oil. The plaster is then applied for a short period of time. While the plaster is in contact with the skin, the blood rushes to the area of application. The additional blood supply serves to produce an anti-inflammatory response, relax muscles, and in general provide relief from muscle strains and similar ailments. It must be pointed out that the mustard plaster should not be allowed to remain in contact with the skin for any prolonged period of time, or it will result in the formation of blisters. The blisters are very painful and there is always a possibility that infection will result. However, mustard plasters, applied externally for periods up to 15 minutes, will usually not result in blistering and are quite safe and effective for those whose skin is of normal sensitivity.

Mustard oil itself is used in many proprietary ointments intended for external application for the relief of minor aches and pains, much the same as mustard plaster.

Mustard encompasses various species, with the seeds and greens being the most commonly

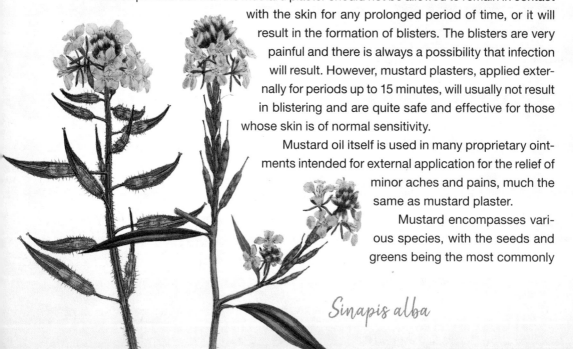

Sinapis alba

used parts. Mustard seeds are a staple in many kitchens, celebrated for their culinary versatility and pungent flavor. They are a key ingredient in various condiments and culinary applications, offering a combination of heat and depth to dishes. Mustard greens, on the other hand, are prized for their tender leaves and a peppery, earthy flavor. Beyond their culinary use, they are rich in nutrients, including vitamins A, C, and K, making them a valuable addition to a balanced diet.

MYRRH
Commiphora myrrha

Parts used: Oleo-gum-resin from stem. *This ancient aromatic resin is an excellent decongestant.*

TRADITIONAL USAGES

Myrrh is a gummy substance exuded from a small tree of eastern Africa and Arabia. In Greek mythology, Myrrha, the daughter of the king of Syria, was punished by Aphrodite, who caused her to disguise herself and commit incest with her father. When her father discovered her identity, he attempted to kill her, but the gods intervened, turning Myrrha into a myrrh tree. The gum resin is said to be her tears. The gum's name comes from the Arabic word meaning "bitter."

Myrrh has been used for thousands of years as an ingredient in incense and perfumes. The gum resin was used by the ancients for embalming. Its use is mentioned in an Egyptian papyrus from about 2000 B.C. There are numerous biblical references to myrrh, including in the Song of Solomon: "A bundle of myrrh *is* my well beloved unto me; he shall lie all night betwixt my breasts." The Hasidic prayer book contains a formula for a holy incense containing myrrh that was prepared by the ancient Hebrews. Myrrh was also one of the wise men's gifts to the baby Jesus.

As a medicinal, myrrh is a stimulant tonic and expectorant, and was most commonly administered to patients suffering from chest problems in order to stimulate mucus secretions and promote their drainage.

A second major area of usage concerned the female reproductive organs. Myrrh was taken to stimulate the menstrual flow or to bring

Commiphora myrrha

it on, even when the patient had never menstruated. In this connection, it was often combined with aloes for the laxative properties contributed by the latter. Myrrh was also applied to spongy gums and mouth ulcers. For centuries, myrrh has been used by the Chinese to treat menstrual difficulties and hemorrhoids.

A gentle rubefacient in external application, myrrh was employed to make a plaster where it was desirable to produce blisters slowly and with a minimum of pain.

RECENT SCIENTIFIC FINDINGS

Myrrh gum contains several volatile oils, rendering this herb an excellent promoter of free breathing during congestive colds. Myrrh acts on the mucous membranes of the respiratory tract.

Myrrh is an aromatic resin obtained from the bark of certain tree species. This resin has a storied history in traditional medicine and cultural practices, particularly in regions of the Middle East and Africa. Myrrh is recognized for its potential antimicrobial and anti-inflammatory properties. It has been used topically and orally to address various health concerns, such as wound healing, gum health, and inflammation. Myrrh resin has also been used in incense, perfumes, and oral hygiene products, adding a layer of sensory richness to cultural and spiritual practices.

NETTLE
Urtica dioica

Parts used: Roots, leaves, and seeds. *Ironically, this stinging plant is sometimes used in cosmetics as a facial.*

TRADITIONAL USAGES

Nettle has been used medicinally either to excite the skin locally or to affect the nervous system generally. The poisonous stinging hairs of fresh nettle will produce intense itching and stinging. However, both Pliny and homeopathic physicians applied the juice to cure its own sting! The leaves will stimulate, irritate, and cause blisters, so they are used where a rubefacient is desired, such as to heal wounds and burns.

In the second and third centuries B.C., several practitioners referred to the medicinal properties of nettle. It was used as an antidote for hemlock, a counterpoison for henbane, and as a cure for snakebite and scorpion sting. It was reputedly an aid for gout, asthma, and tuberculosis. Other recorded applications of the plant are as a diuretic and to arrest uterine hemorrhages. Nettle juice at one time formed the main component (93%) of a preparation known as Brandol, which was commercially marketed. Nettle seeds are sometimes used in home remedies for hair troubles, coughs, and shortness of breath.

The tops of the plants, boiled, are eaten as greens in soups by many people. It is recommended as an emergency food plant and has been suggested as a possible source of chlorophyll for commercial purposes.

RECENT SCIENTIFIC FINDINGS

Extracts of nettle have been tested in animals and show anti-inflammatory effects and also lower the amount of sugar in the blood. Nettle is sometimes used in hair products and facials.

Nettle is a versatile herb with serrated leaves and tiny stinging hairs. It is celebrated for its potential health benefits and versatility. Nettle has a rich history in traditional herbal medicine, where it has been used as a nutritive tonic due to its impressive nutrient content. It is especially high in iron, making it a valuable addition to diets, particularly for individuals dealing with anemia or low iron levels. Additionally, nettle is known for its anti-inflammatory properties and its role in alleviating allergies and arthritis symptoms. It has a long-standing reputation as a gentle diuretic and is used to promote detoxification and support kidney health.

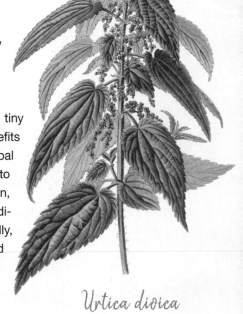

Urtica dioica

OAK (White)
Quercus alba

Parts used: Bark. *There is renewed interest in the inner bark of this stately tree due to its high tannin content.*

TRADITIONAL USAGES

Of the more than 50 species of oak in the United States, the white oak has been the most important medicinal, both to Native Americans and whites. The acorns formed the staple of the diet of many tribes, especially in California. After leaching the bitter tannins, the nuts were ground into a meal that was made into bread.

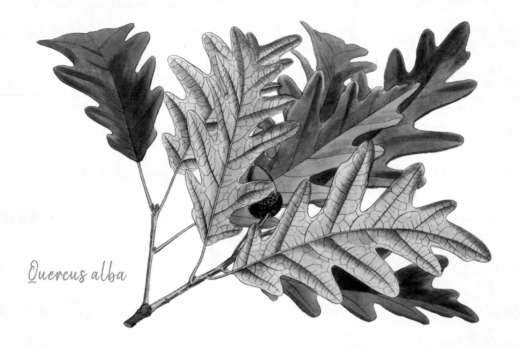

Quercus alba

The Menominees treated hemorrhoids by squirting an infusion of the scraped inner bark into the rectum with a syringe made from an animal bladder and the hollow bone of a bird. This type of syringe was reputedly made by many tribes. The Iroquois and Penobscots also boiled white oak bark and drank the liquid to treat diarrhea.

In my antique copy of the *Dispensatory of the United States* (1834), white oak bark is accorded all the respect that a major pharmaceutical would receive in a current textbook of pharmacology. The inner bark was listed in the *U.S. Pharmacopoeia* from 1820 to 1916. Oak bark was taken in the form of a powder, extract, or decoction, primarily for its high tannin content. It was not used internally to a great extent, but a decoction of the bark has been found useful in treating chronic diarrhea, advanced dysentery, and other conditions. The bark's principal use has been for external application, as an astringent wash, especially for flabby ulcers, as a gargle, and internally via injection for leucorrhea and hemorrhoids.

RECENT SCIENTIFIC FINDINGS

The inner bark of white oak is known to contain about 10% of a tannin complex, often referred to as quercitannic acid. As with all tannins, it predictably exerts an astringent and mild antiseptic action, the latter effect being due primarily to the phenolic nature of the tannin complex. Thus, as reported in folklore accounts, decoctions or infusions of *Quercus alba* bark, when applied locally, would have an astringent effect that tends to shrink hemorrhoids and accelerate the healing of flabby ulcers.

It is not known whether tannins kill parasites directly or if they act to protect an invaded intestinal wall by this mechanism. That they do work is attested to by the fact tannins are going through a revival owing to their medicinal properties. With the proliferation of intestinal parasites, this class of plant-derived substances is receiving the respect once seen in older books on pharmacognosy and botanical medicine. Tannins precipitate proteins from solution and act to protect injured tissues by precipitating their proteins to form an antiseptic, protective coat under which the regeneration of new tissues may take place. They are utilized in medicine as astringents in the GI tract, on burns, on skin abrasions, for bleeding or infected mouth sores, as a local application for hemorrhoids, and as a douche for vaginal and cervical discharges.

It should be noted, however, that tannins should not be taken for prolonged periods. An increased incidence of cancer of the esophagus and buccal cavity has been noted among habitual chewers of betel nut (*Areca catechu*) in India and South Africa. This is linked to the high content of condensed catechin tannin found in the nuts, which are chewed for their stimulant drug content.

White oak is a hardwood tree known for its strong, ridged bark. This bark has astringent properties, and it has been used in traditional herbal medicine, particularly for its topical applications. White oak bark has been employed to create poultices and ointments used on the skin to address a range of concerns, including minor cuts, burns, bruises, and inflammatory skin conditions. Its astringent nature is believed to help tighten and tone tissues, making it a valuable herb for promoting wound healing and skin health.

OAT STRAW
Avena sativa

Parts used: Straw. *This popular grain has been shown to lower cholesterol.*

TRADITIONAL USAGES

This annual grass has been cultivated as a primary food source for centuries. It is a rich nutritive addition to the diet, and that has been its primary use. Oats are thought to promote healthy skin, hair, nails, and teeth.

Oat baths have long been popular in Europe for rheumatism as well as kidney and bladder problems.

Oat straw consists of the dried stems of the oat plant. It is celebrated for its rich nutrient content and soothing properties.

RECENT SCIENTIFIC FINDINGS

Oat straw is rich in the element silicon, which is necessary to build the outer layer of skin, hair, and fingernails.

Researchers in the United States and in Israel have shown oats to have both estrogenic and antiestrogenic effects in rats and mice.

Oat bran has been shown to lower cholesterol, reducing cholesterol levels in the blood by about 20%. It has also been found to reduce fecal pH, which may be a risk factor for colorectal cancer.

Oat straw consists of the dried stems of the oat plant. It is celebrated for its rich nutrient content and soothing properties.

Oat straw is often used in herbal teas and infusions, where it is known for its role in promoting relaxation and supporting the nervous system. It contains a variety of essential nutrients, including B vitamins, minerals such as calcium and magnesium, and avenanthramides, which contribute to its reputation as a nourishing and calming herb.

The gentle and nutritive qualities of oat straw make it a favorite choice for those seeking a natural remedy to help manage stress and anxiety, and support overall well-being.

OPIUM
Papaver somniferum

Parts used: Seed capsules. *This has been called the most important and valuable medicine in the whole materia medica.*

TRADITIONAL USAGES

Although we consider this the mother of medicinal plants, the Latin name *Papaver* is thought to be derived from the Celtic *papa* (whence "pap," the soft food given to children), a food in which opium seeds were formerly boiled to induce sleep.

The use of opium as a medicine can be traced back to the time of Hippocrates. It has been called the most important and valuable medicine of the whole materia

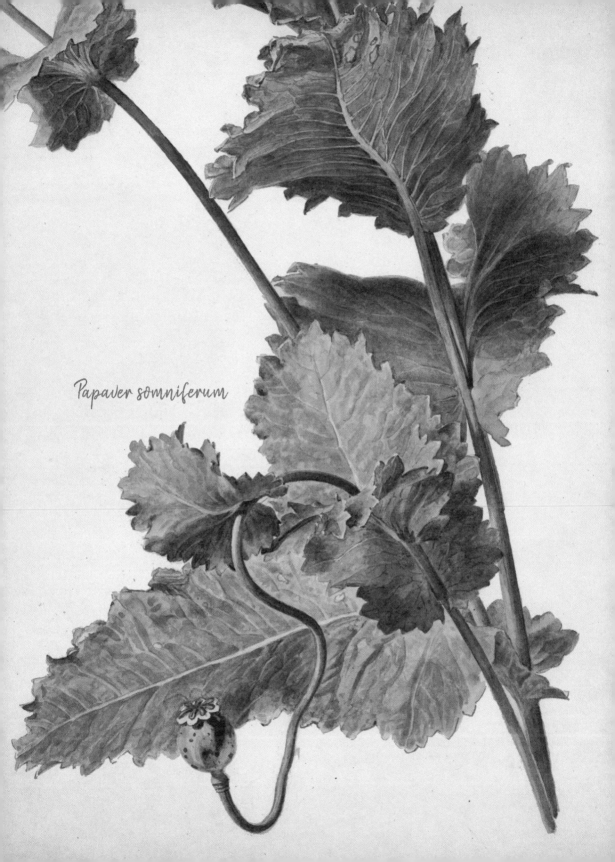

Papaver somniferum

Opium is a potent and highly regulated substance derived from the opium poppy. It has a long history of use in medicine, particularly for its potential pain-relieving properties.

medica, and "the source, by its judicious employment, of more happiness, and by its abuse, of more misery, than any other drug employed by mankind." Pereira Laudanum (tincture of opium) was regularly given to infants and small children to treat colic during the 19th century.

RECENT SCIENTIFIC FINDINGS

The gummy latex of this annual herb contains many alkaloids, including morphine, codeine, narcotine, laudenine, and papaverine. Various medicines made from opium alkaloids are used for their sedative, hypnotic, narcotic, antispasmodic, and analgesic effects. The highly addicting synthetic heroin is made by modifying morphine.

There is no substitute for the narcotic abilities of opium. Many terminally ill cancer patients in this country whose major concern is dying with dignity, where drug addiction is not a problem of any concern whatever, are denied this most efficacious painkiller, to suffer out their last weeks and months in needless agony for themselves—and for their families, who must stand by helplessly.

It is the author's fervent hope that opium and its derivatives will once again be made available in this country to ease the suffering of the terminally ill, and with proper controls, for use in place of the synthetic tranquilizers. Ultimately, we would like to see this plant regain its status as the valued natural drug it is.

Opium is a potent and highly regulated substance derived from the opium poppy. It has a long history of use in medicine, particularly for its potential pain-relieving properties. The opium poppy contains alkaloids such as morphine and codeine, which have been isolated and used for their analgesic effects. However, opium is a controlled substance due to its highly addictive and narcotic nature. Its use is regulated and is typically administered under strict medical supervision for the management of severe pain, such as in cases of surgery or terminal illness.

ORCHID (Wild)

Orchis spp.

Parts used: Tubers. *The tubers of these beautiful flowers are the source for salep.*

TRADITIONAL USAGES

Orchids have enjoyed a widespread reputation as restoratives, rejuvenants, and aphrodisiacs, seemingly more because of the splendid and opulent flowers than from any specific excitant or stimulant properties.

A product known as salep is prepared from the tubers of various *Orchis* species. The tubers are strung on strings, scalded to destroy their vitality, then dried to a hard consistency; after maceration in water they regain their original form and volume. These strings of dried tubers, or salep, are highly prized in India, Persia, and Turkey for restoring the strength of debilitated or aged people, and especially as an aphrodisiac. One writer has speculated that it is the odor and appearance of the salep, and the tubers from which it is derived, that suggested its application as an aphrodisiac, on the basis of the doctrine of signatures.

RECENT SCIENTIFIC FINDINGS

Fundamentally, the tubers are nutritive and compare favorably with tapioca and sago in the convalescent's diet. Salep has also been used to treat diarrhea, dysentery, and nervous fevers.

Wild orchids are a diverse and captivating group of flowering plants known for their exotic and often fragrant blossoms. While many wild

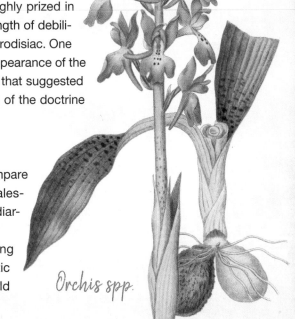

Orchis spp.

orchids are admired for their aesthetics and are integral to cultural traditions and rituals, certain varieties have been used in traditional herbal medicine, particularly in Asia. They are appreciated for their potential aphrodisiac properties and have been employed in various traditional remedies for their medicinal benefits.

OREGON GRAPE
Berberis aquifolium

Parts used: Root. *At one time, these roots were a major trade item.*

TRADITIONAL USAGES

Oregon grape is the state flower of Oregon. The Kwakiutls made a bark tea to offset the digestive disorder characterized by an excess of bile. In California, many tribes boiled the roots to make a tea they drank as an aperitif.

Soon adopted for domestic uses, the roots became such a major trade item that at the beginning of the 20th century, the species was almost exterminated around larger towns and cities. The roots, which are rich in berberine, were official in the *U.S. Pharmacopoeia* from 1905 to 1916.

Oregon grape has also been used to treat jaundice, chronic hepatitis, syphilis, and scrofula. It was believed to have specific action on the spleen and was administered in cases of malaria where the spleen was dangerously enlarged; this was a risky procedure, however, since the ability to produce contraction was so strong that there was a possibility of rupture and fatal hemorrhage if the herb was taken by a person whose spleen was dangerously softened.

The plant has also been considered a diuretic, mild tonic, and gentle laxative. It has been applied topically for various minor skin irritations.

RECENT SCIENTIFIC FINDINGS

All *Berberis* species are quite similar in chemical composition and hence would give rise to similar pharmacological effects. See remarks in the section on barberry (*Berberis vulgaris*) for further details.

Oregon grape is native to North America and is known for its striking, holly-like leaves and clusters of small, yellow flowers. The roots of the Oregon grape have been utilized in traditional herbal medicine for their antimicrobial and digestive properties. The root contains berberine, a potent compound with potential immune-boosting and antibacterial effects, which has led to its use in herbal remedies for infections and digestive discomfort. Oregon grape's presence in traditional healing practices reflects the rich botanical diversity of North America and the cultural significance of indigenous plants.

ORRIS

Iris germanica and other *Iris* species

Parts used: Rhizome. *No longer used as a medicinal, the root and oil are common ingredients in cosmetics.*

TRADITIONAL USAGES

Orris root is prepared by stripping away the outer layer of the rhizome and the roots. The remainder of the root is distilled to yield a solid oil. This oil (one part diluted with 3–4 parts alcohol) has a scent resembling the smell of violets. Consequently, it is valued in the perfume and cosmetics businesses.

Medicinally, orris is reputedly cathartic and diuretic, and in stronger doses it has been reported to be emetic. It was felt to be useful in treating dropsical conditions (water retention of tissues and/or organs). The root was also chewed as a coverup for bad breath.

Blue flag (*Iris versicolor*), another herbaceous perennial found in the eastern United States, was once used for its emetic, diuretic, and cathartic effects.

This rhizome contains an acrid resin and essential oil.

RECENT SCIENTIFIC FINDINGS

At this time, orris is not used for medicinal purposes. However, orris root is a common ingredient in talcum powders and is a contact allergen.

Orris root, derived from the iris plant, is a botanical gem known for its delicate and sweet scent reminiscent of violets. This fragrant herb is valued for its role in perfumery and cosmetics, where it serves as a natural fixative. Orris root plays a crucial role in fine fragrance creation, where it helps to stabilize and enhance the aromatic compounds of other botanical extracts, allowing scents to linger and evolve over time. Orris root adds a touch of floral elegance to

Iris germanica

various fragrances and cosmetic products, making it a prized ingredient in the world of aromatics and personal care.

PANSY (Wild)
Viola tricolor

Parts used: Herb, flowers, and root. *Used both internally and externally, this lovely flower has a long history of treating certain skin conditions.*

TRADITIONAL USAGES

The pansy's use in medicine can be traced back to ancient herbalists. In the 17th century, it was reported that a North American tribe treated boils and swellings with a yellow-flowered pansy. It is not clear whether the Indians learned this plant remedy from the newly arriving Europeans. By the late 1800s, wild pansy was being ground up for application for a variety of skin diseases, such as scabies.

The herb, which contains mucilaginous material, functions as an external soothing lotion for boils, swellings, and skin diseases of various kinds. It is also a good and gentle laxative, also because of the mucilage. This part of the pansy has been utilized to treat pectoral and nephritic diseases.

The flowers also have demulcent properties, again because of the mucilage, and are made into syrup and administered as a laxative for infants. The root is both emetic and cathartic.

Sweet violet (*V. odorata*) is much used as a flavoring and in candy making, while a leaf tea is a good cough remedy. The wonder violet (*V. mirabilis*) is used in decoction in Ukrainian folk medicine to treat heart ailments, palpitations, and shortness of breath.

RECENT SCIENTIFIC FINDINGS

Wild pansy contains saponins. Reports describe a tea made from the plant as effective on certain skin conditions. Given both as a tea internally and as compresses externally, it has been found useful in cases of eczema and other skin complaints in infants.

Wild pansy is a charming flowering herb with a rich history in traditional herbal medicine. It is valued for its potential to soothe and heal. Wild pansy has been used in remedies for various skin

Viola tricolor

conditions, such as eczema and acne, thanks to its mild anti-inflammatory properties. Additionally, it has been employed to address respiratory discomfort. This herb showcases nature's capacity to offer gentle, multifaceted support for health and well-being.

PAPAYA
Carica papaya

Parts used: Leaf and latex. *The dried latex of this delicious fruit contains an enzyme that has been experimentally successful in cases of slipped discs.*

TRADITIONAL USAGES

Although papaya is best known for its delicious fruit, fresh papaya leaves were used medicinally as a dressing for wounds by the Indigenous people in the tropical areas where the plant grows. People also wrapped meat in these leaves to make the flesh more tender.

In Fiji, a filtrate of the inner bark is used to treat toothaches, while the fresh milky white sap (latex) is applied directly on large boils and also utilized to treat wounds.

RECENT SCIENTIFIC FINDINGS

The dried latex of papaya is marketed under the names papayotin, papain, or papoid, and is given to treat dyspepsia and gastric catarrh. In powder form, it is applied to treat skin diseases, including warts and tubercle swellings. Much of this medicinal product is supplied from Sri Lanka and the West Indies. It is still employed as a meat tenderizer and is contained as an additive in one brand of beer to dissolve excess proteins, thereby making the beer clearer.

The enzyme chymopapain, a derivative of the latex of papaya, has been used on an experimental basis by neurosurgeons to dissolve herniated ("slipped") intervertebral discs in patients complaining of back pain.

Preliminary research has also revealed cardiac depressant activity when given orally to human adults and cardiotonic activity.

Carica papaya

Papaya is a tropical fruit tree celebrated for its juicy, vibrant orange fruit and nutrient-rich properties. Beyond its culinary appeal, papaya offers numerous health benefits. It is a rich source of digestive enzymes, including papain, which aids in digestion and eases digestive discomfort. Papaya is also abundant in vitamins A, C, and E, along with antioxidants, making it a nourishing addition to diets. Its nutritional value and digestive support role make it a tropical treasure that promotes overall health and vitality.

PARSLEY
Petroselinum sativum

Parts used: Leaf, root, and seeds. *This popular cooking herb contains apiol, which has been marketed in Russia to promote uterine contractions during labor.*

TRADITIONAL USAGES

This popular cooking herb also has a long history of use as a medicinal. It was believed to be invigorating to the blood. Parsley was used to regulate menstrual flow with the oil of the seeds reputedly an abortifacient.

Parsley was employed for a variety of abdominal ailments, including liver and spleen complaints, such as jaundice and gastritis. It was also considered a digestive aid that promoted urination and helped expel gallstones.

RECENT SCIENTIFIC FINDINGS

A great deal of research has been conducted on parsley's effect on cells and DNA. Some of the medical implications involve the enzymes that are integral to disease resistance response. In vitro studies have shown parsley has antibacterial and anti-fungal effects. Unfortunately, little research has occurred to confirm or deny parsley's folkloric claims as a remedy for liver ailments.

One of parsley's chemical constituents, apiol, is a uterine stimulant, as to a lesser extent is another constituent, myristicin. At one time, apiol was used in capsules as an abortifacient. Apiol and myristicin also contribute to parsley's effectiveness as a diuretic.

Parsley is rich in nutrients, including vitamins A, B, C, and K, as well as protein and potassium.

Caution: Use of parsley should be avoided during pregnancy.

Parsley is a versatile culinary herb known for its fresh and vibrant flavor. Beyond its role in enhancing the taste of dishes, parsley is a nutritional powerhouse. It provides essential vitamins, including vitamin C and vitamin K, and is a rich source of antioxidants. Parsley is believed to offer potential health benefits, such as supporting bone health and providing immune-boosting properties. Its culinary and nutritional contributions highlight how herbs can elevate both the flavor and health quotient of a meal, embodying the synergy between good taste and good health.

PASSIONFLOWER
Passiflora incarnata

Parts used: Plant and flowers. *Native Americans used this flower as a natural tranquilizer, and modern research is confirming its superior effects.*

TRADITIONAL USAGES

All but about 40 species of the nearly 400 known species of *Passiflora* are native to the Americas; the other 40 are native to Asia, South Pacific islands, and Madagascar. Early European travelers in tropical America gave the strange flower the name "passionflower," as it suggested to them the passion of Christ: the 10 equal sepals and petals represented the crown of thorns; the five stamens, the five wounds; the three styles, the three nails; the tendrils, the cords or scourges; the leaves, the hands of the persecutors. The white color symbolizes purity; the blue, heaven.

In the Yucatan, it is an old remedy for insomnia, hysteria, and convulsions in children. Interestingly, the early Algonquins brewed this woody vine to soothe their nerves. The Houmas believed it was a systemic tonic and added the pulverized root to their water. However, passionflower was largely ignored in conventional North American medicine until the late 1800s. The flowering and fruiting tops were used to relieve insomnia and to soothe nerves. They were official in the *National Formulary* from 1916 to 1936.

Passiflora incarnata

Passionflower is known to promote relaxation and tranquility, making it a valuable natural solution for those seeking emotional balance and restful sleep.

RECENT SCIENTIFIC FINDINGS

The state wildflower of Tennessee appears to be a useful bridge between traditional medicine and modern ills, especially anxiety states. Physicians could well recommend this plant to patients who want to wean themselves from synthetic sleeping pills and tranquilizers.

As a sedative, passionflower has qualities unlike those of any other herb. It is very effective, with a pleasant taste, and yet surprisingly gentle. It is helpful in a variety of ailments, from insomnia, dysmenorrhea, nervous tension, and fatigue to muscle spasms. It can be used with safety even for small children. In Italy, it is used to treat hyperactive children.

Passiflora incarnata may be our best tranquilizer yet. The dried leaves and stems both induce a natural sleep and calm hyperactive people. It is currently being employed as a nonaddictive substitute and natural tranquilizer by physicians in the treatment of tranquilizer-addicted patients. Surprisingly, one kind of passionflower (*P. quadrangularis,* or giant granadilla) was recently found to contain serotonin. Low levels of this compound in the cerebrospinal fluid of patients with chronic depression have led some researchers to speculate that adding it to circulating blood would relieve states of depression. This may be confirmed by the fact that LSD-like compounds that are used to induce clinical psychoses are known to have potent anti-serotonin activity; perhaps passionflower acts as a natural calming agent by promoting the transmission of subtle nerve impulses. It appears to aid concentration, alter perception, and gently shift mood.

Passionflower is celebrated for its calming and sedative properties. It contains compounds such as flavonoids and alkaloids that interact with the nervous system, making it a popular choice in herbal remedies for anxiety and sleep support. Passionflower is known to promote relaxation and tranquility, making it a valuable natural solution for those seeking emotional balance and restful sleep.

PATCHOULI LEAF

Pogostemon patchouli (P. cablin)

Parts used: Herb. *More known for its sexual use, the oil is a common ingredient in perfumes.*

TRADITIONAL USAGES

The Arabs, Chinese, and Japanese believed that the oil of patchouli prevented venereal disease when applied prior to and during sexual intercourse.

It has a valuable property of fixing odors, giving it broad application in the perfumery business as an odor and scent preservative added to other fragrances.

RECENT SCIENTIFIC FINDINGS

Almost all essential oils from plants have inhibitory activity against some type of microorganism. However, they rarely are tested against the organisms responsible for venereal disease, and thus it is difficult to project whether or not the use of patchouli oil as a prophylaxis for venereal diseases is valid.

Although the author has not personally used patchouli oil as an application to the genitalia to prevent venereal disease, we nevertheless pass on a word of caution. Virtually any essential oil, when applied undiluted to any mucous tissue, including the genitalia, produces a rush of heat to the area due to rapid evaporation and dilation of blood vessels in the area. This could produce a very uncomfortable condition if patchouli oil was applied to the sensitive tissue of the penis and/or vagina.

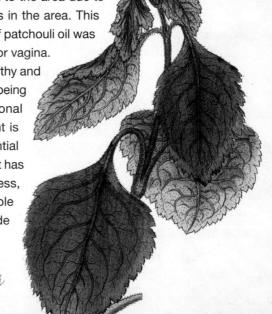

Patchouli is a fragrant herb known for its earthy and slightly sweet aroma. It has a versatile presence, being used in perfumery, aromatherapy, and traditional remedies. Patchouli's rich and grounding scent is attributed to its essential oils, which have potential antimicrobial and anti-inflammatory properties. It has been used to soothe skin conditions, relieve stress, and improve mood. Patchouli is a prime example of how herbs can engage our senses and provide holistic well-being.

Pogostemon patchouli

PAU D'ARCO or Taheebo

Tabebuia impetiginosa and other *Tabebuia* species

Parts used: Inner bark. *This "miracle" bark from South America may have anticancer properties.*

TRADITIONAL USAGES

Traditionally, pau d'arco bark was used as a strengthener for increased energy and endurance.

RECENT SCIENTIFIC FINDINGS

The inner bark of these stately, full-leaved trees of Central and South America have received so much attention for their medicinal properties that sales of nearly $200 million have been reported. This is no doubt in part due to the keen marketing program undertaken by Brazilian and Argentinean suppliers of "taheebo." However, this marketing was based on shoddy reports of the bark's anticancer properties, first published in the 1960s.

The bark is rich (2–7%) in lapachol, a naphthoquinone, and also contains lapachone and xyloidone, both quinoids. Studies in the 1970s showed evidence that lapachol was active against mouse lymphocytic leukemia.

Currently, pau d'arco is widely utilized for its reputed anti-candida properties. While no direct evidence exists to confirm or deny this activity, the anecdotal evidence is quite overwhelming. Moreover, a carefully controlled animal study published by a researcher at the prestigious Naval Medical Research Institute in Bethesda, Maryland, demonstrated that dietary intake of lapachol is protective against penetration and infection by another deadly parasite, *Schistosoma mansoni*.

From the available evidence, it appears that this "miracle" bark from South America, which has gained wide acceptance for its antifungal properties, will continue to gain in its applications, most notably against intestinal parasites.

Pau d'arco is a revered herb with a history of traditional use in South American herbal medicine. It is valued for its potential antimicrobial and immune-enhancing properties, largely attributed to compounds like lapachol. Pau d'arco is used to address infections, from bacterial to fungal, and to support overall immune health. This herb showcases the remarkable healing potential of botanicals and their role in holistic health.

PENNYROYAL

Hedeoma pulegioides (American), *Mentha pulegium* (European)

Parts used: Whole plant. *The pleasant tea of this herb is an aromatic calmative.*

TRADITIONAL USAGES

The Onondagas, one of the divisions of the Iroquois, steeped pennyroyal leaves and drank the resulting tea to cure headaches. A related species (*H. reverchonii*) was also used by the Mescalero Apaches as a headache remedy by crushing the twigs and inhaling the mint-like odor.

In the Thomsonian system of medicine, pennyroyal was utilized to check nosebleed; the patient sat with feet immersed in a tub of quite warm water while drinking a tea made from the plant.

This was thought to equalize circulation and alleviate pressure to the head. From 1831 to 1916, the dried leaves were official in the *U.S. Pharmacopoeia.*

It is a gentle stimulant, and as an aid in relieving the common cold, a draught was often drunk at bedtime to promote perspiration, again with the feet soaking in hot water. It was also used the same way to bring on suppressed menstruation.

RECENT SCIENTIFIC FINDINGS

The two species both have the medicinal properties of the official mints, possessing stimulant, aromatic, calmative, and stomachic properties. The volatile oil has similar properties to the herb and is frequently used in domestic practice to promote the menstrual flow. Pennyroyal is considered inferior in its medicinal qualities to peppermint, which largely superseded it in regular medicine, but pennyroyal has continued to be popular in domestic practice. The alcoholic infusion has been utilized to treat fainting, asphyxia, paralysis, asthma, hysteria, atonic gout, and flatulence. Experimentally, extracts of pennyroyal are known

Mentha pulegium

to stimulate the uterus in test-tube studies, which could account for the menses-inducing effect.

It is a very soothing tea and produces a nice sense of comforting warmth.

Caution: Large doses of this plant are known to produce nausea, vomiting, and possible toxic effects. One death was found to be the result of the ingestion of pennyroyal essential oil, not an infusion of the herb.

Pennyroyal is a fragrant herb known for its potential insect-repellent properties. It has a complex history of use in herbal remedies, but its use is highly cautioned against due to potential toxicity. Pennyroyal contains pulegone, a compound known for its toxic effects on the liver and nervous system. Historically, it was used for its potential to induce menstruation and manage digestive discomfort. However, due to safety concerns, it is essential to approach this herb with extreme caution or avoid it altogether, highlighting the importance of informed and responsible herbal practices.

PEPPERMINT
Mentha piperita

Parts used: Leaves and flowering tops. *This remains one of our most refreshing carminatives.*

TRADITIONAL USAGES

The genus name, *Mentha,* originated in Greek mythology; the nymph Mintha was metamorphosed into this plant. It is recorded that peppermint was cultivated by the ancient Egyptians, and its usage is documented in the Icelandic pharmacopoeia of the 13th century. The most agreeable and powerful of the mints, it possesses aromatic, carminative, stimulant, antispasmodic, and stomachic properties.

Peppermint is frequently used to allay nausea, relieve stomach and bowel spasms and griping, and promote the expulsion of flatus. It is often drunk after mealtime as an aid to digestion. The volatile oil, which has been similarly used in medicine, is also employed as a flavoring and scenting agent in cordials and candles and has also been added to less palatable medicines to mask disagreeable odors and/or tastes.

Mentha piperita

RECENT SCIENTIFIC FINDINGS

Peppermint tea is one of the most common herbal remedies, used primarily as a carminative and intestinal antispasmodic. These effects are all explained on the basis of animal experiments using the essential oil from peppermint, or purified essential oil constituents, the results of which mimic the effects claimed in humans. This essential oil has a high menthol content. Menthol both stimulates the flow of bile to the stomach and is an antispasmodic.

Peppermint is a widely recognized herb celebrated for its refreshing flavor and potential digestive and soothing properties. It contains menthol, a compound known for its cooling and calming effects. Peppermint is used in teas, culinary applications, and aromatherapy. It helps alleviate digestive issues, ease headaches, and promote relaxation. Peppermint's invigorating taste and versatile qualities make it a popular choice for enhancing both taste and overall well-being.

PERIWINKLE (Tropical)
Catharanthus roseus, Vinca rosea

Parts used: Herb. *This lovely ornamental plant is the source of the potent anticancer drugs vinblastine and vincristine.*

TRADITIONAL USAGES

Tropical periwinkle is a pantropical plant that is often cultivated in temperate climates as an ornamental. However, in the Philippines, periwinkle has long been taken orally as a folkloric remedy for the treatment of hyperglycemia. A leaf extract was used to treat diabetes.

RECENT SCIENTIFIC FINDINGS

Tropical periwinkle is an extremely important example of a traditional folk medicine whose use was investigated by a major pharmaceutical company, resulting in the discovery of two alkaloids with practical application in the treatment of cancer.

In 1953, Dr. Faustino Garcia reported at the Pacific Science Congress on periwinkle's use in the Philippines to treat hyperglycemia. Researchers at the Lily Company, conducting a general survey of many folk remedy plants through preliminary testing in a cancer-screening program, found that periwinkle showed striking anticancer activity in test animals.

In the early 1960s, it was discovered that extracts of the leaves of *C. roseus* would significantly prolong the life of mice in which leukemia had been clinically induced. This finding eventually led to the discovery of two potent anticancer drugs, vincaleukoblastine (vinblastine, VLB) and leurocristine (vincristine, VCR), both of which are now available on a worldwide basis for the treatment of human cancer. While nearly identical structurally, these two alkaloids each effect different types of tumors.

Vincristine is one of our most important anticancer drugs, being most useful for the treatment of childhood leukemias. Vinblastine is of lesser importance but is effective in treating certain types of Hodgkin's disease.

Since vincristine doses have neurotoxic side effects, and vinblastine can cause a marked decrease in the number of white blood cells, these must be considered as very potent drugs. Thus, it cannot be recommended that tropical periwinkle be used as an herbal remedy, since the danger of potential life-threatening complications is very real.

The leaves have also been used most extensively as an oral insulin substitute. Proprietary products have been sold in Africa and the Philippines for this purpose. At least seven or eight scientific publications are available in which investigators have reported no effect on blood sugar levels in normal, as well as diabetic, animals, when aqueous extracts of periwinkle leaves were administered orally. Other studies have been published in which hot water extracts of the leaves of this plant were given to diabetic patients, but in every instance, there was no significant benefit to the patients.

Both *Vinca major* (greater periwinkle) and *Vinca minor* (lesser periwinkle) are often confused with tropical periwinkle (*Catharanthus roseus*), and although *Vinca* and *Catharanthus* are related in being members of the Dogbane (Apocynaceae) family, they are chemically and pharmacologically quite different.

Although greater periwinkle and lesser periwinkle are somewhat different in chemical makeup, they have both been used externally to stop hemorrhages, such effect most likely being due to astringent tannins present in both plants. Any effect of preventing menstrual hemorrhaging (menorrhagia) could be due to vincamine, an indole alkaloid present in both species, which has been shown to contract uterine muscle in test-tube experiments.

Catharanthus roseus

Neither of these effects has been confirmed, however, by direct experiments involving the use of extracts from these plants.

Vincamine has also been found to affect the flow of blood in the brain. A series of ECG studies and double-blind trials found that vincamine improved the cerebral vascular system.

PINEAPPLE
Ananas comosus

Parts used: Enzyme (bromelain). *This delicious fruit contains an enzyme that may have anticancer properties.*

RECENT SCIENTIFIC FINDINGS

Pineapple contains bromelain, an enzyme whose exact chemical structure is currently being investigated. However, bromelain has exhibited some interesting pharmacological possibilities. It appears to interfere with the growth of malignant cells, inhibit platelet aggregation, and possess fibrinolytic, anti-inflammatory, and skin debridement properties. These properties therapeutically might prove effective in treating tumor growth, blood coagulation, inflammatory changes, debridement (removal of unhealthy tissue) of third-degree burns, and enhancement of the absorption of drugs. Animal experiments with rats indicated that pineapple enzymes rapidly effect debridement of skin burns.

Pineapple is a tropical fruit celebrated for its sweet and tangy taste. It is a rich source of vitamins, particularly vitamin C, minerals, such as manganese, and enzymes, such as bromelain. Pineapple is known for its potential antioxidant and anti-inflammatory effects. It offers digestive support, aids in wound healing, and promotes immune function. Pineapple's nutritional profile and delightful flavor make it a delicious and healthful addition to diets, showcasing the interplay between taste and well-being.

Ananas comosus

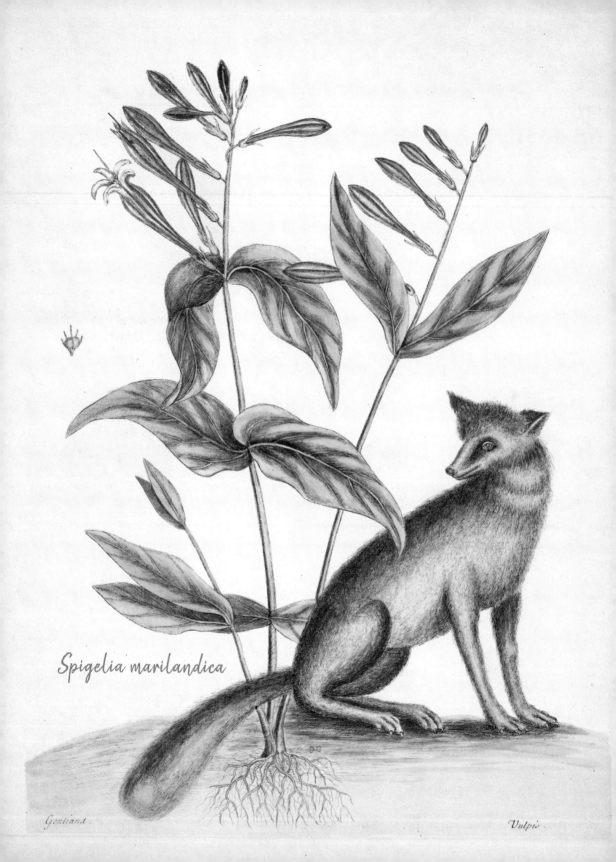

Spigelia marilandica

Gentiana.

Vulpis.

PINKROOT
Spigelia marilandica

Parts used: Rhizome and roots. *Native Americans discovered this root's ability to treat intestinal worms.*

TRADITIONAL USAGES

Overdose can be fatal, but use of pinkroot has rarely been reported to produce ill effects so long as it is eliminated. For this reason, it is commonly prescribed in combination with calomel, senna, or some other cathartic.

Pinkroot is one of the clearest examples of acceptance of a Native American remedy by the medical profession. The Cherokees prepared a worm medicine by boiling a large quantity of the freshly dug root in water. In the early 1700s, two physicians from Charleston, South Carolina, learned about pinkroot from Native Americans. Quickly spreading to the general public, pinkroot was praised as a worm treatment, particularly roundworms, and commonly used for the next 200 years. In the early 1900s, pinkroot fell into disuse when greedy herb dealers adulterated or substituted other plants.

The 23rd edition of the *Dispensatory of the United States* lists the prescribed adult dose of the powdered root as four or eight grams each morning and evening for several days, then to be followed by a strong laxative.

A preparation sold under the name Worm Tea contained pinkroot and senna. It was mixed in different strengths by the apothecary to suit individual needs.

RECENT SCIENTIFIC FINDINGS

The roots contain spigeline, which resembles coniine (found in hemlock) and nicotine, which explains its stimulant effects.

PIPSISSEWA
Chimaphila umbellata, C. maculata

Parts used: Leaves and herb. *This Native American remedy remains a first-rate medicinal for urinary tract infections.*

TRADITIONAL USAGES

Why the generic name of these plants is formed of two Greek words for "winter" and "love" remains a mystery, although their use in folk medicine is readily explained. This

Native American remedy for rheumatism and scrofula (a type of tuberculosis) was also used by the settlers for the same purposes. Both groups also took the plant as a tea to induce sweating. The Mohegans and the Penobscots steeped the plant in warm water and applied the liquid externally to draw out blisters. The Thompsons of British Columbia pulverized the entire fresh plant and applied the mass in the form of a wet dressing to swellings of the lower legs and feet.

Pipsissewa was a popular home remedy among the early settlers of the United States, especially the Pennsylvania Germans, who used it as a tea to induce sweating. From 1820 to 1916, it was official in the *U.S. Pharmacopoeia* as an astringent or tissue-drying agent.

Chimaphila umbellata

It is credited with tonic, astringent, and diuretic properties, and was administered in the treatment of cystitis and was held to be a diuretic and antiseptic to the urinary tract. A decoction was applied externally for blisters and scrofulous sores and swellings, but pipsissewa remains a first-rate folk remedy for miscellaneous urinary tract infections.

RECENT SCIENTIFIC FINDINGS

The leaves of this half-shrub contain ericolin, arbutin, chimaphilin, urson, tannin, and gallic acid. Chimaphilin, as well as extracts of this plant, show antibacterial properties in test-tube experiments. This can explain the use of this plant in scrofula and in treating cystitis.

Pipsissewa is an herb known for potential diuretic and antimicrobial properties. It contains arbutin, a compound with mild diuretic effects and potential antimicrobial action. It has a history of use in herbal remedies to support urinary tract health and address conditions like urinary infections and kidney stones. Pipsissewa exemplifies the targeted and effective solutions certain herbs offer for specific health concerns.

PLANTAIN

Plantago major, P. lanceolata, and various other species

Parts used: Seeds and leaves. *Called "white man's foot" by Native Americans, the leaves are an effective treatment for poison ivy rash.*

TRADITIONAL USAGES

Plantain has been used medicinally since antiquity. Formerly this common weed was utilized to relieve thirst and reduce fever, to remove obstructions within the system, and as an astringent. Later it was seldom used internally but remained a popular external stimulant application to boils, sores, and wounds. The leaves were bruised and applied whole to the affected area in poultice form. To relieve bee stings, the fresh leaves are rubbed on.

Native Americans named plantain "white man's foot" due to the plant's trait of growing in the footsteps of the white man; the plant was commonly introduced wherever a settlement developed. The Shoshoni heated the leaves and applied them in a wet dressing for wounds. In early American domestic medicine, the leaves were employed as an antidote to the bites of venomous snakes and insects, while the seeds were used as a worm remedy. Herman Boerhaave, an 18th-century botanist, recommended that plantain leaves be bound to aching feet after long hikes to relieve pain and fatigue. In Ayurvedic medicine, plantain is used to treat ulcers.

RECENT SCIENTIFIC FINDINGS

P. media, the hoary plantain, and *P. lanceolata,* the narrow-leaved plantain (rib grass), possess the same properties as *P. major* and may be utilized interchangeably. A European species, *P. psyllium,* also known as fleawort, has seeds that are used medicinally due to their mucilaginous nature. They have demulcent and emollient properties and were used for the same purposes as flax seed (see section on flax).

The seeds of most *Plantago* species contain high concentrations of mucilage and thus will have a demulcent and emollient effect externally and will act as a laxative if taken internally due to the swelling of the seeds.

An Italian study found that plantain served effectively in contributing to weight loss in conjunction with a prescribed diet. Researchers in Russia and Italy found plantain reduced intestinal absorption of lipids.

A study published in the *Lancet* described several people who contracted poison ivy rash. They were immediately treated with plantain leaf. The itching subsided and did not return.

Plantain is a common herb with broad leaves and small, inconspicuous flowers. It is celebrated for its potential skin-soothing and wound-healing properties. Plantain contains compounds like allantoin, which

Plantago major

promote tissue repair, and tannins, with astringent properties. It has been traditionally used in herbal remedies to address various skin irritations, including insect bites, minor wounds, and eczema. Plantain is a versatile and valuable botanical ally for skin health, embodying nature's ability to provide remedies for common ailments.

PLEURISY ROOT
Asclepias tuberosa

Parts used: Root. *In both Native American and domestic American practice, this root was used to treat respiratory ailments.*

TRADITIONAL USAGES

Pleurisy root derives its name from its effectiveness as an expectorant, helping to expel phlegm from the bronchial and nasal passages. It was employed in a variety of respiratory ailments besides pleurisy, including cough, tuberculosis, and bronchitis. Because of its claimed antispasmodic properties, the dried and powdered root was administered to cure infant colic. Adults, likewise, drank an herb tea of the root as an aid in eliminating flatulence.

The Natchez drank a tea of the boiled roots as a remedy for pneumonia. The same preparation was used by the Catawbas for dysentery. The fresh root was chewed by the Omahas for bronchitis and other respiratory complaints.

Prior to the advent of synthetic drugs, pleurisy root was widely employed by medical practitioners in the United States. Medical journals frequently carried scientific articles on the effectiveness of pleurisy root preparations as a diaphoretic, expectorant, emetic, and cathartic. The specific effect was dependent on the amount of the preparation used. Pleurisy root was in the *U.S. Pharmacopoeia* from 1820 to 1905 and in the *National Formulary* from 1916 to 1936. The active principle responsible for these effects, however, remains unknown.

RECENT SCIENTIFIC FINDINGS

Pleurisy root is a flowering herb recognized for its potential respiratory benefits. It contains beneficial compounds such as saponins, which have expectorant properties,

Asclepias tuberosa

Pleurisy root derives its name from its effectiveness as an expectorant, helping to expel phlegm from the bronchial and nasal passages.

making it valuable for addressing lung and chest discomfort. Pleurisy root is used to alleviate respiratory issues, particularly those involving congestion and inflammation. It highlights how certain herbs play a pivotal role in supporting respiratory well-being and overall health.

Pleurisy root has yet to have a fair trial in the laboratory and would appear to be a good candidate for renewed research.

POMEGRANATE
Punica granatum

Parts used: Bark, rind, and fruit. *This tasty fruit's root bark has long been an effective remedy for intestinal worms.*

TRADITIONAL USAGES

The fruit of this small shrubby tree is eaten and its juice is used to make refreshing drinks, particularly in the Middle East. In Israel, the fruit has been cultivated for 5,000 years. The powdered root rind was held to be astringent and was utilized to treat diarrhea, for excessive perspiration, as a gargle for sore throats, for intermittent fevers, and for leucorrhea. The root bark was administered by the ancients to rid the intestines of worms. This medicinal usage was overlooked by Europeans until 1804, when a practitioner in India who had cured an Englishman of a tapeworm was persuaded to share his secret remedy.

Nausea and vomiting sometimes accompanied the purgative action of this plant; consequently, patients were advised to fast for 12 hours prior to treatment. Two hours after administration of the remedy, a brisk cathartic was given to expedite discharge of the remains of the worm. The remedy was repeated day after day, sometimes as many as four times, until success was achieved.

RECENT SCIENTIFIC FINDINGS

Of all types of intestinal worm infestations, pomegranate root bark is most useful in cases of tapeworm. The active principle, discovered in 1878, is the liquid alkaloid pelletierine, which was used in human medicine for a number of years and then became relegated to veterinary use. Thus, it is well established that root bark preparations of pomegranate would be effective when used to expel worms from the intestinal tract.

Punica granatum

Anyone who has bitten into the peel of a pomegranate fruit can testify to the highly astringent nature of this material. In fact, it is known that the fruit peel contains about 30% tannin, which is the active astringent substance.

Pomegranate is a remarkable fruit-bearing tree with vibrant, ruby-red arils. These arils are prized for their juicy, sweet-tart taste and are packed with essential nutrients and antioxidants. Pomegranate is celebrated for its potential health benefits, particularly its rich content of polyphenols, such as anthocyanins and ellagic acid. These compounds have strong antioxidant and anti-inflammatory properties, making pomegranate a superfood known for supporting heart health, improving digestion, and potentially reducing the risk of chronic diseases. Pomegranate's unique combination of flavor and health-promoting properties underscores the synergy between culinary delight and well-being.

POPLAR

Populus nigra, P. balsamifera

Parts used: Leaf buds. *At one time, the leaf buds were used to make a popular European ointment.*

TRADITIONAL USAGES

Poplar leaf buds are covered with a resinous exudate; their smell is balsamic and pleasant, the taste bitterly aromatic. Poplar buds have been used for the same purposes as the turpentines and other balsams. Macerated in oil, they were applied externally as a liniment for the treatment of rheumatism. A popular salve was made in France of equal parts (100 grams) of poppy, belladonna, and black nightshade, moistened

> *Poplar bark, in particular, is recognized for its potential therapeutic properties in herbal medicine.*

with 400 grams of alcohol, rested for 24 hours, then heated with 4,000 grams of lard for three hours, after which 800 grams of crushed poplar buds were added and the mixture was heated for 10 more hours, then strained. This anodyne ointment was used to treat painful local afflictions, including sores and burns. Known as Pommade de Bourgeons de Peuplier, it was widely used throughout Europe. There were several different ways to concoct this ointment, using the same plant materials.

In tincture form, the buds have been given for chest complaints and in the treatment of inflammation of the kidneys.

RECENT SCIENTIFIC FINDINGS

Poplar buds are rich in chemical substances having actions similar to aspirin, such as salicin and mixtures of phenolic acids. Thus, poplar buds taken internally would be useful in minor rheumatic pains. The phenolic acids would contribute to the effectiveness of extracts being used for coughs as well. We can find no rationale for the application of poplar bud extracts externally to relieve rheumatism symptoms, since the active chemicals are not known to be absorbed through the skin.

Poplar trees are a group of hardwood trees with a diverse range of species. While poplar trees are primarily valued for their timber and wood products, they have cultural and traditional significance in various regions. Poplar bark, in particular, is recognized for its potential therapeutic properties in herbal medicine. It contains salicin, a natural compound similar to aspirin, which can be used for its anti-inflammatory and pain-relieving effects. The historical use of poplar bark in traditional remedies reflects the deep-rooted connection between nature's offerings and human health.

PRICKLY ASH

Aralia spinosa, Zanthoxylum clava-herculis, Z. fraxineum

Parts used: Bark and berries. *This was called the "toothache tree," and the dried bark was in the U.S. Pharmacopoeia as a rheumatism treatment.*

TRADITIONAL USAGES

Numerous Native American tribes employed the pulverized root and/or the bark for toothaches. In domestic American medicine, the bark was simply chewed raw or inserted into cavities.

Prickly ash was also a popular remedy for chronic rheumatism and was utilized extensively in the United States for this purpose. This plant is a stimulant and was also used to produce perspiration.

The bark and roots were boiled in water and the decoction drunk as a cure for venereal disease. Jonathan Carver's *Travels Through the Interior Parts of North America* includes an account of a Winnebago chief who cured a white trader of gonorrhea. During the 19th century, prickly ash bark was used to treat typhoid pneumonia. The dried bark was official in the *U.S. Pharmacopoeia* from 1820 to 1926 as a treatment for rheumatism. The berries were listed in the *National Formulary* from 1916 to 1947 for their antispasmodic, stimulant, and antirheumatic purposes.

Prickly ash bark was also employed in the treatment of flatulence and diarrhea. The berries are aromatic in addition to these properties and were used medicinally only in this connection.

RECENT SCIENTIFIC FINDINGS

Prickly ash has been the subject of only limited laboratory or clinical testing. To date, it has exhibited analgesic and diaphoretic properties as well as promoting saliva. It also may prove useful as an insecticide.

Prickly ash is a deciduous shrub known for its prickly stems and aromatic bark. It has a long history of use in traditional herbal medicine, particularly by Indigenous cultures in North America. Prickly ash bark is valued for its potential circulatory and digestive benefits. It contains compounds such as alkaloids and terpenes, which give it a tingling or numbing sensation when chewed. It has been used to stimulate digestion, relieve pain, and promote blood circulation.

Aralia spinosa

PSYLLIUM

Plantago ovata

Parts used: Seeds. *These seeds have exhibited some extraordinary effects as a dietary supplement.*

TRADITIONAL USAGES

Psyllium was esteemed by Indian, Persian, and Arab physicians of the Middle Ages as a lubricating agent for the lower intestinal tract. It also was used as an emollient.

RECENT SCIENTIFIC FINDINGS

Psyllium proves to have a remarkable variety of positive applications as a dietary supplement.

Psyllium is commonly used to manage diarrhea, not only in the short-term but also for long-term management of irritable bowel syndrome. For instance, in one clinical trial conducted over a several month period, patients undergoing treatment remained in remission. Interestingly, patients on placebo who had relapsed became asymptomatic upon resumption of the treatment. Also, those for whom treatment was curtailed relapsed but then recovered upon resumption.

Recent research has found that psyllium's ability to manage diarrhea may also be useful for patients in intensive care who are being fed intravenously. Diarrhea is a major complication for tube-fed patients. In one study involving 49 patients at a large medical center, psyllium significantly reduced diarrhea.

Psyllium's hypocholesterolemic effects are well established. Hypercholesterolemia is a significant risk factor for coronary heart disease. There are numerous clinical trials attesting to psyllium's cholesterol-lowering effects. One double-blind study of 163 men and women with high serum cholesterol levels supplemented the American Heart Association's recommended diet with psyllium. The results showed that psyllium "significantly enhances the American Heart Association diet effects." Another study involving 59 subjects came to the same conclusion regarding psyllium supplementation to the Phase I diet.

A randomized double-blind, placebo-controlled study involving 58 male patients confirmed that psyllium cereals are "an effective and well-tolerated part of a prudent diet in the treatment of mild to moderate hypercholesterolemia." Another double-blind study involving 75 patients as well as a two-stage study with 14 individuals also concluded that psyllium was an effective adjunct to diet. An eight-week study of

26 men stated that "the reductions in total cholesterol and LDL cholesterol became progressively larger with time, and this trend appeared to be continuing at the eighth week. Psyllium treatment did not affect body weight, blood pressure, or serum levels of high-density lipoprotein cholesterol, triglycerides, glucose, iron, or zinc."

In a longer-term study conducted over a one-year period, 176 ambulatory elderly patients used psyllium hydrophilic mucilloid (PHM), while 741 patients did not use PHM. The researchers concluded that "the dose of PHM administered was significantly correlated with the change in serum cholesterol."

While it is not known exactly how psyllium reduces cholesterol, preliminary findings indicate that psyllium lowers cholesterol absorption and increases the rate of cholesterol transformation to bile acids.

Psyllium added to the diet has also been found to possibly be helpful for diabetics. In a crossover study, 18 non-insulin-dependent diabetics were given psyllium before breakfast and dinner. The results showed that psyllium reduced glucose levels following the meals.

Preliminary research raises the possibility that psyllium may also indirectly protect the colon from cancer by providing protection for colonocytes.

Caution: Severe allergic reactions to psyllium have occurred, especially among individuals sensitized by occupational exposure, such as healthcare workers.

Psyllium is an herbaceous plant known for its tiny seeds, particularly the husk of these seeds. Psyllium husk is a rich source of soluble fiber, primarily mucilage. It has been used as a dietary supplement and in traditional remedies for its potential to support digestive health. Psyllium is known to relieve constipation, improve bowel regularity, and reduce cholesterol levels. Its gentle yet effective properties make it a valuable addition to promote digestive well-being.

Plantago ovata

PUMPKIN
Cucurbita pepo

Parts used: Seeds. *For centuries, pumpkin seeds have been used to remove intestinal worms.*

TRADITIONAL USAGES

Pumpkin seeds have been used in almost every culture in the world for centuries as an aid to remove intestinal worms (vermifuge) from the body, or more specifically, to rid the body of tapeworms (taeniafuge).

In 1820, a Cuban physician reported that three ounces of fresh flesh of pumpkin would accomplish the death and expulsion of the tapeworm exactly as the recommended dose of one ounce of seeds. Medicinal knowledge of pumpkin was first introduced into the United States in 1851 by Richard Soule.

RECENT SCIENTIFIC FINDINGS

The amount of pumpkin seeds used for vermifuge purposes ranges from 10 to 200 grams per dose in humans. Studies in China, Russia, and elsewhere have shown that pumpkin seeds are very effective in removing worms from both animals and humans. The active anthelmintic agent in pumpkin seeds has been known for some time: it is an unusual amino acid known as cucurbitin. Cucurbitin is present in pumpkin seeds in quantities ranging from 0.18 to 0.66%.

Purified cucurbitin was studied in 150 patients with various types of intestinal worm infestations. It was shown to be unusually safe when given by mouth, especially against tapeworm and pinworms. No contraindications were recommended for the use of cucurbitin as a result of the study. A small number (3%) of the patients (5/150) had mild side effects from the drug, including nausea, dizziness, and weakness.

Other studies in the United States have shown that when 30–65 grams of pumpkin seeds are taken by mouth daily, a slight decrease in the amount of urine excreted occurs. On the other hand, daily elimination of urea and uric acid in the urine was increased. Thus, we can once again point out a rational basis for the use of a centuries-old herbal remedy, based on animal and human studies.

Pumpkin also exhibited interesting results as a psychological treatment. L-tryptophan had been long-established as a safe, effective treatment for anxiety, depression, and sleep disorders when it was abruptly withdrawn from the market, for capricious reasons.

A 1988 study reported on a 44-year-old man successfully treated with an alternate source of this amino acid, pumpkin seeds.

The patient suffered from "recurrent unipolar depressions." He could not tolerate pharmaceutical antidepressants; in 1985, he was put on L-tryptophan as an alternative. He was so sensitive that on 4.5 grams per day he became hypomanic. When the dose was reduced to 1.5 grams per day, he was stabilized and discharged from the clinic. For five years the man remained well, "apart from a bout of depression with biological features every three months or so. At these points he took about 1.5 grams of L-tryptophan over two days and found that this quickly restored his wellbeing." Unfortunately, the patient was unable to self-treat his latest bout of depression due to this product's withdrawal from the marketplace.

Seeking an alternative, this innovative psychiatrist drew on the work of another patient, a physician who had cured his own sleep problem with L-tryptophan from pumpkin seeds. This patient was given about 200 grams of these seeds, equal to about 1 gram of L-tryptophan, and "within 24 hours . . . he felt quite transformed. He was no longer anergic or depressed and happily returned to work the following day."

Pumpkin is a nutritious and versatile squash celebrated for its vibrant color, flavor, and potential health benefits. It is rich in essential nutrients, including vitamins A, C, and E, as well as dietary fiber and antioxidants like beta-carotene. Pumpkin is known for its potential to support immune health, improve vision, and enhance skin health. Additionally, its seeds are a source of healthy fats and protein, making them a popular choice for snacks and culinary use. Pumpkin embodies the synergy between delicious taste and nutritional value, offering both culinary delight and wellness support.

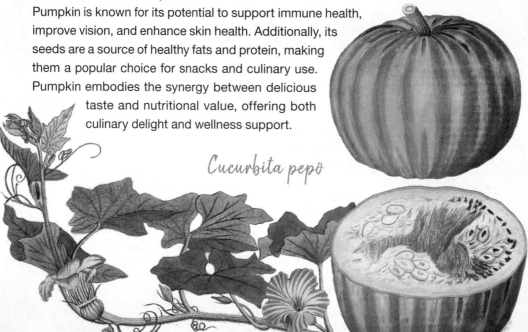

Cucurbita pepo

QUERCETIN
(a bioflavonoid)

Parts used: Bioflavonoid found in many plants. *This common bioflavonoid possesses remarkable anti-inflammatory properties.*

RECENT SCIENTIFIC FINDINGS

Here we briefly look at a bioflavonoid found in many, many plants. In my many years of searching the tropical jungles for new plant remedies, I've often watched local healers as they prepared and administered various folk cures. Seeing cases of badly inflamed skin treated with plant medicine made me wonder if the almost instantaneous anti-inflammatory effects were due to the flavonoids found in the various salves and infusions.

Quercetin achieves these "blocking" actions by inhibiting IgE-mediated allergic mediator release from mast cells. In simpler terms, this type of naturally occurring flavonoid acts as an antihistamine. Quercetin works best when combined with vitamin C. Like quercetin, substantial evidence supports the use of vitamin C in allergic diseases.

In addition, quercetin inhibits lipoxygenase, an enzyme involved in the metabolism of arachidonic acid (AA) in cells. Recall that AA is required for the inflammatory response to occur, via the production of prostaglandins and leukotrienes. Bioflavonoids such as quercetin can block the production of leukotrienes and other pro-inflammatory AA metabolites. They also act as antioxidants, scavenging dangerous free radicals and protecting cells.

allium cepa

Suppressing inflammation and allergies are only some of the effects of quercetin. This potent phytopharmaceutical, made by nature and found in many plants, has also been found to stimulate the immune system and kill viruses.

Where can we find this remarkable herbal compound? As we stated, it is widely distributed in the vegetable kingdom. Quercetin (and other flavonoids) is found in fruits, vegetables, seeds, nuts, leaves, flowers, roots, and bark. It is celebrated for its antioxidant properties and potential health benefits. Quercetin is known for its potential to reduce inflammation, support heart health, and boost the immune system. It is often used as a dietary supplement to promote overall well-being and address conditions such as allergies, cardiovascular health, and immune function.

RASPBERRY (Red)

Rubus spp.

Parts used: Leaves. *The leaves of this tasty fruit are the source of a tea often drunk during pregnancy to relieve morning sickness.*

TRADITIONAL USAGES

Five varieties and one form have been distinguished of this common plant that is found in dry or moist woods, fields, and roadsides, north to Alaska, south to New England, Pennsylvania, Indiana, and Iowa, and in the west to Arizona.

The Pawnee, Omaha, and Dakota tribes used a boiled decoction of black raspberry roots for dysentery. The fruit was listed in the *U.S. Pharmacopoeia* from 1882 to 1905 as a flavoring.

RECENT SCIENTIFIC FINDINGS

Red raspberry leaves contain high concentrations of tannins, which is most likely responsible for the antinauseant, antivomiting, antidiarrheal, and astringent effects of this plant. Vast literature exists supporting the numerous folkloric claims for this interesting plant genus. Various species of raspberry have been shown to induce ovulation, relax the uterus, act as a diuretic, stimulate immunity, kill viruses (including herpes), control glucose-induced high blood sugar, promote insulin production, kill fungi, and stimulate interferon induction.

Red raspberry leaf or root tea is an excellent astringent remedy for diarrhea and will also allay nausea and vomiting. The leaf tea is also drunk during pregnancy to facilitate childbirth and, as mentioned previously, will help with morning sickness.

As the scientific evidence indicates, many species of raspberry are "super-useful" for a myriad of women's problems. One study showed that raspberry leaf prevented the typical hypergrowth effects of chronic gonadotropin on ovaries and uterus, while another study demonstrated that raspberry leaf relaxes uterine muscles. In the latter study, tea concentrates were tested on several species of animal. If the smooth muscle of the uterus was "in tone," the water extract of raspberry leaf relaxed it. If the muscle was relaxed, the herb caused contractions.

Rubus spp.

Other studies have found antiviral activity in cell cultures against vaccinia virus and strong antiviral activity (in cell culture) against herpes virus II; also antiviral activity has been found against coxsackie virus, influenza virus, polio virus I, and reovirus I.

Red raspberry is a flavorful and nutritious berry with a wide range of potential health benefits. These berries are packed with vitamins, minerals, and antioxidants. They are known for their potential to support digestion, reduce inflammation, and promote women's health, particularly during pregnancy. Red raspberries are a delectable and healthful addition to diets, offering both delightful taste and nutritional support.

REISHI MUSHROOM
Ganoderma lucidum, G. japonicum

Parts used: Cap and stem. *This "lucky fungus," which has been eaten in Japan for at least 3,000 years, now is being discovered by Americans.*

TRADITIONAL USAGES

The Japanese names for this member of the basidiomycetes are *mannentake,* meaning "tens-of-thousand-year fungus," *saiwaitake,* "happy fungus," or *kisshotake,* "lucky fungus." Originally utilized in China as a food "to lengthen life," reishi mushrooms have been eaten in Japan for at least 3,000 years.

In traditional Chinese medicine, this almost magical fungus has long been prized to "prevent serious damage or recover quickly from disease." In other words, reishi is able to work both as a preventive herb as well as to treat seriously ill people.

RECENT SCIENTIFIC FINDINGS

Long regarded with suspicion by Americans, the mushrooms are now receiving renewed attention owing to the health-promoting compounds found in several species. While most of the results reported thus far are based on animal studies, the historical reverence assigned reishi mushrooms by the Japanese tends to support the contention that human studies will produce equally exciting results.

Reishi mushrooms are commercially available in several varieties. *G. lucidum,* the red variety, is the type preferred in Japan. *G. japonicum,* which is darker and softer, as well as cultured varieties are also sold. Chinese herb doctors tend not to distinguish these species, using them all. However, only *G. lucidum* has been the subject of intensive research.

A recent study from Korea showed that *Ganoderma* elicited immunopotentiation in mice. Antitumor activity in mice of polysaccharide fractions of these mushrooms was reported from Japan, while Chinese scientists described adaptogenic activity, again in mice. According to this Chinese study, a hot water extract was found to enhance a self-protecting mechanism of the central nervous system, improve heart function, and correct parasympathetic nerve function. Perhaps most interestingly, this study also demonstrated an anti-radiation effect from a polysaccharide fraction.

The immune-enhancing effects ascribed to reishi mushrooms by the Korean scientists noted here were described as enhancing macrophages and polymorphonuclear leucocytes (two types of fighting cells). Many studies have reported potent antiallergic activity, including antihistamine actions. And it is now well-established that mushrooms such as reishi can significantly reduce serum cholesterol and "thin" the blood in a manner similar to aspirin by reducing agglutination of platelets.

A 1990 study involved 15 healthy volunteers and 33 patients with atherosclerotic diseases. When a watery soluble extract was added to the platelets in vitro, the healthy volunteers showed platelet inhibition in relation to dosage.

From this documentation, it appears that the claims of healing properties in these (and other) mushrooms are based on fact not myth. Fears of toxicity should be allayed by the finding that reishi has an LD50—the dose required to cause death in fifty percent of the population—of greater than 5,000 mg/kg, with no toxic effect at this high level of consumption even after 30 days. No toxic effects in humans are to be expected even if a person were to eat 350 grams a day, between 40 and 300 times the therapeutic dose.

Reishi mushroom is a revered fungus with a long history of use in traditional Chinese medicine. It is celebrated for its potential immune-boosting and adaptogenic properties. Reishi contains bioactive compounds, including beta-glucans and triterpenoids, which contribute to its reputation as a medicinal mushroom. It is often used to support immune function, reduce stress, and enhance overall vitality. Reishi mushroom highlights how certain fungi play a pivotal role in holistic well-being and have been revered for centuries for their potential health benefits.

Ganoderma lucidum

ROSE

Rosa gallica

Parts used: Unexpanded petals and buds. *Since ancient times, the petals of these beautiful flowers have been employed for their astringent properties.*

TRADITIONAL USAGES

The use of rose petals dates from very ancient times. Early writers considered the petals purgative, astringent, and tonic, and used them for chronic catarrh, hemoptysis, diarrhea, and leucorrhea. Avicenna and other physicians after him recommended the petals in pulmonary phthisis.

The medicinal properties of the petals were generally considered very mild. The buds and petals have a pleasantly astringent and bitter taste and were formerly prepared as a simple tonic. Their medicinal application ultimately dropped off entirely, and they remained in use only as an elegant vehicle for tonic and astringent medicines, due to their coloration and flavor qualities. The essential oil, because of its powerful aroma, has been believed since early times to exert an effect on the nervous system. Hippocrates recommended the oil in diseases of the uterus.

RECENT SCIENTIFIC FINDINGS

It is known that rose buds and petals are a rich source of vitamin C, astringent tannins, and related phenolic compounds. They are thus used to advantage as tonics and astringents.

Rose petals are used to create fragrant and soothing teas, essential oils, and topical products. Rose is celebrated for its potential to relax the mind, uplift the spirit, and support skin health. Its aroma and properties make it a beloved botanical in both wellness and perfumery.

ROSEMARY

Rosmarinus officinalis

Parts used: Leaves and flowers. *Once a subject of superstition, it is official in the U.S. Pharmacopoeia.*

TRADITIONAL USAGES

Rosemary's history is rich with superstitions concerning its power. Ancient Greek students wore rosemary to improve their memory. During the Middle Ages, it was

> *Rosemary is used to enhance the taste of dishes and support digestion, and may improve memory and cognitive function.*

believed that rosemary warded off evil spirits. Medicinally, the flowers were steeped in water and drunk as a tonic. The legendary rosemary water was reputed to cure paralysis. The burning of rosemary branches was thought to prevent the plague. More recently, herbalists prescribed rosemary leaves as a stomachic, astringent, and expectorant. Externally, an ointment from oil of rosemary is used for rheumatism and minor wounds and bruises.

RECENT SCIENTIFIC FINDINGS

Rosemary's volatile oil is used in rubefacients and carminatives. It is official in the *U.S. Pharmacopoeia.* A recent study suggested that a rosemary extract may be a chemo-preventive agent for breast cancer. A dietary supplement of the extract "resulted in a significant (47%) decrease in mammary tumor incidence compared to controls."

Rosemary is a fragrant and flavorful herb with a multitude of culinary and medic-inal uses. Its aromatic leaves contain essential oils, including rosmarinic acid, known for their potential antioxidant and anti-inflammatory effects. Rosemary is used to enhance the taste of dishes and support digestion, and may improve memory and cognitive function, highlighting its role in both the kitchen and holistic well-being.

SAFFLOWER
Carthamus tinctorius

Parts used: Flowers. *The flowers of this herb are the source of safflower oil, which is a healthy vegetable oil rich in linoleic acid, an essential fatty acid.*

TRADITIONAL USAGES

Safflower is an annual herb with bright yellow or red flowers. Safflower oil is used in cooking and is considered heart-healthy due to its ability to reduce cholesterol levels. Additionally, safflower has been used as a medicinal herb in traditional Chinese medi-cine to treat conditions such as menstrual pain and promote blood circulation. In large doses, safflower is thought to have laxative value and when given as a warm infusion to have a diaphoretic effect. *Carthamus* flowers are sometimes fraudulently mixed in commerce with much more costly saffron, which they resemble in color, but they may be distinguished by their tubular form and by the yellowish style and filaments that they enclose. Like Spanish saffron (*Crocus sativus*), *Carthamus* is used in treating measles, scarlet fever, and other inflammatory eruptions of the skin, including those of viral origin, in order to promote and hasten eruption. Saffron, in addition, was extensively employed by the ancients and by medieval physicians as a highly stimulant antispasmodic and to relieve menstrual cramping and pain. The fruits are edible and when fried are used to make chutney.

RECENT SCIENTIFIC FINDINGS

Numerous animal studies have been conducted recently comparing safflower oil with other fatty oils. In one study, safflower oil was not as beneficial as perilla oil in suppressing carcinogenesis, allergic hyperreactivity, thrombotic tendency, apoplexy, and hypertension.

A comparison of groundnut, coconut, mustard, and safflower oils found that rats fed safflower and mustard oils had higher cholesterol content and a higher degree of unsaturation in the membrane fatty acid composition. The researchers believe the higher cholesterol levels with safflower oil are due to its linoleic and arachidonic acid content.

In a dietary study with rabbits, plasma cholesterol levels doubled after two weeks and remained elevated when their diet was supplemented with a mixture of corn, palm, and safflower oils. A rat study found that oral administration of safflower oil significantly increased awake systolic blood pressure. Interestingly, evening primrose oil prevented this increase.

Carthamus tinctorius

SAGE
Salvia officinalis

Parts used: Leaves and flowering tops. *Believed by the ancients to promote longevity, the Chinese variety of this herb may be an ideal tranquilizer.*

TRADITIONAL USAGES

Sage is a fragrant perennial herb with gray-green leaves that are widely used in culinary applications. It imparts a savory and slightly peppery flavor to dishes, making it a popular choice for seasoning poultry, stuffing, and various Mediterranean dishes. Beyond its culinary use, sage has been used for its potential health benefits. It contains compounds that may help improve memory and cognitive function. It is also employed as a natural remedy for sore throats, mouth ulcers, and digestive discomfort. In traditional practices, sage is associated with wisdom and is used in spiritual cleansing rituals.

An ancient Arabian proverb said, "How shall a man die who has sage in his garden?" Since ancient times, sage was believed to promote longevity. During the Middle Ages, sage was one of the main ingredients of longevity tonics. As late as the 17th century, the English botanical writer John Evelyn claimed that the use of sage would render a man immortal.

California sage was used by Native Americans to prevent drying of the nasal mucus. The ground seeds were stirred in water, and the resulting mucilate was slowly sucked. On the East Coast, the Catawbas pounded wild sage roots into a salve to be applied to sores. From 1842 to 1916, *Salvia officinalis* was official in the *U.S. Pharmacopoeia,* where it was recommended for its tonic, astringent, and aromatic properties.

The mint-like Asian variety of this herb is classified as a "blood regulator" in Chinese medicine and is said to "facilitate blood circulation, dissolve clots, and keep the blood vessels soft and supple." *Salvia*

Salvia officinalis

As late as the 17th century, the English botanical writer John Evelyn claimed that the use of sage would render a man immortal.

miltiorrhiza, a member of the Labiatae family, has a long history in Chinese folk medicine as a treatment for insomnia, cerebrovascular diseases, and coronary heart diseases.

RECENT SCIENTIFIC FINDINGS

"Minor" tranquilizers such as Valium and Librium, classified as benzodiazepines, have been widely prescribed since 1960 to treat epilepsy, muscle spasms, sleep problems, and anxiety. They are very effective but quite addictive, with physical dependence demonstrated in humans who have used these agents repeatedly.

If only humankind could have that "perfect" antianxiety agent! It would calm without sedating, be nonaddictive, and not induce strong muscle relaxation. Does this sound like soma, the mythic perfect drug sought for ages?

According to a team of Japanese scientists, the common Chinese variety of sage may contain the perfect tranquilizing compound within its roots. A single compound found in this plant may become the source of a new tranquilizing agent, acting like Valium without the troublesome side effects.

The benzodiazepines act at pharmacologically specific sites in the central nervous system, the central B2 receptors, to inhibit nerve transmission by enhancing the neurotransmission of GABA (an inhibitor of neurotransmission). The plant-derived compounds also interact with the central B2 receptors. Determined to be diterpene quinones, so-called tanshinones, they chemically differ from all the other known natural and synthetic B2 receptors yet discovered.

The most potent of these tanshinones is miltirone. In experiments with mice, it was found to diminish anxiety without producing sedation or muscle relaxation, and without diminishing performance or producing addiction.

Other studies have found sage to be of some use in soothing and regulating menopausal problems, possessing antibacterial activity in vitro against several human pathogens, and exhibiting anti-yeast activity in vitro against *Candida albicans* and antiviral activity in cell culture against herpes simplex virus II, influenza virus A2, vaccinia virus, and polio virus II.

ST. JOHN'S WORT
Hypericum perforatum

Parts used: Tops and flowers. *At one time ascribed magical properties, this herb is the source of hypericin.*

TRADITIONAL USAGES

St. John's wort was valued by the ancients and continued to enjoy a good reputation among the earlier modern physicians. Galen and Discorides recommended St. John's wort as a diuretic, as an emmenagogue, and for killing internal worms. The famous herbalist John Gerard wrote, "St. John's Wort, with his flowers and seed boyled and drunken, provoketh urine, and is right good against stone in the bladder." It is possible that the employment of St. John's wort as a remedy for wounds was originally suggested, according to the doctrine of signatures, by the red juice of its capsules, which was taken as a signature of human blood.

The plant's name came about because the peasantry of Europe assigned the plant magical powers. They gathered it on St. John's Day, June 24, for special cures.

At one time, it was believed that this plant could be used to drive the devil out of a person possessed; however, this may have been based on the observation of its usefulness in treating hypochondriasis and insanity. The plant was a popular charm against witchcraft and evil spirits.

RECENT SCIENTIFIC FINDINGS

Although the USFDA has included this plant in their (out-of-date) March 1977 "unsafe herb list," it has been used beneficially for thousands of years, especially for wounds and bruises, administered both internally and externally. Evidently, the FDA included St. John's wort on the list based on reports of toxic reactions in cattle, not humans.

An oil extract is recommended as a good external salve for burns, sores, bruises, and skin problems. German scientists applied an ointment containing St. John's wort to burns and reported that first-degree burns healed in 48 hours and second- and third-degree burns healed three times faster than burns treated conventionally. St.

Hypericum perforatum

John's wort's chemical constituents include tannins, flavonoids, xanthones, terpenes, phloroglucinol derivatives, and carotenoids. An extract, hypericin, has been found to be an antidepressant. A 1984 clinical trial with this extract involved six depressive women between the ages of 55 and 65. The researchers measured metabolites of noradrenaline and dopamine in urinalysis. After taking the hypericin extract, there was a significant increase in 3-methoxy-4-hydroxyphenylglucol, which is a chemical marker for antidepressive reactions. These same researchers conducted another study with 15 women. Results showed an improvement in symptoms of depression, anxiety, insomnia, dysphoric mood, and self-esteem. No side effects were reported.

Caution: It has been firmly established that hypericin is a phototoxic constituent. After taking the plant or its extracts, and following exposure to sunlight, light skinned individuals may suffer dermatitis, severe burning, and possibly blistering of the skin. The severity of these effects will depend on the amount of plant consumed and the length of exposure to sunlight. Therefore, individuals with fair skin should avoid sunlight while taking St. John's wort. Some authorities recommend that all individuals avoid sunlight when using hypericin, especially when taking large quantities. Considering the extensive use of hypericin extracts in Europe, consumers should not be in danger as long as they confine their use to moderate doses and restrict their exposure to sunlight.

St. John's wort is a yellow-flowered herb native to Europe, but it has been naturalized in many parts of the world. It is known for its potential antidepressant properties. The active compounds in St. John's wort, such as hypericin and hyperforin, may influence serotonin levels in the brain, which can help alleviate symptoms of mild to moderate depression and anxiety. It has been used in herbal medicine for centuries and is still a popular natural remedy for mood disorders.

SARSAPARILLA
Smilax aristolochiifolia, S. medica, S. officinalis

Parts used: Root. *At one time a popular remedy for a variety of ailments, the root is now considered a mild diuretic.*

TRADITIONAL USAGES

Sarsaparilla was used extensively by various Native Americans, who transmitted their knowledge to white settlers. The Penobscots made a cough remedy from pulverized sarsaparilla roots in combination with sweet flag roots. In the Pacific Northwest, the Kwakiutl prepared a cough medicine with the pulverized root and an unspecified oil.

> *Sarsaparilla is a woody vine with aromatic roots that have been traditionally used as a natural remedy in various cultures.*

The cough remedy of the Pillager Ojibwas was a decoction of pulverized root boiled in water. While Native Americans generally utilized sarsaparilla by itself, popular commercial drinks featured sarsaparilla root mixed with the roots of several other plants..

Sarsaparilla was introduced into European medicine in the mid-16th century as a treatment for syphilis and subsequently discarded for that purpose. Thereafter it was utilized for many chronic diseases, such as rheumatism and scrofula. The smoke of sarsaparilla was even inhaled by asthmatic patients.

Mexican sarsaparilla (*S. aristolochiifolia*), one of the commercial sources of the "drug," is utilized extensively in that country. Some tribes use a root decoction to lower fevers and for kidney troubles, while it is also generally used externally for skin diseases and rheumatism.

RECENT SCIENTIFIC FINDINGS

Commonly regarded as a tonic, diaphoretic, and diuretic, sarsaparilla in actuality is probably no more than a mild gastric irritant due to its saponin content. Sarsasapogenin and smilagenin are steroidal aglycones with potential use as precusors for the synthetic production of cortisone and other steroidal drugs. The plant possesses diuretic action, stimulating the excretion of uric acid. Sarsaparilla root extracts have been observed to have anti-tubercle bacillus activity in culture studies. Sarsaparilla is a woody vine with aromatic roots that have been traditionally used as a natural remedy in various cultures. It is considered a blood purifier and has been used for skin conditions like psoriasis and rheumatoid arthritis. Sarsaparilla root contains saponins, which may have anti-inflammatory and immune-boosting properties. It is believed to support overall health and wellness.

Smilax aristolochiifolia

SAW PALMETTO

Serenoa repens

Parts used: Berries. *Research has confirmed the berries' folkloric use for prostate problems.*

TRADITIONAL USAGES

The tea made from the berries of saw palmetto has a long history of use for genitourinary conditions. In the early 20th century, it was commonly employed to treat prostate problems and as a mild diuretic. Saw palmetto earned the nickname "plant catheter" due to its tonic effect on the bladder neck, which helped increase the breakdown of DHT in the prostate.

Saw palmetto also was used as an aphrodisiac as well as to increase sperm production, and by women to enlarge breasts. It was also used as a nutritive tonic and for respiratory diseases. Enslaved people in the South fed saw palmetto to livestock and the practice was copied by whites.

Saw palmetto was official in the *U.S. Pharmacopoeia* from 1905 to 1926 and *The National Formulary* from 1926 to 1950. It was most commonly prescribed for frequency of urination and excessive night urination due to inflammation of the bladder and prostate enlargement.

RECENT SCIENTIFIC FINDINGS

Saw palmetto was generally considered by the scientific community to have no therapeutic value. Recent studies have contradicted this earlier skepticism. Several extracts from the berries have been the subject of research, exhibiting estrogenic activity and inhibiting the enzyme testosterone-5-alpha-reductase in mice experiments. The dried berries of saw palmetto contain high amounts of sitosterols.

Serenoa repens

Also, the folkloric claims of benefits for prostate problems have been substantiated. Benign prostatic hyperplasia (BPH) is considered to be caused by testosterone accumulating in the prostate. The testosterone is then converted to dihydrotestosterone (DHT), which causes the cells to multiply too quickly and leads to enlargement of the prostate. The saw palmetto extract prevents testosterone from converting to dihydrotestosterone. It also inhibits DHT from binding to cellular receptors and excretion.

Several double-blind trials have been conducted. One study involved 110 patients with each receiving either a placebo or a hexane extract of saw palmetto for a period of one month. The researchers found a statistically significant improvement for those patients receiving the extract. Despite the improvement, the reduction in residual urine was not enough to remove the symptoms.

A randomized, double-blind, placebo-controlled study of 30 patients suffering from prostate adenoma also found statistically significant differences between the treated group and placebo. However, once again the improvement was only minimal. So, while saw palmetto may provide some relief from prostate symptoms, it does not seem to be meaningful enough to be an effective treatment. For this reason, in 1990, the FDA refused to grant the drug OTC status.

There is preliminary evidence that saw palmetto aids those suffering from thyroid deficiency.

SCHISANDRA
Schisandra chinensis

Parts used: Berries. *This is the source for several Oriental medicines and a registered medicine in Russia.*

TRADITIONAL USAGES

Schisandra is the source of several Oriental medicines, including *gomishi* in Japan, where it is utilized for tonic and antitussive purposes. Classed as an adaptogen (like ginseng), schisandra has a long history of folkloric use in China and Tibet and more recent folk applications in Russia.

Throughout the ages, various groups of people have enjoyed the benefits of schisandra. For example, in Northern China, there lives a hunting tribe known as the Nanajas. Their hunting lifestyle means that they often set out on long and exhausting hunting trips under harsh conditions. But they always take along dried schisandra fruit. A handful of the small red berries gives them the strength to hunt all day without eating. To this day, hunters in the wilds of eastern Siberia use the berries, stalks, and roots of this plant in the form of tea to provide them with extra energy when hunting.

This amazing fruit helped Russian pilots to withstand lack of oxygen in their flights during the forties. In more recent years, schisandra has contributed to the successes of the Swedish skiing team. In Russia, schisandra is a registered medicine for vision difficulties, e.g., short-sight and astigmatism, etc.

RECENT SCIENTIFIC FINDINGS

This interesting plant has many biological activities, including antibacterial (with equivocal results), sympathomimetic (stimulant), resistance stimulation, liver-protective, antitoxic, antiallergenic, antidepressant, and glycogenesis stimulation.

In addition, and perhaps most interesting from the point of view of it being a folkloric "tonic," this herb protected against the narcotic and sedative effects of alcohol and pentobarbital and exposure to highly toxic ether, in mice. As a result of these data, the authors concluded that schisandra may be a useful clinical agent for reversal of central nervous system depression.

They based this antidepressant activity on the reasoning that depression may be due, in part, to adrenergic exhaustion following severe psychogenic stress. It is known that MAO (monoamine oxidase) inhibitors, as well as other selected compounds that increase noradrenergic neurotransmission within the central nervous system (such as imipramine), have proven beneficial in treating depression.

This herb is also being promoted for its stimulating effect on the nervous system without being excitatory like amphetamine or caffeine. There are some proponents who claim that "the higher the degree of exhaustion, the greater the stimulating effect."

A very interesting study on performance in racehorses tends to confirm the folkloric claims. Polo horses given the berry extract of this species showed a lower increase in heart rate (during exercise), a quicker recovery of respiratory function, a reduction of plasma lactate, and improved performance.

A 1990 study reported that a lignan component of schisandra fruit suppresses the arachidonic (AA) cascade in macrophages. The AA cascade pushes the production of leukotrienes, which may play a role in inflammatory diseases. By inhibiting the arachidonic acid cascade, schisandra both protects the liver and stimulates the immune system—two key roles of an ideal adaptogen.

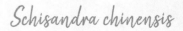

Schisandra chinensis

An interesting non-Western 1991 study tested the "tonifying and invigorating yang" powers of schisandra and other herbs in mice. The researchers measured the animals' body weight, thymus weight, leukocyte count, and other parameters of "yang." They observed a direct correlation between the amount of herb ingested (as hot water extracts) and improved immunocompetence. They also noticed a distinct anti-fatigue quality, which was measured by reduced excitability of the parasympathetic nervous system. No toxicity was reported.

It appears that this creeping herb from the Far East has valid claims to the title of a "new" anti-fatigue agent that possibly helps to accelerate restorative processes within the human body. Traditional Chinese nedicine continues to offer new candidates to the annals of world medicine. As we in the West are slowly learning, "traditional" or "folk" medicine really is the medicine of the people.

Caution: While schisandra is a very safe herb with much historical usage, one supplier of a standardized extract recommends that this herb be avoided by epileptics, those with high intracranial pressure or severe hypertension, and those with "high acidity."

Schisandra is a climbing vine native to Northern China and parts of Russia. It is distinguished by its vibrant red berries, which are known for their unique combination of five flavors. Schisandra is considered an adaptogen in traditional Chinese medicine, helping the body adapt to stress and increase endurance. It is also known for its potential liver-protective and antioxidant properties, making it a popular choice in herbal medicine for promoting overall vitality.

SCULLCAP or Skullcap
Scutellaria lateriflora

Parts used: Whole plant. *At one time, this was named "mad dog scullcap" and was used to treat rabies, and recent studies indicate promising action against pulmonary infections.*

TRADITIONAL USAGES

Scullcap is a delicate herb with small, helmet-shaped flowers. It is traditionally used for its mild sedative properties, making it an effective herbal remedy for conditions like anxiety, insomnia, and nervous tension. Scullcap is often prepared as an herbal tea or tincture. It is considered a natural way to calm the nervous system and promote relaxation.

Employed rather commonly as a tonic and general relaxant in times of excitement, Scullcap tea was a very mild and safe nervine. In the Thomsonian system of medicine, it was used in the treatment of delirium tremens, St. Vitus' dance, convulsions, lockjaw, and tremors, and was given to teething babies.

Beginning with a series of experiments in 1772 by Dr. Van Derveer, the sedative and antispasmodic properties of this perennial herb were applied widely in the treatment of rabies. This use earned the plant its nickname "mad dog scullcap." The dried herb was entered into the *U.S. Pharmacopoeia* in 1863 and remained until 1916 when it was shifted to *The National Formulary*.

Scutellaria lateriflora

RECENT SCIENTIFIC FINDINGS

Scullcap contains the flavonoid glycosides scutellarin and scutellarein. Scullcap preparations have been shown to have a relaxant effect on uterine tissue in test-tube studies.

A survey of 60 patients with pulmonary infection (mainly pneumonia) compared the effect of a scullcap compound with a placebo. The patients were randomly divided into two groups of 30 with no difference in clinical data prior to beginning the treatment. The total effective rate was over 70%. The researchers concluded that their results indicate that further investigation is warranted.

Animal studies have demonstrated *Scutellaria* species to have diuretic, bile-stimulating, anti-fever, and depressant activity, and lowers blood pressure. In Chinese studies, a root extract demonstrated central nervous system depressant activity in humans.

SEAWEEDS

Gelidium, Gracilaria, and *Pterocladia* spp. (agar-agar); *Lyngbya lagerheimii* and *Phormidium tenue* (blue-green algae); *Laminaria* spp. (brown algae, kelp); *Chlorella* spp. (chlorella); *Chondrus* (Irish moss)

Parts used: Whole plant.

Seaweeds are marine algae that come in various types, including nori, kelp, and dulse. These underwater plants are not only used extensively in culinary traditions worldwide but also offer a range of health benefits. Seaweeds are rich in essential minerals like iodine, vitamins, and antioxidants. They are commonly used in Asian cuisines, such as sushi, miso soup, and seaweed salads. Beyond their culinary applications, they play a role in supporting thyroid health, providing a source of essential nutrients and contributing to overall wellness. Used in Oriental medicine for centuries, these sea vegetables are yielding some fascinating discoveries.

TRADITIONAL USAGES

Seaweeds, especially brown kelp, have been used in Oriental medicine for centuries. They were applied externally for skin diseases, burns, and insect bites. Internally, they are most widely known for their use as a cancer treatment, but a host of ailments were also treated. These include bronchial problems, disorders of the digestive and urinary systems, and rheumatic diseases.

Agar-agar is the dried mucilaginous substance extracted from marine algae. It has been widely used to treat chronic constipation. It has also been employed for its emollient and demulcent properties.

Irish moss was used by the New England colonists as a bulk laxative.

RECENT SCIENTIFIC FINDINGS

Marine flora is shown to possess numerous medicinal properties, including antibiotic, antiviral, antimicrobial in general, and antifungal.

Japanese food is in vogue in Western nations, primarily because of the low fat, low calorie, high-fiber aspects. Wakame (a brown kelp, *Undaria*), kombu (*Laminaria*), and nori (*Porphyra*), which is used to wrap around rice for sushi, all contain active antitumor compounds.

These sea vegetables protect us against cancers of the digestive tract due to at least four known factors:

- The alginic acid content swells in the intestine thus diluting potential carcinogens.
- Some contain beta-sitosterol, a potent anticancer compound.
- They may contain antibiotic compounds that inhibit the growth of several different gram-positive and gram-negative bacteria known to potentiate carcinogens in the colon.
- They may possess antioxidant activity.

AGAR-AGAR

Recently, Dr. K. R. Gustafson and others have discovered that agar contains a high concentration of polysaccharide mucilage, which swells and becomes very slimy when

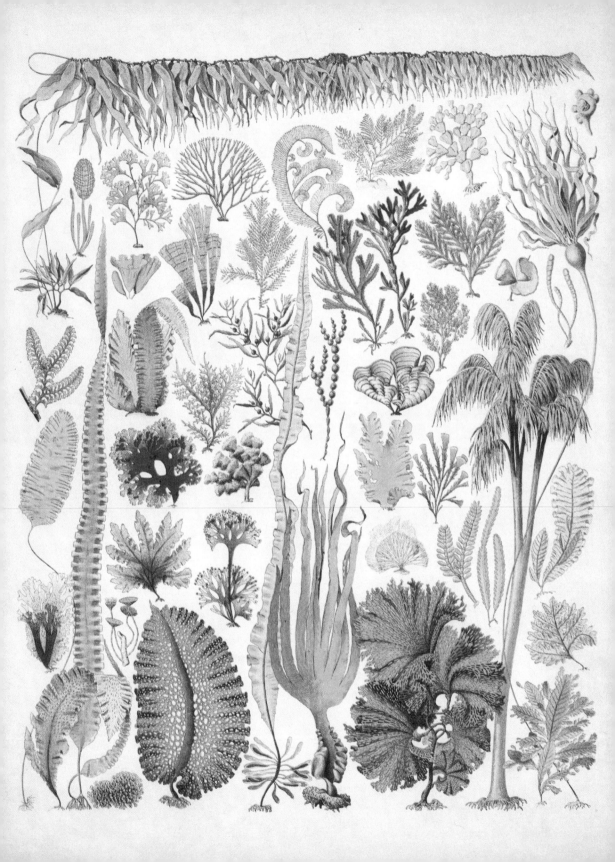

moistened. This mucilage is responsible for the laxative effect of agar, as it exerts a lubricating effect.

When used as a laxative, agar should be taken with large amounts of water, and never dry. It usually will not produce a laxative effect with a single dose but must be used regularly. Its function is very similar to that of vegetable cellulose foods and of bran. As a good bulk laxative, it may also be added to cereals, soups, cakes, or any other food without altering its effect. If the constipation is stubborn, cascara (see section on cascara sagrada) bark is added to precipitate action.

BLUE-GREEN ALGAE

Dextran sulfate is created when dextran is boiled with chlorosulfonic acid. It is a sulfate ester not a sulfonic acid. Dextran sulfate has been used for more than 30 years in Japan, primarily as an intravenous drug that reduces clotting and lowers blood cholesterol. Dextran sulfate also inactivates the herpes simplex virus.

In a 1987 letter to *The Lancet,* two Japanese researchers reported that dextran sulfate blocked the binding of HIV-1 to T-lymphocytes as well as blocked the transfer of HIV from cell to cell by cell fusion. Scientists at the National Cancer Institute (U.S.) reported that cellular extracts from cultured blue-green algae protected human T cells from infection with the AIDS virus. In test-tube experiments, pure compounds extracted from these algae also proved to be "strikingly active against HIV-1."

These algae were originally collected in Hawaii and the Palau Islands (Micronesia) and then cultured. The original technique for culturing such marine organisms and producing an extract (which later proved to be cytotoxic) was pioneered by my first professor of pharmacology, Dr. T.R. Norton. It was in 1968 in Dr. Norton's basement laboratory at Leahi Hospital of the University of Hawaii School of Medicine where I was first introduced to the search for medicines from plants.

BROWN ALGAE

I first learned of the anticancer and antithrombotic effects of brown algae from a Japanese colleague. True, I had long believed that mankind would once again "return to the sea" by adding the aquatic plants to his armamentarium of terrestrial medicinals. But my attention was not galvanized until I learned about fucoidan.

Research has shown that the main active component with antitumor activity in edible seaweeds is likely a type of sulphated polysaccharide, fucoidan. The same compound has been shown to be responsible for anticoagulant and fibrinolytic activities in animal studies.

Another researcher, utilizing epidemiological and biological data, speculates that the brown kelp seaweed *Laminaria* is "an important factor contributing to the relatively low breast cancer rates reported in Japan."

Brown algae also contains dextran sulfate. See the previous discussion about blue-green algae for further information.

CHLORELLA

These microscopic species of algae possess distinct biological activities and are certain to take their place among the better-known marine organisms. All that has been said about the other species of seaweed is also applicable to the various unicellular marine algae, especially species of *Chlorella.*

Numerous animal studies have demonstrated antitumor activity, antiviral activity, and interferon-inducing effects. The antitumor activity was observed specifically against mammary tumors, leukemia, ascitic sarcoma, and liver cancer. A glycolipid fraction was tested that showed immune-enhancing effects in mice; most likely it was chlorellin.

An extract of chlorella was found to have antiviral activity against cytomegalovirus (in mice) and against equine encephalitis virus (horse).

Immune stimulation by extract of chlorella was observed due to induction of interferon production in mice infected with estomegalovirus (murine), and enhanced natural killer cell production was observed in mice infested with estomegalovirus as well as in mice with lymphoma-YAC-1.

Antihypertensive and antihyperlipedimic activity were observed with the protein fraction derived from chlorella.

IRISH MOSS

Irish moss is commonly used as a stabilizer in various foods, especially dairy products.

Experimental results have shown that Irish moss may reduce high blood pressure.

A product has been patented containing an extract of Irish moss. The manufacturers claim the extract treats ulcers.

Other promising areas that have been observed in preliminary testing and warrant further investigation include Irish moss's properties as a demulcent, an anti-inflammatory, an immune-stimulant, an antibacterial against *Streptococcus mutans*, and a lymphocyte blastogenesis stimulant.

SENEGA SNAKEROOT

Polygala senega

Parts used: Root. *As its name indicates, this was a popular remedy for rattlesnake bites in the 18th century.*

TRADITIONAL USAGES

Senega snakeroot, also known as Virginia snakeroot, is a perennial herb native to the eastern United States. The roots of this plant have been historically used by Native American tribes and early settlers for medicinal purposes. It is believed to have potential benefits for the digestive and urinary systems. Senega snakeroot has been used to treat conditions such as indigestion, fevers, and urinary tract issues. However, it's important to note that some species of *Aristolochia contain compounds that may be harmful, so careful identification and usage are necessary.*

It is said that senega was originally introduced into practice as a remedy for rattlesnake bites. Like most snakebite remedies, the roots were chewed and then applied directly to the bite. In 1735, a Scotch physician, John Tennent, noted that the Senecas successfully employed this plant for rattlesnake bites. He persuaded the Senecas to show him the root. Since the symptoms of snakebite were similar in certain aspects to pleurisy and latter stages of peripneumonia, Tennent tried the root on those diseases. After successful experiments, he wrote an epistle that was printed in Edinburgh in 1738, leading to the drug's acceptance in Europe and the beginning of cultivation in Britain in 1739. However, it came to be recognized of questionable value in treating venomous bites. The primary application of senega has been as an expectorant, to help the expulsion of mucus from the respiratory tract in cases of bronchitis, asthma, and where otherwise indicated in similar pulmonary conditions. The 23rd edition of the *Dispensatory of the United States* describes the plant's use in bronchitis and asthma, attributing the therapeutic value to the saponins contained in the dried root. It was official in the *U.S. Pharmacopeia* from 1820 to 1936.

Polygala senega

In larger doses the plant has been used as an irritant poison to produce vomiting and purging of the intestinal tract, but this usage was very infrequent, there being more desirable plants available for this purpose.

RECENT SCIENTIFIC FINDINGS

Extracts of senega snakeroot have been shown experimentally to have expectorant properties when administered orally to a variety of animals, including cats, guinea pigs, and rabbits. It is thus reasonable to believe that tea prepared from the roots of this plant would have a similar beneficial effect in humans.

SENNA

Cassia senna, C. acutifolia (Alexandrian Senna),
C. angustifolia (Indian Senna)

Parts used: Leaves. *For over a thousand years, this has proven to be an effective gentle laxative.*

TRADITIONAL USAGES

Senna is an Arabic name, and the first recorded medical uses appear in Arabic writings from the ninth century. Its Chinese name, *fan-hsieh-yeh,* means "foreign country laxative leaf;" most likely it was introduced to the Orient by Arabic traders. Senna is highly valued as a cathartic, working particularly on the lower bowel. It is consequently utilized on cases of chronic constipation. Senna was official in the *U.S. Pharmacopoeia* from 1820 to 1882.

American senna was utilized by Native Americans in a variety of ways, none of them as a laxative. The Cherokees drank a decoction to reduce fevers and applied the root to sores. Other tribes employed senna as a sore throat remedy.

RECENT SCIENTIFIC FINDINGS

The leaflets and pods of *Cassia acutifolia* and *C. angustifolia* are popular laxative preparations that have the advantage over most other laxatives of being less "harsh," or producing less "intestinal griping." The reason for the laxative effect is that the leaves and pods

Cassia acutifolia

contain varying amounts of complex anthraquinones known as sennosides (sennoside A and B are the two major active constituents). Many laxative preparations combine sennosides with a stool softener, but the combination has not proved more effective than the sennosides alone to the best of our knowledge.

Senna is recommended for people suffering from looser stool constipation who only need to increase frequency of bowel movements. Senna is often combined with aromatics such as anise, fennel, ginger, nutmeg, and peppermint to further reduce the tendency to produce intestinal griping. Its nauseous taste can be removed by preparing the plant as an alcoholic extract.

Caution: Not for use by people suffering from "tension-related" or "nervous" constipation; may cause dehydration if over-used.

Senna is a natural herb primarily known for its laxative properties. Derived from the leaves and pods of various *Cassia* species, senna has been utilized for centuries to address constipation and promote bowel regularity. The active compounds in senna, called sennosides, stimulate the muscles in the intestines, leading to increased bowel movements. This herb is often used in traditional and over-the-counter laxative preparations, typically in the form of teas or capsules.

SHEPHERD'S PURSE

Capsella bursa-pastoris

Parts used: Herb. *This common plant may have anti-ulcer properties.*

TRADITIONAL USAGES

This insignificant-looking little plant, which grows so plentifully almost everywhere, has long been a popular medicinal.

It was used in English domestic medicine for diarrhea.

Shepherd's purse was administered for the alarming symptom of blood in the urine (hematuria). This condition can be caused by a lesion of the urinary tract, contamination

Capsella bursa-pastoris

during menstruation or during the six weeks following childbirth, prostate disease, tumors, poisoning, and toxemia.

RECENT SCIENTIFIC FINDINGS

Shepherd's purse extracts have been shown to prevent duodenal ulcer formation induced by stress in rats and to have marked anti-inflammatory activity under a variety of test conditions in animals. Extracts of this plant have also shown significant antitumor activity against several experimental tumor systems in laboratory animals.

One study showed that extracts of this plant inhibit the growth of bacteria in test-tube experiments. There is also reasonable evidence, in animals and humans, that this plant has hemostatic properties. To date, high quantities of vitamin C have not been reported present in shepherd's purse, and thus, although it has been used as a remedy for scurvy, this antiscorbutic claim may not be warranted.

Shepherd's purse is an herb with a rich history in herbal medicine. It is renowned for its heart-shaped seed pods and is often employed as a remedy for conditions such as heavy menstrual bleeding. It is believed to have hemostatic properties, helping to reduce excessive bleeding. Additionally, shepherd's purse is used as a mild diuretic to support kidney and urinary tract health.

SHIITAKE MUSHROOM

Lentinus edodes

Parts used: Caps and stem. *This fungus has been found to possess antitumor and antiviral properties.*

TRADITIONAL USAGES

Shiitake mushrooms are not only a popular culinary ingredient but also a valued medicinal herb. These mushrooms are recognized for their immune-boosting effects due to compounds like beta-glucans. Shiitakes are also believed to have potential health benefits, including supporting cardiovascular health, reducing inflammation, and enhancing overall immunity.

Shiitake mushrooms traditionally were utilized in the diet as a strengthener.

RECENT SCIENTIFIC FINDINGS

When I first studied medical mycology, over 20 years ago, Wilson and Plunkett's classic text provoked such fear and revulsion through the color

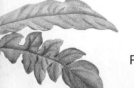

photos of rare fungal diseases of man that I vowed to never eat another mushroom! All fungi became a source of dread for me.

Within the past few years, I have since changed my view of these "lower" plants. The mushrooms are not only acceptable to me but have become highly coveted, owing to their documented immunostimulant, cholesterol-lowering, and antitumor activities.

Extracts of shiitake have been shown to inhibit a number of different cancerous tumors in animal experiments. A principle antitumor compound isolated from this species, lentinan, does not appear to kill tumor cells directly but inhibits tumor growth by stimulating immune function.

Lentinan appears to function by activating macrophages that then engulf cancerous cells. This activation is again via an indirect route—T-helper cells are stimulated, which increase the effectiveness of macrophages.

The AIDS epidemic fostered interest in any helpful compounds, and lentinan became a high priority item. A highly publicized letter to the prestigious medical journal *The Lancet* (October 20, 1984) was signed by Robert Gallo, one of the co-discoverers of HIV, and two French researchers from the Pasteur Institute. In it, the authors concluded that lentinan "may prove to be effective in AIDS or pre-AIDS or for HIV carriers." After intravenous administration of lentinan with two Japanese patients, HTLV-1 and HTLV-III antibodies disappeared.

Unfortunately, despite repeated requests to subject this drug to human trials, based on its long history of usage for cancer treatment in Japan, nothing much has been done by governmental authorities in the U.S.

This is odd considering the long list of studies showing lentinan's antiviral properties: interferon inducing, natural killer cell enhancing, phagocytosis rate enhancing, as well as numerous antitumor studies. The in vitro inhibition of HIV by an extract of this mushroom is not, of itself, highly significant owing to the many substances known to kill this virus. However, taken together with all of the evidence, it is safe to assume that shiitake is all that it is claimed to be.

Caution: Skin and respiratory allergic reactions have been observed in workers involved in the commercial production of shiitake.

Lentinus edodes

SKUNK CABBAGE
Symplocarpus foetidus (Spathyema foetida)

Parts used: Root, rhizome, and seeds. *In the 19th century, the rootstock was official in the U.S. Pharmacopoeia.*

TRADITIONAL USAGES

Skunk cabbage is a wetland plant known for its peculiar odor, which is often described as resembling that of a skunk. It has a history of use in traditional medicine, particularly by Native American communities. Skunk cabbage has been applied as a poultice for external use, helping to soothe various skin conditions and relieve joint discomfort. Additionally, it has been used as a remedy for respiratory issues due to its potential expectorant properties.

Skunk cabbage is a very curious plant, the only one of the genus to which it belongs. Credited with antispasmodic, emetic, diuretic, and narcotic properties, skunk cabbage has been used to treat asthma, chronic dry coughing spells and other upper respiratory problems, chronic rheumatism, nervous affections, muscular spasms and twitching, hysteria, and dropsy (water retention). Externally, it has been utilized as an ointment or salve for skin irritations.

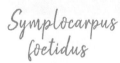

Symplocarpus foetidus

The Menominees boiled skunk cabbage root hairs and applied them to stop external bleeding. The leaf bases were applied in a wet dressing for bruises by the Meskwakis. The Winnebago and Dakota utilized skunk cabbage to stimulate the removal of phlegm in asthma. As employed in respiratory and nervous disorders, rheumatism, and dropsy, the rootstock was official in the *U.S. Pharmacopoeia* from 1820 to 1882.

The roots are an excellent emergency food, especially good baked or fried.

SLIPPERY ELM
Ulmus fulva

Parts used: Bark. *The bark continues to be a useful treatment for sore throats.*

TRADITIONAL USAGES

The demulcent properties of slippery elm bark led to its application in a number of ailments. The Ojibwas of North America made a tea from the inner bark to treat sore throats. The tea is also reportedly helpful for coughs. One pint of warm tea, administered as an enema, was given to babies to soothe the bowels after they had been cured of constipation or colic by repeated enemas. The bark was also eaten after convalescence, both for its soothing effects on the stomach and intestines, and for its nutritional value. Drunk combined with milk, it was easily digested, assimilated, and eliminated.

Used as an ointment, slippery elm sap was employed in Thomsonian medicine during labor as a lubricant for the midwife's hand when she ascertained the presentation of the infant internally. The Thomsonian system also used a poultice of slippery elm, lobelia, and a little soft soap as a means of bringing abscesses and boils to a head. These were then lanced and drained. Mausert considered this one of the most mild and harmless laxatives for children, causing no pain.

Slippery elm sticks were used in some North American tribes to provoke abortion by inserting them into the cervix.

RECENT SCIENTIFIC FINDINGS

All of the effects indicated for slippery elm bark are explained on the basis of an abundance of mucilage-containing cells surrounding each fiber of the bark. When the bark, in strips or powdered form, comes into contact with water, the mucilage cells swell enormously and thus produce a lubricating, demulcent, emollient, and/or laxative effect when administered locally or by mouth. Powdered slippery elm bark is especially useful to soothe sore throats, and it has a pleasant, aromatic odor and taste as well.

Narrow strips of slippery elm bark, when soaked in water for a few minutes, become very slippery and pliable. For this reason, it has been reported that some pregnant women have attempted to induce abortion by inserting a long strip of moistened bark into the cervix. This is an extremely dangerous practice, since many deaths have resulted due to uncontrollable hemorrhaging. Serious infections can also be expected due to the unsanitary conditions under which this type of practice is carried out.

In some states in the United States, the law requires that slippery elm bark be broken into pieces no longer than 1.5 inches in length before being sold. The intent of such laws is obviously to discourage the use of slippery elm bark for the induction of abortion.

Ulmus fulva

SOAPWORT
Saponaria officinalis

Parts used: Root and leaves. *Named for its lathering action, soapwort may possess anticancer properties.*

TRADITIONAL USAGES

Soapwort is an herb that has been used traditionally for its natural cleansing properties. It contains saponins, which create a soapy lather when mixed with water. This quality has led to its historical use in creating gentle, natural soaps and skin care products for cleansing and treating various skin conditions.

Many Native Americans pounded the root and mixed it with water as a hair shampoo. The Kiowa considered it an effective treatment for dandruff and skin irritations. The Pomos prepared a lotion of the soapy juice and rubbed it on poison oak rash. Soapwort was prescribed by medieval Arab physicians for leprosy and other skin complaints. The leaves, soaked for a short time, yield an extract that has been used to promote sweating, as a remedy against rheumatism, and to purify the blood.

RECENT SCIENTIFIC FINDINGS

The active principle responsible for soapwort's lathering effect is saponin, which carries the detergent as well as the medicinal properties of this plant. In 1917, in China, there were reportedly eleven species of trees that contained saponins that were utilized in the formation of detergents for the purpose of laundry washing.

A 1991 study examined the effect on human breast cancer cells of saporin 6, a protein purified from soapwort seeds. The results showed that the breast cancer cells were highly sensitive to saporin 6. Another 1991 study conducted by a different research team investigated saporin 6 for its effect on leukemia cells.

Saponaria officinalis

SOLOMON'S SEAL

Polygonatum officinale

Parts used: Root. *The roots contain allantoin, an anti-inflammatory agent.*

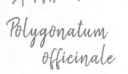

Polygonatum officinale

TRADITIONAL USAGES

Solomon's seal is a plant with unique rhizomes resembling the biblical seal of King Solomon. This herb has been used in traditional herbal medicine for its potential anti-inflammatory and soothing effects. It is often applied topically as a poultice to support joint health and relieve skin irritations.

The root was formerly used for its emetic properties and externally for bruises, especially near the eyes, as well as for treatment of tumors, wounds, poxes, warts, pimples, etc. Taken internally, it was thought to be effective in assisting the knitting of broken bones.

In 16th century Italy, Solomon's seal was esteemed as a cosmetic wash that would maintain healthy skin and prevent freckles, sunburn, pimples, and the mottling of old age.

RECENT SCIENTIFIC FINDINGS

The roots of Solomon's seal contain allantoin, a substance well known for its healing and anti-inflammatory effects. Extracts of the root of this plant lower blood sugar levels in rabbits, lower blood pressure, and have a cardiotonic action, indicating possible usefulness in heart conditions.

SPEARMINT

Mentha spicata

Parts used: Leaves and flowering tops. *Like the other mints, this is one of our most pleasant carminatives.*

TRADITIONAL USAGES

Spearmint is a widely recognized herb, known for its refreshing, minty flavor. Beyond its culinary applications, spearmint has been used for its potential digestive benefits. It may help alleviate indigestion, reduce nausea, and promote overall relaxation, often consumed as a soothing herbal tea.

Mentha spicata

Much the same as peppermint, without the cooling sensation in the mouth that accompanies the ingestion of the plant, spearmint is an aromatic stimulant. It is used for mild indigestion, to cure nausea, to relieve spasmodic stomach and bowel pains, help the expulsion of stomach and intestinal gas, and to otherwise remedy the deleterious effects of too much food or an improper diet. Spearmint is also combined with other less palatable medicines to make them more agreeable or to allay their tendencies of producing nausea or griping effect.

RECENT SCIENTIFIC FINDINGS

The leaves and flowering tops of spearmint owe their pleasant and aromatic properties, as well as characteristic taste, to a volatile oil. The major active principle in the oil is a simple terpene derivative, carvone.

Refer to the section on peppermint for further information. This plant is the same in action, only weaker due to the fact it does not contain menthol. Its use is largely a matter of taste preference.

SPINDLE TREE or Wahoo

Euonymus atropurpureus

Parts used: Bark, root, fruit, and seeds. *Though this is an extremely toxic plant, it was at one time a popular remedy for a variety of ailments.*

TRADITIONAL USAGES

Spindle tree is a plant admired for its vibrant autumn foliage and unique pink fruits.

Despite its toxicity, all parts of this tree have been employed at one time or another in traditional medicine. Native Americans used the wahoo for a variety of purposes, including uterine problems, as an eyewash, and as a physic. The bark became a popular diuretic soon after its introduction to early settlers. The dried root bark was believed to be a stimulant, laxative, and diaphoretic (producing sweating). As a result of this latter characteristic, it was employed in the treatment of dropsy (water retention).

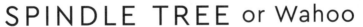

The oil expressed from the seeds was utilized for its emetic and purgative properties. The fruits were held to be diuretic. However, in light of their toxicity in even small quantities, the dosage must have been minute. The inner bark was utilized in treating eye diseases.

In 1912, a report was published that this species effects a digitalis-like action on the heart, which caused wahoo to become a popular heart medicine in domestic practice.

RECENT SCIENTIFIC FINDINGS

Caution: This is one plant that deserves its place on the USFDA 1977 unsafe herb list. The fruits are terribly toxic; ingestion of as few as three or four can prove fatal to a child and can cause an adult extreme pain and discomfort, as they function as a drastic purgative.

Wahoo fruit and seeds contain cardiac glycosides, which would be expected to produce a diuretic effect in people with cardiac insufficiency. Large amounts would also be predicted to cause emesis. These cardiac glycosides, however, are not present in other parts of the plant.

Euonymus atropurpureus

SQUAW VINE
or Partridge Berry

Mitchella repens

Parts used: Vine. *Used by Native Americans to facilitate childbirth, this vine was in the National Formulary from 1926 to 1947.*

TRADITIONAL USAGES

Squaw vine is an herb traditionally associated with women's health, particularly during pregnancy and childbirth. It is believed to possess uterine-toning properties, helping to strengthen the uterine muscles. Squaw vine has been employed to facilitate easier labor and alleviate discomfort associated with the female reproductive system.

Also called partridge berry, squaw vine was administered by Native American women as a tea to facilitate childbirth. As was common for plants employed for "female troubles," Native Americans were reluctant to provide much information about their methods of preparation and specific applications of squaw vine. The Cherokee informed one investigator they used a tea made from the leaves. The Penobscots of Maine used the same preparation. In the weeks prior to the expected date of delivery, frequent doses of the tea were taken. All aspects of labor, delivery of the child and the afterbirth, stimulation of the uterus, and so forth, were thought to be assisted by drinking tea brewed from this plant. (Pipsissewa and squaw vine are thought to have similar properties.)

Squaw vine became quite popular as a home treatment to speed labor. It was admitted into the *National Formulary* in 1926, where it remained until 1947. The leaves were used for their tonic, astringent, and diuretic properties.

RECENT SCIENTIFIC FINDINGS

Experimentally, squaw vine fluid extract has been tested for uterine stimulant activity in guinea pigs and was without effect. Thus, most likely the claims for this plant to be useful in facilitating parturition are unfounded. The plant contains tannins, which probably account for its beneficial effects as a local astringent. We have found no experimental basis for the use of squaw vine as a diuretic.

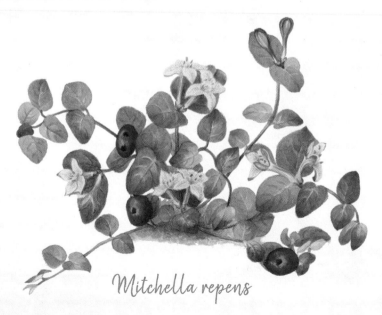

Mitchella repens

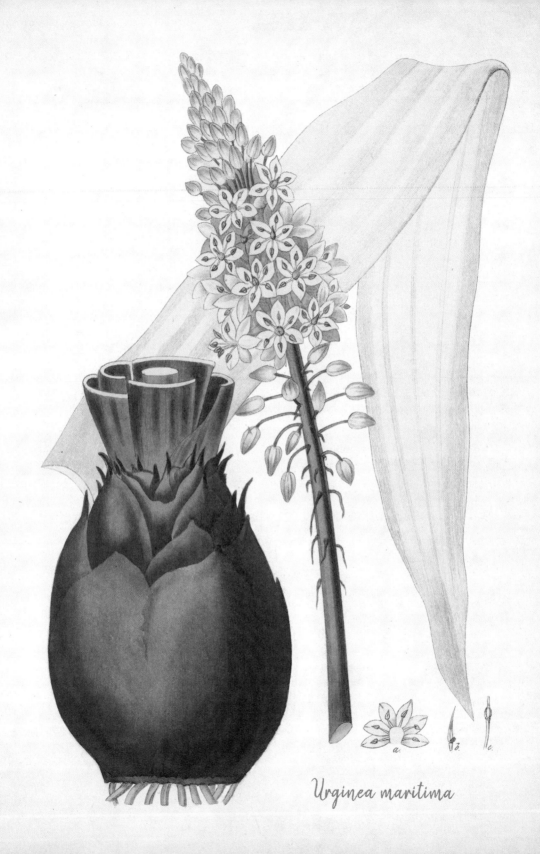

Urginea maritima

SQUILL
Urginea maritima (U. scilla)

Parts used: Bulbs, divested of outercoats and centers. *An ancient Egyptian papyrus described the cardiotonic effects that have been substantiated in this popular European heart medicine.*

TRADITIONAL USAGES

Squill is a bulbous plant with a history of use in traditional medicine. It contains toxic compounds, including cardiac glycosides, and requires careful preparation. Squill has been used to address respiratory and cardiac conditions, but its use should be strictly supervised by a healthcare professional due to its potential toxicity.

The Ebers Papyrus (14th century B.C.) is the first indication that the bulb of squill has cardiotonic effects. Squill was used by Greek physicians to treat dropsy, which is a manifestation of congestive heart failure.

In small doses, squill reportedly acted as an expectorant and diuretic, in large doses as an emetic and purgative, and in overdose as a poison. There are two varieties of squill: white squill and red squill.

RECENT SCIENTIFIC FINDINGS

Squill is quite a dangerous plant and makes an excellent rat poison. This herb belongs on the USFDA unsafe herb list, but it is not to be found there! Obviously not for home use, squill may prove valuable in the hands of the skilled herbalist-physician for its digitalis-like effect on the heart. It can be useful in treating heart disease, but overdose will cause death due to heart paralysis.

White squill contains active cardiac glycosides similar in structure and action to those present in foxglove (see remarks on *Digitalis purpurea* in section on foxglove). The major active substances are scillaren A and scillaren B. Currently, squill preparations are used in medical practice in Europe, but not in the United States. Squill has essentially the same effects as digitalis on the heart, and the only advantage over digitalis is that squill can be used in those people who cannot tolerate the other drug. Red squill has been used as a raticide; 250,000 kilograms were imported annually into the United States prior to World War II. It is curiously toxic to rats; other animals either refuse to eat it, or they apparently always vomit and are thus otherwise unaffected by it (unless the herb is disguised in a mixture!). Since rats do not vomit, they retain the plant material, and it eventually kills them. Red squill is 500–1,000 times more toxic to rats than white squill. The active poison in red squill is called scilliroside.

SQUIRTING CUCUMBER

Ecballium elaterium

Parts used: Juice sediment from fruit. *The juice has been called the most powerful known cathartic.*

TRADITIONAL USAGES

Squirting cucumber is a distinctive plant known for its explosive fruit dispersal mechanism. Historically, its fruit juice has been used as a strong purgative to induce vomiting and relieve constipation. This plant's use is highly specialized and should be approached with caution.

The wild or squirting cucumber owes its name to its fruit. Shaped like a small oval cucumber, the fruit separates from its peduncle when ripe and expels its juice and seeds with considerable force through an opening at its base. The sediment from the juice of the fruit, known as elaterium, traces its name back as far as Hippocrates, who used the term to signify any active purge. The plant was known to the ancients for its purgative effects and was also used by them to stimulate menstruation. In Turkey, the juice is a well-known folk remedy for sinusitis.

RECENT SCIENTIFIC FINDINGS

Elaterium has been called the most powerful hydragogue cathartic known, effective in extremely small doses. The fruit juice of the squirting cucumber is well known to cause

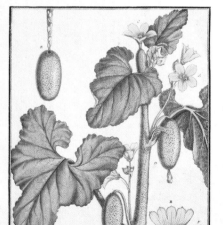

a powerful hydragogue cathartic effect in humans. This effect is caused by the major principles in the juice, a mixture of compounds referred to as cucurbitacins.

There is evidence from animal experiments that the juice of the squirting cucumber has an effect on the heart that would suggest a useful application in humans to treat dropsy (congestive heart failure). However, human experiments are lacking to support this contention. Further, the toxicity of the cucurbitacins must be taken into account when considering the use of squirting cucumber for any condition requiring long-term use, such as in dropsy.

We have found no experimental evidence that this plant would be useful in treating mania and melancholy,

Ecballium elaterium

as reported by some herbalists. In large doses, it would probably have an emetic effect due to the cucurbitacins, but experimental evidence to support this is lacking.

Cucurbitacin B, an extract isolated from the juice, showed significant anti-inflammatory activity in a 1988 animal study.

Ecballine, a compound derived from the fruits, is used in treating baldness as well as a cure against scalp diseases.

STAR ANISE
Illicium verum

Parts used: Fruit. *Used in Chinese medicine for centuries, this aromatic fruit is a satisfying carminative.*

TRADITIONAL USAGES

Star anise is both a culinary spice and a medicinal herb. It has a licorice-like flavor and is used to flavor various dishes, especially in Asian cuisine. Medicinally, it has been employed for digestive relief and reducing bloating and gas, and may have antimicrobial properties. Star anise is also a source of the compound shikimic acid, which is used in the production of antiviral medications.

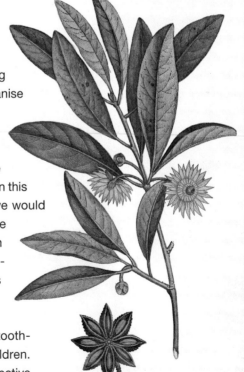

The fruit of the Chinese star anise is remarkable among the herbal remedies for its unusual appearance and its characteristic aroma. If we were to stumble upon this plant without being aware of its medicinal virtues, we would undoubtedly try it out. It has been employed in Chinese medicine for centuries, particularly to cure rheumatism and lumbago. The seeds and oil have stimulant, carminative, diuretic, and digestive properties; star anise is also used to soothe inflamed mucous membranes of the nasal passages.

In China, the seeds are applied locally to treat toothaches, while the essential oil is given for colic in children. Experimentally, alcoholic extracts of the fruit were effective against gram-positive and gram-negative bacteria and against twelve species of fungi.

Illicium verum

RECENT SCIENTIFIC FINDINGS

Star anise owes much of its therapeutic effect to the essential oil present in the fruits. About 90% or more of the essential oil is comprised of anethole, which produces a carminative and mild internal stimulant effect, if taken internally. Thus, there is ample justification for the use of star anise infusions or decoctions as a carminative or mild stimulant.

The fruit is now popularly employed in several commercial brands of herbal tea.

STROPHANTHUS

Strophanthus kombe, S. hispidus

Parts used: Seeds. *The seeds are a potent cardiac medicine similar to digitalis.*

TRADITIONAL USAGES

Strophanthus is a plant known for its seeds, which contain compounds that have been historically used in traditional medicine and as a source of cardiac glycosides. These compounds are employed to treat various heart conditions, particularly heart failure, and to increase cardiac contractility

Strophanthus was originally used by native people in the region of Lakes Tanganyika and Nyasa in Africa for arrow poison.

RECENT SCIENTIFIC FINDINGS

Strophanthus is formally recognized as a cardiac stimulant. Its action is very similar to that of digitalis, but it exerts its effect more rapidly, diminishes its action in less time, and does not reduce the pulse rate to the same levels as does digitalis. All parts of these two species, particularly the seeds, are known to contain cardiac glycosides quite similar in chemical structure and also in their effects on the body to the *Digitalis* glycosides. Strophanthus preparations thus exert a strengthening action on the heart by causing it to slow down and function with stronger force. This confirms the usage long reported in folklore. Strophanthus is less dependable than digitalis due to its irregular absorption through the intestinal tract. A reported side effect of strophanthus

Strophanthus kombe

is diarrhea, produced by increased peristalsis of the intestines. The plant was also felt to be a diuretic and has therefore been widely used in cases of chronic heart weakness coupled with dropsy (water retention).

Because it functions more rapidly than digitalis, Strophanthus is of great benefit during an emergency heart failure. In such cases, it has been administered intravenously by injection.

SUMAC
Rhus glabra

Parts used: Bark and fruit. *The berries contain high concentrations of tannins and are an excellent gargle for sore throats.*

TRADITIONAL USAGES
Of this genus, there are several species that possess poisonous properties and should be carefully distinguished from that here described. This species of *Rhus*, called variously smooth sumac, Pennsylvania sumac, and upland sumac, is an indigenous shrub from 4 to 12 feet high. The leaves are smooth petioles and consist of many pairs of opposite leaflets, with an odd one at the extremity, all of which are lanceolate, acuminate, acutely serrate, glabrous, and green on their upper surface and whitish beneath. In autumn, their color changes to a beautiful red. The flowers are greenish-red and disposed in large, erect, terminal, compound thyrses, which are succeeded by dusters of small crimson berries covered with a silky down.

Rhus glabra

Sumac berries were given as a gargle in decoction form and believed to be helpful during attacks of angina pain. The decoction was also gargled for throat irritations, or by people suffering from any inability to breathe easily, such as asthmatics. The high tannin content of the bitter berries made them valuable in the alleviation of diarrhea. The root was chewed by some North American tribes for mouth sores.

RECENT SCIENTIFIC FINDINGS
Sumac berries contain high concentrations of tannins, which as indicated previously have an astringent effect on mucous membranes. Thus, when water extracts of sumac

berries are used as a gargle, or applied to other mucous membranes, the medicinal effect that is experienced has a rational explanation.

Sumac is a group of flowering plants known for their vibrant red berries. While some species are used in culinary applications to add a tart, citrus-like flavor to dishes, in traditional medicine, sumac has been applied for its potential astringent and anti-inflammatory properties. It can be used topically to alleviate skin conditions.

SWEET FERN
Polypodium vulgare

Parts used: Root. *Its flavor lives up to its name.*

TRADITIONAL USAGES

Sweet fern is a North American shrub known for its aromatic leaves. These leaves have a history of use in herbal remedies, including as an herbal tea. Sweet fern tea is believed to have mild astringent and digestive properties and has been used traditionally to alleviate various gastrointestinal discomforts and skin irritations.

Not surprisingly, the taste of this fern is sweet; the rhizome is reminiscent of the licorice root in shape. Its medicinal virtues are rather mild, although it was lavishly praised by the ancients for melancholic conditions and visceral obstructions. While the resin is considered anthelmintic, sweet fern is also a useful purgative. Its demulcent properties prevent it from being a strong medicine. A very strong decoction is necessary for the expulsion of intestinal parasitic worms. Sweet fern is reportedly useful in alleviating coughs and other chest complaints and is a useful tonic in dyspepsia and loss of appetite.

RECENT SCIENTIFIC FINDINGS

Aqueous extracts of sweet fern root have produced central nervous system depressant activity.

Polypodium vulgare

TAMARIND

Tamarindus indica

Parts used: Fruit. *This refreshing fruit is one of nature's most gentle cathartics.*

TRADITIONAL USAGES

The Tamarind tree is the only species of this genus. Tamarind's medicinal and nonirritant properties were first discovered by Arab physicians. The Arabs imported tamarind stock from India to Europe, where it became extensively cultivated.

Mildly cathartic, tamarind has long been considered a beneficial addition to the convalescent diet. It is often mixed with senna and chocolate and administered to infants when a gentle cathartic is necessary. Tamarind is therefore a useful drink in feverish conditions, as well as being a popular cooking beverage in hot countries.

RECENT SCIENTIFIC FINDINGS

The pulp of the fruit contains citric, tartaric, and malic acids, which give it cooling properties. The fruit of tamarind owes its laxative, mild cathartic, and refrigerant effects almost totally to a high sugar concentration. The types of sugars are not absorbed to a high degree when in the intestinal tract. Because of this, they cause water to migrate from the surrounding tissues into the lumen of the intestines. This causes the intestines to expand, which results in a nonirritant type of bowel movement.

Tamarindus indica

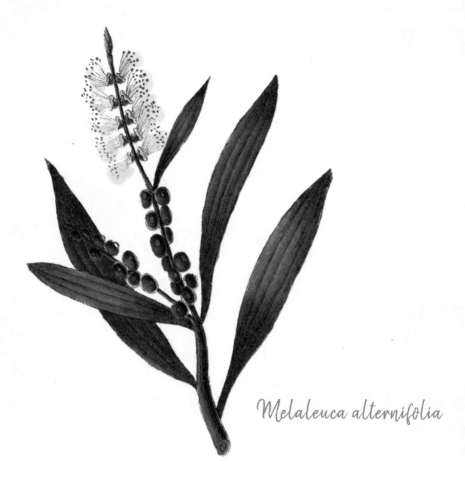

Melaleuca alternifolia

TEA TREE
Melaleuca alternifolia

Parts used: Leaf oil obtained from steam distillation. *This has become a very well-respected major ingredient in many preparations used to treat a variety of external skin complaints ranging from dandruff and herpes to acne and fungal infections.*

TRADITIONAL USAGES

The tea tree is native to Australia, where it was well respected for its many applications for a variety of ailments, most notably ailments affecting the skin. It was thought to be an antiseptic as well as an antifungal and to possess rejuvenating properties.

RECENT SCIENTIFIC FINDINGS

The active constituents of *Melaleuca* are cineole and terpinol. The balance of these two constituents determines the efficacy of the plant oil. It is desirable to have a cineole level below 15% and a terpinol level above 30% to achieve the best results. (The Australian government standard requirement mandates these specifications as well.)

Aching muscles, diaper rash, sore throat, gingivitis, burns, heat rash, acne, ear infections (antiseptic), cuts and abrasions, mouth ulcers, athlete's foot, yeast infections (antifungal), dandruff, sunburns, and sinus and bronchial congestion—all are among the list of potential validated scientific applications of *Melaleuca*.

Tea tree is celebrated for its essential oil, which offers exceptional antibacterial and antifungal properties. The oil extracted from the tea tree is highly regarded for its wide range of applications in skin care and aromatherapy. Renowned for its natural efficacy in addressing skin concerns, tea tree oil is a popular choice for combating issues like acne, fungal infections, and other dermatological conditions, contributing to improved overall well-being.

THYME
Thymus vulgaris

Parts used: Herb. *This common spice contains thymol, which has disinfectant and anti-inflammatory properties.*

TRADITIONAL USAGES

This popular spice has also been used as a medicinal since ancient times. The Greeks Pliny, Dioscorides, and Theophrastus all make reference to this tasty herb.

It has been utilized for coughs, bronchitis, asthma, and whooping cough; for flatulence; for colic in infants; to produce sweating to break a fever; for anemia; and for all kinds of stomach upsets.

The oil, applied locally to carious teeth, has been used as a means of relieving toothaches. The herb has also been employed as an antiseptic against tooth decay.

Thymus vulgaris

Externally, the leaves have been applied in fomentation (cloth or towels dipped in infusion or decoction and applied locally) for aches and pains.

RECENT SCIENTIFIC FINDINGS

The active principle, a simple terpene, thymol or thymic acid, has been shown to have disinfectant properties equal to those of carbolic acid. Thymol has been shown to have antiseptic value and expectorant and bronchodilator effects in animal as well as human experiments. Thymol additionally releases entrapped gas in the stomach and relaxes the smooth muscle of that organ. This explains the use of thyme to alleviate the symptoms of colic and flatulence.

Externally, thymol and thymol-containing plants act as rubefacients. That is, thymol causes an increased blood flow to the area of application, which then results in relief of inflammation and pain.

Thyme, a versatile herb with a fragrant aroma and a warm, earthy flavor, is a beloved culinary favorite in many cuisines around the world. Beyond its culinary applications, thyme has garnered attention for its potential medicinal properties. It has a rich history of use in traditional medicine, where it is believed to support respiratory health by relieving coughs and congestion. Thyme is valued for its antioxidant properties, which may help combat oxidative stress and promote overall wellness.

TOADFLAX

Linaria vulgaris

Parts used: Herb and leaves. *This was once used for a variety of ailments.*

TRADITIONAL USAGES

A very common herb, toadflax was valued for its external and internal usages. To treat hemorrhoids, a poultice or fomentation of the fresh plant was applied locally. This method was used on various skin diseases. In addition, the flowers were sometimes mixed with vegetable oils to make a liniment.

Taken internally, an infusion of the leaves was used to eliminate kidney stones, the effects being diuretic and cathartic. This remedy was often given to treat dropsy and jaundice, being a favored herb for disorders of the pneumo-gastric region.

Linaria vulgaris

Toadflax is an enchanting wildflower that graces gardens with its colorful blossoms. While not as commonly used in contemporary herbalism, some herbal practitioners have explored the use of toadflax for its potential soothing properties. Its delicate flowers and leaves contain various natural compounds, some of which are believed to have mild calming and anti-inflammatory effects. Toadflax may be employed in infusions, tinctures, or poultices, with the aim of addressing minor discomforts or skin irritations.

TORMENTIL
Potentilla tormentilla, P. erecta

Parts used: Root. *The roots' high concentrations of tannins make them a powerful astringent.*

TRADITIONAL USAGES

Tormentil is a powerful astringent and has been used primarily to treat diarrhea and hemorrhage. Additionally, it was considered by the ancients to promote sweating and was thought helpful in curing plague. It was administered to treat syphilis, fevers, smallpox, measles, and a vast list of other disorders. As a treatment for warts, a piece of linen was soaked in a strong decoction of tormentil, placed on the wart, and repeated frequently until success was achieved. The decoction was also gargled to cure mouth ulcers and spongy gums. The herbalists Gerard and Culpepper both employed tormentil for toothache, comparing it favorably with cloves. In Europe, a tincture is frequently utilized for intestinal disorders and in brandy for stomach disorders.

As is the case with most strong astringents, the root was also utilized for tanning leather, in this case in the Orkney Islands of Scotland. The masticated root was used to dye leather red by the Laplanders.

Potentilla tormentilla

RECENT SCIENTIFIC FINDINGS

The dried root contains chinovin, tormentilic acid, and chinova acid. However, the antidiarrhetic and antidysenteric effect of this perennial herb is due to the astringent and mildly antiseptic action of the tannins present in the rhizomes of virtually all *Potentilla* species.

Tormentil is recognized for its astringent properties, which have earned it a respected place in the realm of herbal medicine. Its historical use revolves around addressing issues related to digestion and mucous membrane health. Often, it has been used to soothe digestive discomfort and alleviate symptoms associated with conditions like diarrhea. The herb's astringent qualities are believed to help tighten and tone tissues, contributing to its potential for gastrointestinal relief.

TURMERIC
Curcuma longa

Parts used: Rhizome. *This common spice of Indian cuisine may be a potent antimutagenic agent.*

TRADITIONAL USAGES

The wisdom of ethnic diets continues to amaze me. Time-tested, authentic ethnic foods and food combinations evolved slowly and would not have survived as part of a culture were it not for the health benefits experienced through trial and error. In the case of East Indian cuisine, it has long been the unique use and preparation of freshly ground seasonings that set these dishes apart; the *vasana*, or aroma, of food is key.

Turmeric, ginger, pepper, and chili are the major spices found in Indian food. But the list of all the spices used is quite large: cardamon, cloves, cinnamon, mace, nutmeg, saffron, various peppers, dill, cumin, fennel, bay leaf, mustard, coriander, and, of course, garlic.

The turmeric rhizome, or underground rootlike stem, is also widely utilized in traditional medical systems, mainly for treating various inflammatory conditions such as arthritis. In Ayurvedic medicine, turmeric was prized for its aromatic, stimulant, and carminative properties.

RECENT SCIENTIFIC FINDINGS

Currently, in India, turmeric is used to treat anorexia and liver disorders, as well as to alleviate coughs and reduce inflammation. Modern science is now confirming what traditional healers have known for centuries, which includes its effectiveness in managing diabetic wounds and rheumatism, and the use of fresh juice from the rhizome to

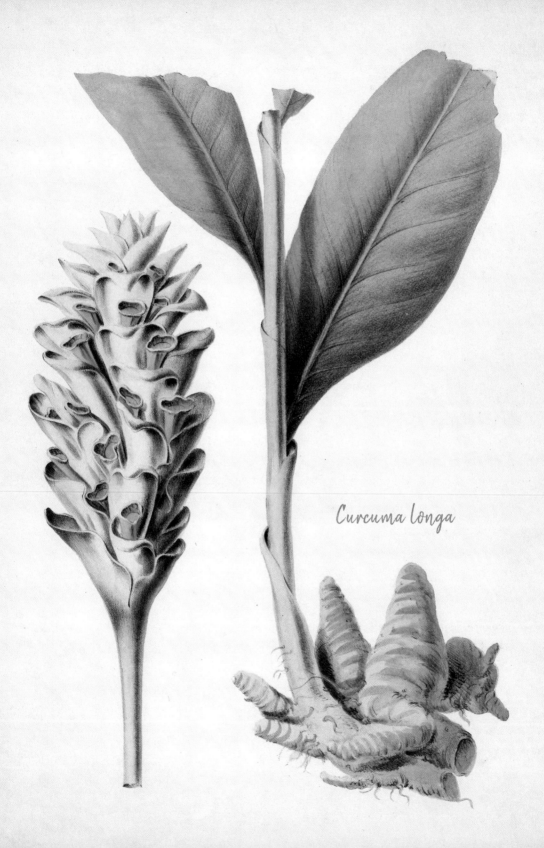

Curcuma longa

Turmeric, a vibrant yellow spice derived from the root of Curcuma longa, is celebrated for its versatile culinary applications and an impressive array of potential health benefits.

reduce inflammation. In one study, tumeric extract was tested for its anticarcinogenic and antimutagenic properties. Laboratory (nonhuman) experiments found that this ancient spice reduced both the number of tumors in mice and the mutagenicity of benzo[a]pyrene (BP) and two other potent mutagens, NPD and DMBA.

Preventing cancer now receives the attention it has long deserved. Numerous biochemical and epidemiological studies have demonstrated diet's role in modulating the development of cancer. Laboratory experiments have established that the active principle of turmeric (curcumin) is a potent antimutagenic agent.

For those interested in how curcumin may act to prevent cancer, we turn again to the by now all-pervasive theory of free-radical inactivation. The test carcinogens BP and DMBA are metabolically activated to proximate mutagenic/carcinogenic epoxides, which then bind to macromolecules. One study's authors concluded that since curcumin is a potent antioxidant, it may scavenge the epoxides and prevent binding to macro-swelling in recent bruises, wounds, and insect bites, and that the dried powdered root kills parasites and relieves head colds and arthritic aches. (Interestingly, this spice has sometimes been used to adulterate ginger.) A 1991 pharmacological review confirmed many of turmeric's folkloric effects, including wound healing, gastric mucus protection, antispasmodic activity, reduction of intestinal gas formation, protection of liver cells, increasing bile production, diminishing platelet aggregation (i.e., blood clumping), lowering serum cholesterol (at very high doses), antibacterial properties, antifungal properties, and potential antitumor activity. While most of these effects were demonstrated with intravenous extracts in animals, they do parallel folkloric claims in humans and are not to be dismissed as "experimental" or "trivial." Turmeric's benefits for arthritis treatment have been demonstrated in human clinical trials. An herbal formula of turmeric, ashwagandha, and boswellin was evaluated in a randomized, double-blind, placebo-controlled study. In other words, this spice's cell-protective properties are similar to nutrient antioxidants like vitamins C and E, which inhibit free radical reactions.

This type of herb is known as a nonsteroidal anti-inflammatory drug (NSAID). Curcumin inhibits cyclooxygenase and lipoxygenase enzymes. Curcumin has three main mechanisms of action: (1) antioxidant activity, (2) lipoxygenase inhibition, and (3) cyclo-oxygenase inhibition. By inhibiting the associated biochemical pathways, month evaluation period 12 patients with osteoarthritis were given the herbal formula or placebo for three months. The patients were evaluated every two weeks. After a 15-day wash-out period, the treatment was reversed with the placebo patients receiving the drug and vice versa. Again, results were evaluated over a three-month period. The patients treated with the herbal formula showed a significant drop in severity of pain and disability score.

Turmeric, a vibrant yellow spice derived from the root of *Curcuma longa*, is celebrated for its versatile culinary applications and an impressive array of potential health benefits. Beyond its culinary prowess, turmeric is renowned for its anti-inflammatory and antioxidant properties. Curcumin, the active compound in turmeric, is believed to reduce inflammation and oxidative stress, making it an attractive option for promoting overall well-being and potentially addressing chronic health issues.

TURPENTINE TREE

Pistacia terebinthus and *Pinus, Abies*, and *Larix* spp.

Parts used: Sap. *At one time, "spirits of turpentine" were used as everything from an expectorant to an ointment for rheumatism.*

TRADITIONAL USAGES

The term "turpentine" is now generally applied to certain vegetable juices, liquid, or concrete that consist of resin combined with a peculiar essential oil called oil of turpentine. They are generally procured from different species of pine, though other trees afford products known by the same general title, such as *Pistacia terebinthus*, which yields Chian turpentine.

Pistacia terebinthus is the terebinth, a small tree native to Greece. It flourished in the islands of Cyprus and Chios, the latter giving its name to the turpentine obtained from the tree. The annual production of Chian turpentine was very small. Therefore, the turpentine commanded a high price and very little of it reached North America. It is frequently adulterated with other less costly coniferous turpentines.

White turpentine is the common American variety and is procured chiefly from *Pinus palustris,* partly also from *Pinus taeda* and some other species inhabiting the Southern states. In former times, large quantities were collected in New England. However, the turpentine trees of that area have been largely exhausted, and more recently other parts of the United States have been the source of supply.

"Spirits of turpentine" is the volatile oil distilled with water from the concrete oleoresin. This oil (or "spirit") is locally irritant and feebly antiseptic. It was commonly employed as a stimulating expectorant. As it irritated the mucous membranes, it helped to expel phlegm and was a useful treatment in bronchitis. It stimulates kidney function and was sometimes used in mild doses as a diuretic; in large doses, it is dangerous to the kidneys. It was used as a carminative and was considered one of the most valuable remedies for flatulent colic. Terebinth was also utilized to treat chronic diarrhea and dysentery, typhoid fever, internal hemorrhage, purpureal fever and bleeding, helminthiasis, leucorrhea, and amenorrhea. Turpentine baths, arranged in such a way that the vapors were not inhaled by the patient, were given in cases of chronic rheumatism. Applied externally as a liniment or ointment, it has been used in rheumatic ailments such as lumbago, arthritis, and neuralgias. It was also applied locally to treat and promote the healing of burns and to heal parasitic skin diseases.

RECENT SCIENTIFIC FINDINGS

Unfortunately, research has not been conducted to confirm or deny turpentine's folkloric claims.

Pistacia terebinthus

VALERIAN
Valeriana officinalis

Parts used: Root. *Used since antiquity, this root may be our safest and most effective tranquilizer.*

TRADITIONAL USAGES

Valerian is a popular herb celebrated for its soothing and calming effects. It is often employed in the world of herbal remedies and natural supplements to alleviate stress and anxiety, as well as to promote relaxation and improve sleep quality. Valerian root, known for its distinct aroma, is a time-honored choice for those seeking natural remedies to ease nervous tension and support emotional well-being.

The fresh pulverized roots were applied directly to injured areas, while the dried root was utilized as an antiseptic powder.

Valerian root has been used since ancient times in the treatment of epilepsy, particularly when the seizures are brought on by emotions such as fear and anger. Warriors of the Thompson tribe made several different preparations of American valerian to treat wounds. The fresh pulverized roots were applied directly to injured areas, while the dried root was utilized as an antiseptic powder. In more recent times, valerian has been employed as a stimulant and antispasmodic. Combined with cinchona, it has been given to treat intermittent fevers.

Valerian has been used as a tranquilizing agent since antiquity. It is all too tempting to observe the present frequency of tranquilizer use as indicative of doomed, exhausted populations crushed by machine civilization. Surely the pace and noise of present life create tension in biological man, but what do you make of this curious entry, recorded in 1831 by Samuel Thomson, a practicing botanic family physician.

"This powder [Valerian] is the best nervine known; I have made great use of it and have always found it to produce the most beneficial effects, in all cases of nervous affection, and in hysterical symptoms; in fact, it would be difficult to get along with my practice in many cases without this important article."

Apparently, even then, nervousness was a complaint all too frequently brought before the attention of healers. Thomson recommended half a teaspoon in hot water, sweetened, to promote sleep and leave the patient at ease.

Valeriana officinalis

> *Valerian root has been used since ancient times in the treatment of epilepsy, particularly when the seizures are brought on by emotions such as fear and anger.*

RECENT SCIENTIFIC FINDINGS

In an age of anxiety, when tranquilizing agents reign supreme, it may be wise to reconsider the natural sedatives. Of the many plants employed to calm nervous patients, quiet hysteria, or allay the fears of hypochondriacs, none seems to come forward with such recommendations as this root.

Valerian is clearly a non-narcotic, perfectly safe herbal sedative, highly recommended in anxiety states. While the unground dried root is presently available in most herb stores and very popular (the powdered root is much more potent than the chipped bark), most users are experiencing only a trace, or a remnant of the effects of the fresh root, which is far more potent.

The roots of valerian contain a complex mixture of substances known as valepotriates, which are known to have sedative and tranquilizing properties. Other important chemical constituents, known as esters, are unstable and are lost during the drying process. For this reason, the drug's effects vary considerably, so much so that physicians had largely abandoned it by the end of the 19th century.

A far more potent action is had by using the juice of the fresh root, in dosages of 1 to 3 tablespoonfuls. Of course, in Europe, valerian tincture is freely available and a very popular natural "tranquilizer."

As expected, a remedy so prevalent in ancient and recent usage has proven itself under the sometimes too caustic rituals of the modern pharmacologist. Petkov and associates in Bulgaria recently demonstrated that an extract of the root has central nervous system sedative effects and the ability to steady an arrhythmic heart in lab animals.

Perhaps more interesting is Cavazzuti's work in Italy, which demonstrated that a mixture of valerian, passionflower, chamomile, hawthorn (fluid extract), sucrose, and orange essence was effective in treating children "one- to twelve-year-olds with psychomotor agitation and non-adaptation disorders." By the all too infrequently applied double-blind method (rarely applied in evaluating herbs), this herbal mixture displayed genuine effects in treating hyperactivity and insomnia. Unlike other hyper-activity medications, valerian showed no side effects.

Another research team performed a double-blind study of valerian's effect on poor sleep. Of the patients given the valerian preparation, 44% reported perfect sleep and 99% reported improved sleep. Again, no side effects were observed.

Caution: Valerian may produce sensations of "strangeness" in some individuals. These people should not use valerian.

WALL GERMANDER
Teucrium chamaedrys

Parts used: Tops and leaves. *This was once a major ingredient of a popular patented medicine, Portland Powder.*

TRADITIONAL USAGES

Wall germander was recommended by ancient herbalists for its vulnerary properties (ability to heal wounds) and continues to be a folk remedy for ulcers and sores. It is also recommended for general use as a tonic for digestion. Other ailments that have reportedly been treated with this plant are anemia, asthma, bronchitis, and other chronic respiratory diseases.

It is an astringent, antiseptic, diuretic, and stimulant, and has been used in the treatment of jaundice, dropsy, gout, and ailments of the spleen. The Egyptians utilized the plant for treating intermittent fevers; interestingly, it was given as a preventive, the dose being taken one hour in advance of the parox-ysm that was known to reoccur at four-hour intervals.

At one time, this herb was part of a popular patented medicine for the treatment of gout and arthritis, known as Portland Powder, which contained equal parts *Aristolochia rotunda* root, *Gentiana lutea* root, tops and leaves of germander and *Erythroea centaurium,* and leaves of *Ajuga chamaepitys,* the ground pine.

RECENT SCIENTIFIC FINDINGS

Studies on a closely related species, *Teucrium polium,* showed anti-inflammatory action.

Teucrium chamaedrys

WALNUT (Black)

Juglans nigra

Parts used: Hulls and inner bark. *This tree's inner bark has long been valued as a mild laxative, while researchers have also found it lowers blood pressure.*

TRADITIONAL USAGES

Known in different sections of the U.S. by the various names of butternut, oilnut, and white walnut, the inner bark and the root are the medicinal portions. Walnut root was formerly recommended in the *U.S. Pharmacopoeia.* It should be collected in May or June.

On the living tree, the inner bark when first uncovered is a pure white, which, on exposure, immediately becomes a beautiful lemon color and ultimately changes to deep brown. It has a fibrous texture, a feeble odor, and a peculiar bitter, somewhat acrid taste. Its medical virtues are entirely extracted by boiling water. Gathered in the autumn, the bark contains resins, juglandin, jugloine, juglandic acid, and essential oil.

The bark has been valued as one of the mildest and most certain laxatives given us by nature; it operates without causing nausea, irritation, or pain, and does not impair the digestive function. During the Revolutionary War, it was commonly used as a habitual laxative and was also considered quite valuable in the treatment of liver disorders.

The Menominees ate the syrup of white walnut, or butternut, as a remedy for digestive disorders. A tea from the inner bark was drunk by the Potawatomis for upset stomach, while the Meskwakis used a tea as a mild laxative.

The common European walnut, *J. regia,* is also used medicinally. The hull of the fruit has been utilized as a vermifuge and as a treatment for syphilis and ulcers, and the oil of the fruit is reportedly antiparasitic and has cured tapeworm, as

Juglans nigra

well as being employed as a laxative. The Chinese employed this plant to treat asthma, lumbago, beriberi, impotence, and constipation.

Information on the effectiveness of walnut preparations for hepatic congestion has not been found in the scientific literature. However, folkloric use for liver complaints is reported.

RECENT SCIENTIFIC FINDINGS

The inner root owes all of its pharmacologic effect either to the presence of tannins or the simple quinone compound juglone. These have astringent, antiseptic, and vermifuge properties, especially juglone.

The chemical constituents are iron, iodine, calcium, silica, the quinone juglone, tannins, and ellagic acid. Using large doses, researchers at the University of Missouri in the 1960s found that ellagic acid paradoxically both lowered blood pressure and prevented other agents from lowering blood pressure. This same group of researchers also found that several constituents of black walnut had anticancer properties.

Based on data from mice experiments, the alkaloid fraction of black walnut may prevent tumor formation (specifically in mammary glands).

Black walnut is a tree renowned for its rich, earthy flavor. While its nuts are used in culinary applications, the hulls of black walnuts have been associated with potential health benefits. These hulls are believed to have properties that support digestion and enhance immune function. Black walnut's historical significance and potential health properties make it a valuable addition to the world of herbal remedies and culinary traditions.

WATER LILY

Nymphaea alba and other *Nymphaea* species

Parts used: Rhizome. *These beautiful flowers were once used to treat a variety of skin problems.*

TRADITIONAL USAGES

Water lily, with its elegant floating blooms, adds a touch of beauty to ponds and aquatic environments. The roots of water lily, known as rhizomes, have been used in traditional herbal concoctions for their potential health benefits. These remedies often focus on addressing issues related to the digestive system, such as diarrhea and inflammation. The rhizomes are typically prepared by drying and then grinding them into a fine powder, which can be used in teas, tinctures, or other herbal formulations.

The roots of water lily, known as rhizomes, have been used in traditional herbal concoctions for their potential health benefits.

Although all colors of water lilies were employed in folk medicine, the white water lily in particular was valued, due to its purity, rising out of the often-murky marsh, stream, or pond.

It was used as an anaphrodisiac (depress the sexual function). This concept most likely originated with the romantic notion of the purity of the flower rising from the muck more than any true folkloric belief in such abilities. This power was likely attributed only to the white *Nymphaea.*

Externally, white and yellow water lilies were used to treat various skin disorders, such as boils, inflammation, tumors, and ulcers. It was also employed for diabetes. The rootstocks contain much starch, useful as a food in emergencies.

A 1989 article maintains the water lily was used by the ancient Egyptians as an integral part of shamanistic healing. The author argues that water lily and mandrake were used to induce a shamanistic trance and used both medicinally and ritualistically.

RECENT SCIENTIFIC FINDINGS
No research exists to support the folkloric claims for water lily.

Nymphaea alba

WHEATGRASS or Couch Grass

Agropyron spp.

Parts used: Root and rhizome. *For centuries, herbalists have employed this plant to treat urinary tract disorders.*

TRADITIONAL USAGES

Dogs and cats, when they are ill, will seek out and eat this plant in preference to other field grasses. The roots possess both diuretic and demulcent properties, and have been used by herbalists for centuries to treat inflammation of the bladder, frequent or painful urination, blood in the urine, and other urinary tract diseases.

An old home remedy for coughing, the roasted rootstocks have also long been utilized as a coffee substitute and as a source of bread in times of famine.

RECENT SCIENTIFIC FINDINGS

The roots of couch grass contain mucilage, which accounts for the plant's soothing and demulcent action on mucous membranes. Animal studies in Romania showed that couch grass rhizome preparations had a diuretic effect in rats. In Tanzania, researchers found strong central nervous system depressant activity in mice.

Water extracts of the roots of *A. repens* have been studied in laboratory animals, and when administered orally give rise to pronounced diuretic effects. In addition, the extracts are known to have antibiotic effects against a variety of bacteria and molds.

Couch grass is very valuable in disorders of the kidneys and bladder and in urinary troubles that originate with colds or catarrhal inflammation of these organs. It induces the proper flow of the urine and tends to relieve painful, scanty, but frequent urination. Its blood-purifying properties are also quite pronounced.

Wheatgrass, the young shoots of the wheat plant, is a nutritional powerhouse. Often juiced to harness its nutrient-rich properties, wheatgrass is highly regarded for its exceptional nutrient content, which includes a wide array of vitamins, minerals, antioxidants, and

Agropyron spp.

essential amino acids. It is a rich source of vitamins A, C, E, and K, as well as essential minerals like iron, magnesium, calcium, and potassium. Notably, it is one of the best dietary sources of chlorophyll, a green pigment that plays a crucial role in photosynthesis and is associated with various health benefits. Chlorophyll, the prominent component in wheatgrass, is believed to help the body detoxify by neutralizing toxins and promoting the elimination of harmful substances. This detoxification process is thought to support liver health and boost the immune system.

WILLOW (White)
Salix alba

Parts used: Bark. *For centuries, willow bark has been revered as one of the safest and most effective means for pain relief and lowering fevers.*

TRADITIONAL USAGES

Most of the willows have been utilized for their pain-relieving and fever-lowering properties since antiquity. Ancient Egyptian, Assyrian, and Greek texts refer to willow bark; the Greek physicians Hippocrates and Dioscorides (circa A.D. 60) used it to combat pain and fevers.

Willows were employed throughout their range of growth in the United States. The Pomos boiled the inner root bark of the California willow and drank the resulting tea to promote sweating in cases of chills and fever. In the South, the Natchez used red willow bark in their fever remedies, while the Alabama and Creeks plunged into willow root steam baths to alleviate fever. The use of willow is also reported among tribes from the Pima of Arizona to the Penobscots of Maine. In the mid-1700s, the bark enjoyed immense popularity in colonial America as a fever treatment.

For thousands of years, people were known to chew the leaves or inner bark of willows or other shrubs in the spirea subfamily of plants. All of these contain salicylic acid; in 1838, using willow bark, Raffaele Piria prepared the first pure form of salicylic acid. As obtained from various species of willow, salicin was official in the *U.S. Pharmacopoeia* from 1882 to 1926. Salicylic acid was used to produce acetylsalicylic acid, which was dubbed aspirin (a-spirin) to denote that it did not utilize plants from the spirea sub-family.

RECENT SCIENTIFIC FINDINGS

Willow bark contains salicin, which probably decomposes into salicylic acid in the human system. The structural formulas for acetylsalicylic acid (aspirin) and salicylic

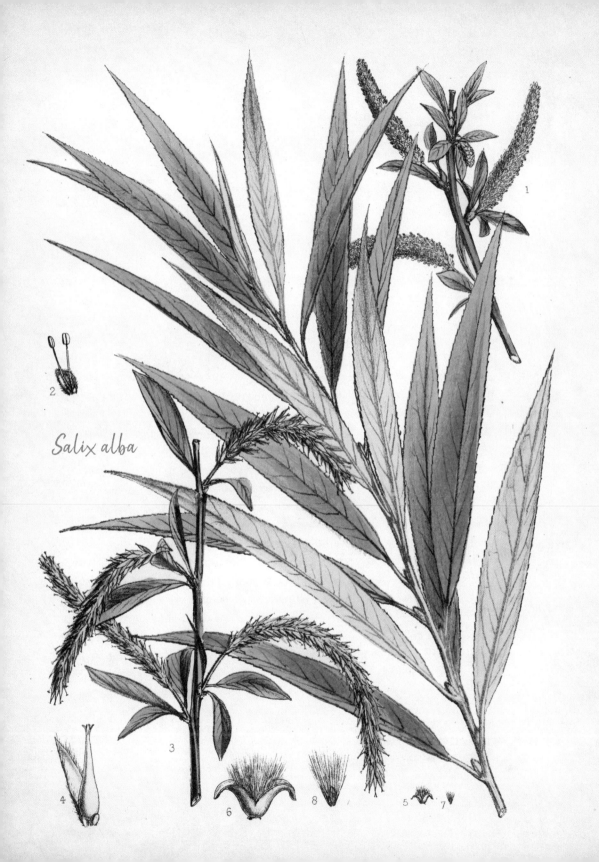

Salix alba

1

2

3

4

6

8

5   7

Most of the willows have been utilized for their pain-relieving and fever-lowering properties since antiquity.

acid are quite similar. Aspirin-like compounds, the nonsteroidal anti-inflammatories (NSAIDs), have been found to inhibit the manufacture of certain prostaglandins (PGs) from their precursor, the fatty acid arachidonic acid (AA). Prostaglandins play a key role in the regulation of immune function.

Aspirin is a prostaglandin (PGE2) inhibitor. When we take aspirin, or similar compounds, we may stimulate our immune system by blocking PGE2 production. Although salicylic acid is only a weak cyclooxygenase inhibitor, its potency within the body is about equal to aspirin. It is speculated that salicin (from willow) does not cause gastric or intestinal upset or bleeding because, unlike acetylsalicylic acid (aspirin), this natural product does not block prostaglandins in the stomach or intestine. Instead, salicin bypasses the stomach or intestine and does not have prostaglandin-blocking effects until it reaches the liver, where the acetyl group is metabolically picked up.

It should be noted, though, that the immune system is not a one-way path. Both enhancement and suppression of immunological functions have been reported for PGs! For the sake of this small discussion, it is sufficient to note that PGs and the metabolites of AA are involved in immune reactions.

Aspirin is now receiving wide usage to prevent heart attacks in men over 50. This may be due to the fact that cyclooxygenase inhibitors prevent platelet aggregation or blood clots. The spread of tumor cells is also thought to be associated with platelet clumping. Several tumor cell types can aggregate platelets and form a metastasis. So, along with preventing heart attacks, the aspirin-like compounds, including salicin, may also help prevent the spread of cancer.

White willow is esteemed for its natural salicylic acid content. One of the most renowned attributes of white willow is its natural salicylic acid content. Salicylic acid, a compound with anti-inflammatory and pain-relieving properties, is the active ingredient in aspirin. White willow's historical use as a pain reliever, fever reducer, and anti-inflammatory agent is well-documented. White willow's analgesic properties have made it a popular choice for alleviating various types of discomfort, including headaches, muscle pain, and joint pain. It is often preferred by those who seek natural alternatives to over-the-counter pain relievers.

In addition to its pain-relieving properties, white willow is known for its potential benefits in reducing fever, which has earned it a place in traditional remedies for managing febrile conditions. White willow's anti-inflammatory effects have also led to its application in managing chronic conditions associated with inflammation, such as arthritis. Regular use of white willow may help reduce joint pain and stiffness.

WINTERGREEN
Gaultheria procumbens

Parts used: Leaves and flowering tops. *This aromatic herb is still listed in the U.S. Pharmacopoeia for its astringent, diuretic, and stimulant properties.*

TRADITIONAL USAGES
Wintergreen is an aromatic herb celebrated for its sweet, minty flavor. Its essential oil is used in various applications, including flavoring candies and offering soothing relief for muscle and joint discomfort.

The name "wintergreen" has been ascribed to many different plants, including *Pyrola, Chimaphila,* and *Moneses.* However, *Gaultheria* is the most popular in domestic American medicine. Henry David Thoreau describes imbibing the leaves as a tea prepared by his Native American guide. The Montagnais of Labrador and southeastern Canada drank wintergreen tea to treat paralysis.

An old favorite, wintergreen tea is diuretic in small doses; large doses are emetic. It is an aromatic stimulant with astringent properties, and consequently is of assistance in cases of chronic diarrhea. It has been used to promote menstruation and increase milk production in nursing mothers. Oil of wintergreen has been used as an external application, in the form of cloths soaked in the aromatic liquid and tied to the painful part, in the treatment of body aches and pains. Wintergreen leaves were official in the *U.S. Pharmacopoeia* from 1820 to 1894. Oil of wintergreen is still listed for its astringent, diuretic, and stimulant properties.

RECENT SCIENTIFIC FINDINGS
Some of the medicinal actions can be explained on the basis of the methyl salicylate contained in the oil, which is closely related to acetylsalicylic acid, or aspirin.

Gaultheria procumbens

WITCH HAZEL
Hamamelis virginiana

Parts used: Bark, twigs, and leaves. *Once ascribed occult powers, this plant is an ingredient in many cosmetic face creams and lotions.*

TRADITIONAL USAGES

This plant was named by those who ascribed occult powers to it. The forked branches were used as divining rods to find water and gold.

North American tribes used this shrub as a sedative application to external inflammations, and so we inherited yet another valuable gift of nature from the Indigenous Americans. A decoction of boiled twigs was employed as a cure for aching backs. The Potawatomi treated muscular aches with a steam created by placing the twigs in water with hot rocks. In 1744, it was observed that the Mohawks treated bruised eyes with a wash of steeped witch hazel bark. In 1850, the American Medical Association listed witch hazel as a treatment for eye inflammations, internal hemorrhages, and piles. Witch hazel leaves were listed in the *U.S. Pharmacopoeia* from 1862 through 1916 and in the *National Formulary* from 1916 to 1955.

Internally, it was at one time recommended as a fluid extract in the treatment of varicose veins and internal bleeding. Itching hemorrhoids were treated with a soothing ointment made of lard and a decoction of apple tree bark, witch hazel bark, and white oak bark.

RECENT SCIENTIFIC FINDINGS

Witch hazel is utilized today largely as described here, and as a liniment for body aches and pains. Witch hazel extracts contain astringent tannins that explain the beneficial effects of water extract in reducing inflammation when applied externally. Commercially available "witch hazel extract," however, does not contain tannins. When the extract is prepared, the plant is mixed with water and distilled. The distillate is a clear, colorless liquid having an aromatic odor. It contains a mixture of aromatic substances

Hamamelis virginiana

that have not been well studied. Yet, that this extract is soothing and refreshing when applied externally can be verified by anyone who has used it.

Many cosmetic face creams and lotions contain witch hazel.

Witch hazel is valued for its astringent properties. It is commonly found in skin care products due to its potential to soothe and tone the skin, making it a staple in the realm of natural skin care. Native to North America, witch hazel is a deciduous shrub known for its striking, spidery yellow flowers and its distinctive seed capsules that "explode" when mature, propelling the seeds some distance from the parent plant. One of the primary traditional uses of witch hazel is in its role as an astringent. Astringents are substances that cause the contraction of tissues, and witch hazel is particularly effective in this regard. It has been used for various skin conditions, including soothing minor irritations, bug bites, and burns. Witch hazel's astringent properties are also valuable for toning the skin, minimizing the appearance of pores, and reducing inflammation, making it a popular ingredient in many skin care products. The herb is rich in tannins, which contribute to its astringent properties. Tannins help to tighten and tone the skin, which can be especially beneficial for those with oily or acne-prone skin. Witch hazel is also recognized for its potential anti-inflammatory properties, which further enhance its use in skin care and as a home remedy for common skin issues. It is often employed to relieve itching and inflammation associated with conditions like eczema, psoriasis, and dermatitis.

WOLFSBANE
Aconitum napellus

Parts used: Root. *Also known as aconite, this plant was adopted by conventional medicine from homeopathic practitioners.*

TRADITIONAL USAGES

Wolfsbane, or aconite, possesses sedative, anodyne, diuretic, and inflammation-reducing properties. But in overdose, it and all its relatives are swift and fatal poisons. Nevertheless, in 1762, a Viennese physician, Baron Storck, published experiments proving the value of this plant in the materia medica, claiming success in treating gout, rheumatism, intermittent fevers, and scrofulous swellings.

By the time the twentieth edition of the *Dispensatory of the United States* was issued (1918), aconite was recognized as a valuable circulatory sedative in heart problems, since it reduced excessive heart action and decreased arterial tension.

Concomitant with the reduction of blood pressure, aconite was also noted for its ability to induce sweating.

Aconite is a highly valued homeopathic remedy; in fact, it originally crossed over into regular medicine from homeopathic practice as a substitute for the widespread and sometimes fatal practice of bloodletting that prevailed through the 19th century. Homeopathic practitioners also used aconite in the treatment of pains, to promote a sense of calm, and, parallel to the observations of the *Dispensatory of the United States,* to produce and increase perspiration.

Used externally as a liniment, the plant has proved useful in the treatment of neuralgia and rheumatic pains.

RECENT SCIENTIFIC FINDINGS

The active principle, aconitine, was discovered in 1833. Although it is exceedingly toxic in even very small quantities, there have been reports of people being able to eat the boiled leaves without harm. We cannot substantiate, however, that boiling destroys the fatally dangerous principle, and it should be noted that a decoction of this herb was employed to execute the condemned in early times.

It is well known that the leaves and roots of wolfsbane contain very potent alkaloids that have been studied in animals and are known to produce sedative and painkilling effects. However, the amount of these alkaloids that will produce these effects is nearly the same as the amount that will produce serious poisonous effects. Thus, one must be cautioned that wolfsbane is a potentially dangerous plant when considered for any use in humans. An overdose will cause adverse effects on the heart (fibrillations).

Aconitum napellus

WOOD BETONY
Betonica officinalis

Parts used: Leaves and root. *Once a very popular remedy, this is now a flavoring for herbal teas.*

TRADITIONAL USAGES

Highly esteemed by the ancients, betony was extolled as a remedy for a wide variety of ailments. The root is both emetic and purgative. It was also used to expel intestinal worms.

The leaves are quite mild, possessing aperient (mildly laxative), cordial, aromatic, and astringent properties. A tea brewed from the plant has been used in the treatment of stomach disorders, gout, headaches, and disorders of the spleen. An infusion was a popular remedy for bladder and kidney problems.

RECENT SCIENTIFIC FINDINGS

Betony's major use today is not as a medicinal but as a flavoring agent in herbal tea blending. It is thought to be a valuable nervine by some people in the herbal tea industry.

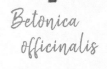

Betonica officinalis

Animal experiments have shown antihypertensive activity and an antihistamine effect (SRSA antagonist).

Wood betony is an herb that has a history of use in herbal remedies. It is primarily known for its potential benefits in relieving headaches and nervous tension.

WORMWOOD or Qinghao
Artemisia spp.

Parts used: Leaves and flowering tops. *This has long been utilized to invigorate the internal organs, and modern research reveals additional uses for this member of the rose family.*

TRADITIONAL USAGES

Wormwood was formerly utilized in several ways, the most important being as an anthelmintic (to expel tapeworms and other intestinal worms), hence the common name for the plant. It was considered a powerful local anesthetic and has been applied externally to relieve rheumatic pains, as well as for sprains, bruises, and local irritations. Taken internally, it was additionally utilized as a tonic and cathartic. Various Native American tribes employed wormwood for bronchial ailments. Before the introduction of quinine (cinchona bark), it was highly regarded as a remedy in intermittent fevers.

In Chinese medicine, sweet wormwood (*A. annua*) has been written about since 168 B.C. and is prescribed for "summer colds," malaria, and "heat excess"; in other words, as an antipyretic, to reduce fevers. It is not used to kill parasites.

Near relatives *A. indica* and *A. chinensis* were utilized in China to produce moxas. These agents are small combustible masses used to cause sloughing following cauterization. They are caustics, used in skin diseases, to destroy infected tissue and to counteract the bites of animals and insects.

Wormwood has gained an unfavorable reputation among many as an herbal remedy because of the toxicity of the essential oil prepared by distilling the above-ground portions of the plant. The liqueur absinthe, made from oils of wormwood, angelica, anise, and marjoram, contains a high concentration of thujone, which is a convulsant poison and narcotic when taken in large amounts. Absinthe is banned in virtually every country in the world. Unlike ordinary alcoholism, absinthism also produces "restlessness at night, with disturbing dreams, nausea and vomiting in the morning with great trembling of the hands and tongue, vertigo, and a tendency to epileptiform convulsions."

RECENT SCIENTIFIC FINDINGS

Species of *Artemisia* are now receiving much attention for their purported anti-parasitic properties. Experimental evidence supporting such claims is weak or non-existent.

We have been unable to find experimental evidence to corroborate the anthelmintic or anti-parasitic effect of wormwood, but water extracts given to animals by mouth have been shown to produce a cathartic action. A tea of wormwood would be bitter, and most bitter substances act as tonics by increasing gastric secretion. Mausert prescribed this herb for liver complaints since it promoted the flow of bile. Being an active medicinal, it must be carefully dosed.

However, a great deal of research has recently been undertaken concerning wormwood's antimalarial properties.

Malarial parasites have developed resistance to synthetic antimalarial agents, leading to a resurgence in the use of quinine.

Artemisia spp.

There's also been renewed attention in finding new antimalarial drugs. A sesquiterpene lactone isolated from wormwood, artemisinin, has been the subject of a great deal of new preliminary research. The World Health Organization has developed artemether, a potent derivative of artemisinin, as the drug of choice.

Wormwood has been used to make an herbal tea containing only a very small amount of absinthe, and hence thujone, in the final beverage. Thujone has a very low water-solubility; thus, it would be difficult to experience the adverse effects of absinthe when the plant is used in the form of a normally brewed herbal tea.

Wormwood, scientifically known as *Artemisia absinthium*, is an herb renowned for its intensely bitter taste and its historical role in the production of the famous alcoholic beverage absinthe. Beyond its use in the world of spirits, wormwood has earned recognition for its potential medicinal properties. It has been traditionally associated with digestive support, with the bitter compounds believed to stimulate digestive secretions and help ease common gastrointestinal discomfort. However, it is essential to exercise caution when using wormwood due to its strong bitterness and potential toxicity in excessive amounts.

YAM (Wild)
Dioscorea villosa

Parts used: Rhizome. *This was once used by enslaved people in the South for rheumatism, and modern research is confirming its anti-inflammatory properties.*

TRADITIONAL USAGES
As the common names (colic root, rheumatism root) clearly indicate, the yam has been considered a remedy for bilious colic, and Southerners once used it as a treatment for rheumatism. The root is diuretic and expectorant, but only in large doses. It is also antispasmodic, which would explain its efficacy in treating bilious colic.

RECENT SCIENTIFIC FINDINGS
All species of wild yam examined to date contain varying amounts of a steroid-like material known as diosgenin. Diosgenin has been shown experimentally to inhibit inflammation in laboratory animals, and thus the wild yam could have beneficial effects in rheumatism, as claimed in folklore.

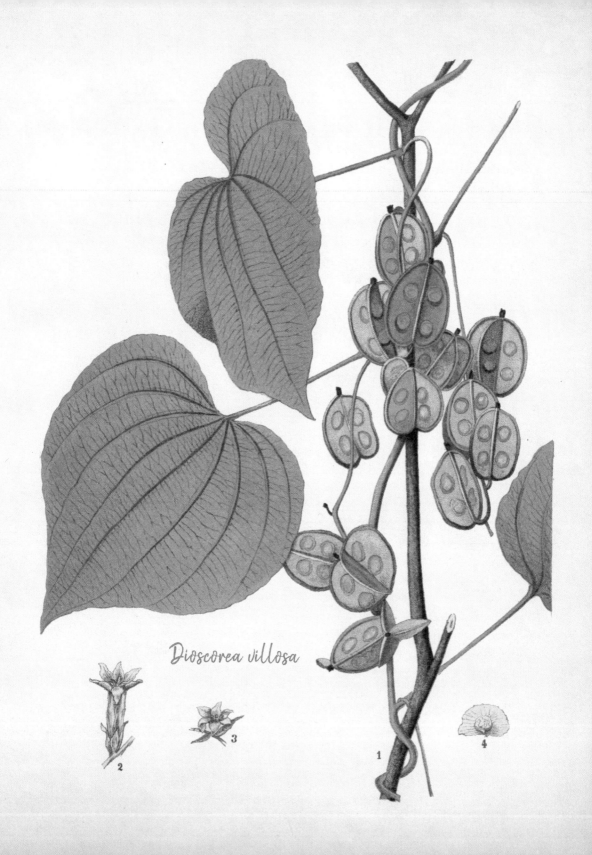

Dioscorea villosa

2   3   1   4

A natural oral contraceptive agent due to a steroidal content of 40% diosgenin and 50–60% of other related sapogenins, yam is utilized as a basis of commercial birth-control product sex hormone production (conversion of diosgenin to progesterone).

Wild yam is an herb celebrated for both its striking, vibrant blooms and its potential effects on hormone balance, especially in the realm of women's health. While wild yam is not a direct source of hormones, it contains compounds known as phytoestrogens that are believed to support hormonal equilibrium. This herb has been traditionally used to address menopausal symptoms and menstrual discomfort, and it remains a subject of interest in the field of natural remedies for women's health.

YARROW

Achillea millefolium

Parts used: Flowering tops and leaves. *Both the ancient Greeks and Native Americans used this plant to heal wounds.*

TRADITIONAL USAGES

The genus name, *Achillea,* is derived from the Greek hero of the *Iliad,* Achilles, who according to mythology healed the wounds of his comrades-in-arms with a relative of this plant. Yarrow was known to the Greeks as a styptic, vulnerary, and astringent, and hence was utilized in hemorrhagic complaints.

Native American warriors also used yarrow to treat cuts, bruises, and other minor injuries. The Ute name for yarrow is translated as "wound medicine." The Zuni used it to treat burns. The dried leaves and tops were listed for promoting menstruation and as a stimulant in the *U.S. Pharmacopoeia* from 1863 to 1882.

Yarrow has been used both locally and internally in the treatment of hemorrhoids and has also been given for bladder conditions such as involuntary urination in children. In weak doses, it has been employed as a mild aromatic, sudorific, tonic, and astringent, the leaves being employed for the latter purpose. Its most noteworthy usage was in menstrual irregularities.

In the Scandinavian countries, yarrow was, at one time, substituted for hops in beer and was probably felt to have sedative properties.

RECENT SCIENTIFIC FINDINGS

The use of decoctions or infusions of yarrow flowers as a tonic has been studied experimentally in humans. It has been confirmed that oral extracts of this plant stimulate gastric juices. This would lead to a tonic effect with improved digestion of foods. The effect is due to the presence of bitter principles (azulenes, sesquiterpenes) in the flowers.

Animal studies have shown that extracts of yarrow can reduce inflammation and have a calming effect. Thus, the use of the juice of this plant for the treatment of ulcers and hemorrhoids has a rational basis. Extracts of yarrow are also known to have antibiotic effects when evaluated in test tubes. Thus, at least for external applications, one would expect that a person suffering from boils or other microbial infections of a minor nature would receive beneficial results by the external application of yarrow preparations.

Yarrow is a versatile herb with a rich history of applications in traditional medicine. Known for its finely divided leaves and umbrella-like clusters of small, white, or pink flowers, yarrow offers a wide range of potential benefits. It is often employed for its capacity to address issues related to digestion, where it may help soothe digestive discomfort and stimulate healthy digestion. Additionally, yarrow is recognized for its potential to promote circulation and is often used in herbal remedies for its ability to stop bleeding, making it a valuable ally for wound healing.

YERBA SANTA
Eriodictyon californicum

Parts used: Leaves. *The "holy herb" may contain chemopreventive compounds.*

TRADITIONAL USAGES

Yerba santa is an herb with a delightful aroma and a reputation for its potential medicinal properties. In herbal remedies, yerba santa is often valued for its role as an expectorant, helping to relieve respiratory congestion by facilitating the removal of mucus from the airways. Its pleasing scent and mild flavor also make it a popular choice for herbal teas and preparations designed to support respiratory health.

Yerba santa was the most highly valued medicinal plant among the Native Americans of Mendocino County, California. The leaves were taken as a tea for colds or smoked and chewed to treat asthma. A natural mouthwash was prepared by rolling the leaves into balls and then allowing them to dry in the sun. After chewing, one drank water. As one user put it, "It makes one taste kind of sweety inside."

Yerba santa was quickly adopted by the Spanish missionaries and then later settlers. V. K. Chestnut in his valuable paper on herb usage describes how it was employed as a cure for grippe, as a blood purifier, and as a cure for rheumatism, tuberculosis, and catarrh.

In 1875, Dr. J. H. Bundy introduced yerba santa to the medical profession. Parke-Davis & Co. researched the drug, and it was official in the *U.S. Pharmacopoeia* first from 1894 to 1905, then again from 1916 to 1947. Since then, yerba santa has been recognized in the *National Formulary.* The leaves of this shrub have been used as a bitter tonic and to disguise the bitterness of quinine. They were particularly valued for their expectorant properties, making this a very popular remedy for asthma, chronic bronchitis, and colds. Yerba santa was also felt to be helpful in cases of chronic genitourinary inflammations. For treating respiratory ailments, the leaves were sometimes smoked, but they could also be administered as an infusion as described previously.

RECENT SCIENTIFIC FINDINGS

The "holy herb" contains a resin, pentatriacontane, and cerotonic acid.

As dietary factors have become more recognized as one of the primary elements in cancer, research on chemopreventive compounds has increased. Chemopreventive compounds include agents that prevent the formation of carcinogens, agents that interfere with the promotion and progression of carcinogens, and what are termed blocking agents, which reduce the activation of carcinogens to react with cells and initiate the induction of cancer. One study (1992) found that a yerba santa extract "exhibited reproducible inhibition" of a potent cancer-causing chemical.

Eriodictyon californicum

YOHIMBE

Corynanthe yohimbe (Pausinystalia yohimbe)

Parts used: Bark. *Though there is no scientific evidence to support it, the bark remains a popular aphrodisiac.*

TRADITIONAL USAGES

Yohimbe bark is one of the most frequently sought-out aphrodisiacs that the world has ever known, and it is still used for this purpose today, particularly in Cameroon.

RECENT SCIENTIFIC FINDINGS

We have carried out an exhaustive search of the scientific literature for publications describing the effects of yohimbe bark extracts on animals or humans in order to confirm or deny its reputed aphrodisiac properties. To our surprise, we were unable to find a single scientific paper that describes any type of effect for this plant in animals or in humans.

However, many papers have been published by scientists attempting to relate the results of experiments in animals with yohimbine (the bark's active derivative) to the alleged aphrodisiac effect of decoctions or infusions of the bark, in man.

To summarize these findings, very clearly yohimbine causes a dilation of the blood vessels in animals and in man, including those in the genitalia. Thus, in man, an increased flow of blood is routed to the penis, which theoretically should result in an erection, following the administration of yohimbine and also yohimbe bark. Unfortunately, yohimbine in doses required to attain this effect also acts as a powerful agent in reducing normal blood pressure due to the dilatory effect on the blood vessels. As would be expected, a person with extremely low blood pressure would no longer have the physical strength to enter into the vigorous sexual experience that would be anticipated as a reason for taking yohimbe bark, and thus the effect would be nullified.

Yohimbine, and also yohimbe bark, are powerful drugs. The effective dose is very close to the toxic dose, and thus one should not experiment with either of them out of curiosity. A person with normal low blood pressure should completely avoid the use of these two substances.

Some investigators have studied yohimbine in animals in order to ascertain whether or not this material affects ejaculation time and/or frequency, and it was found to do neither.

We have never found reference to the use of yohimbe bark as an aphrodisiac in females, which tends to point out the long-standing male-chauvinistic attitudes in scientific work. Presumably, yohimbe bark would also have an aphrodisiac effect in females since it would cause an increased blood flow to the genitalia.

A recent study, however, discovered that yohimbine is a moderately effective weight-loss agent. Yohimbine increased thermogenesis and thus helped obese patients lose body mass. Obese patients who were on a low-calorie diet (1,000 cal/day) were given a daily dose of 20 mg (5 mg, 4 times a day) of yohimbine. The patients were told to take this drug at least 90 minutes before a meal. Yohimbine was found to exert a greater weight-reducing effect than placebo.

The study indicated that yohimbine blocks alpha-2 adrenoreceptors in peripheral tissues. Remember that thermogenesis for weight-reducing purposes can also be achieved by stimulating beta-adrenergic receptors. This has been tried in Denmark using ephedrine (a beta-adrenergic stimulant) in a weight-loss pill. While it increased thermogenesis, the side effects of sleeplessness, tachycardia, and muscular fibrillations precluded the widespread use of ephedrine.

YUCCA
Yucca brevifolia

Parts used: Leaves. *Native Americans valued this both as food and as a cleanser.*

TRADITIONAL USAGES

The dried fruits of this plant were valued as an important food for Navajo warriors, especially during long journeys. The roots were crushed and used for soap.

The Hopi especially prized this natural cleanser, relating, "To cure baldness, wash the hair with yucca root and rub with duck grease because ducks have such heavy feathers."

RECENT SCIENTIFIC FINDINGS

There has been inconclusive research to indicate potential usefulness in the treatment of arthritis.

Yucca, a hardy desert plant, is esteemed for its versatility and valued for various purposes. The root of the yucca plant is rich in saponins, natural compounds that have detergent-like properties and can be used for various purposes. Yucca is used in culinary applications, such as in traditional Native American cuisine, where it is prized for its mild, nutty flavor. Additionally, it has a history of use in traditional herbal remedies for its potential benefits in promoting overall well-being, such as supporting joint health and inflammation reduction. Whether used in the kitchen or for its potential health benefits, yucca reflects the adaptability and diverse uses of natural herbs.

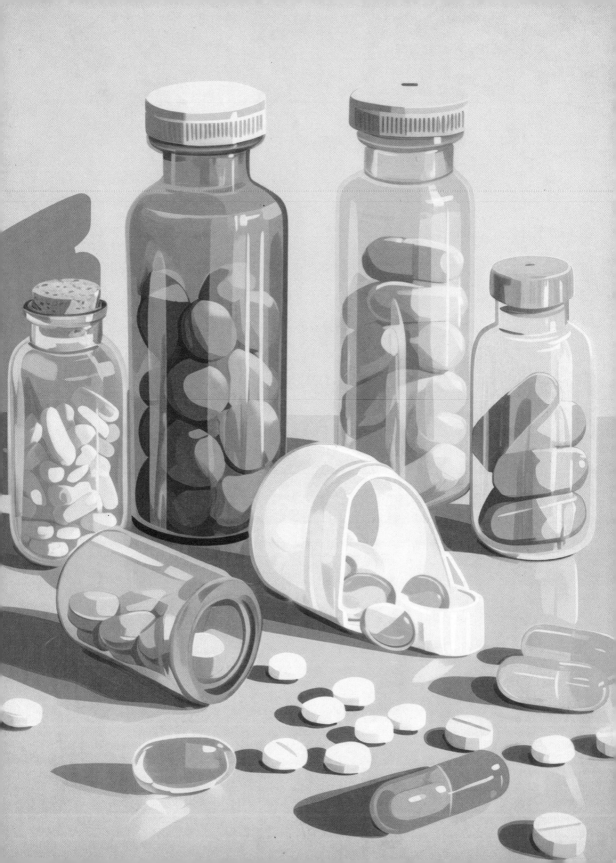

TWO

QUESTIONS & ANSWERS
from the FDA on Dietary Supplements

What is a dietary supplement?

Congress defined the term "dietary supplement" in the Dietary Supplement Health and Education Act (DSHEA) of 1994. A dietary supplement is a product intended for ingestion that, among other requirements, contains a "dietary ingredient" intended to supplement the diet. The term "dietary ingredient" includes vitamins and minerals; herbs and other botanicals; amino acids; "dietary substances" that are part of the food supply, such as enzymes and live microbials (commonly referred to as "probiotics"); and concentrates, metabolites, constituents, extracts, or combinations of any dietary ingredient from the preceding categories. Dietary supplements may be found in many forms, such as pills, tablets, capsules, gummies, softgels, liquids, and powders. They can also be in the same form as a conventional food category, such as teas or bars, but only if the product is not represented as a conventional food or as a "sole item of a meal or the diet." To be a dietary supplement, a product must also be labeled as a dietary supplement; that is, the product label must include the term "dietary supplement" or equivalent (e.g., "iron supplement" or "herbal supplement"). DSHEA places dietary supplements in a special category under the general umbrella of "foods," unless the product meets the definition of a drug (e.g., because it is labeled to treat or mitigate a disease).

Generally, the dietary supplement category excludes articles approved as new drugs, licensed as biologics, or authorized for clinical investigation under an investigational new drug (IND) application that has gone into effect, unless the article was previously marketed as a dietary supplement or as a food. In the case of articles authorized for clinical investigation under an IND application, the exclusion from the dietary supplement definition applies only if "substantial clinical investigations" have been instituted and the existence of such investigations has been made public.

What is a "new dietary ingredient" in a dietary supplement?

The Dietary Supplement Health and Education Act (DSHEA) of 1994 defined the terms "dietary ingredient" and "new dietary ingredient." To be a "dietary ingredient," an ingredient in a dietary supplement must be one of the following:

- A vitamin
- A mineral
- An herb or other botanical
- An amino acid
- A dietary substance for use to supplement the diet by increasing the total dietary intake
- A concentrate, metabolite, constituent, extract, or combination of any dietary ingredient from the other categories listed here

A "new dietary ingredient" is an ingredient that meets the definition of a "dietary ingredient" and was not marketed in the United States before October 15, 1994.

Should I check with my doctor or healthcare provider before using a dietary supplement?

Yes. The FDA advises consumers to talk to their doctor, pharmacist, or other healthcare professional before deciding to purchase or use a dietary supplement. For example, some supplements might interact with medicines or other supplements.

Please see the FDA's "Information for Consumers on Using Dietary Supplements" for additional educational materials.

What is the FDA's role in regulating dietary supplements versus the manufacturer's responsibility for marketing them?

The Dietary Supplement Health and Education Act (DSHEA) amended the Federal Food, Drug, and Cosmetic Act (FD&C Act) to create a new regulatory framework for dietary supplements. Under DSHEA, the FDA does not have the authority to approve dietary supplements before they are marketed. Generally, a firm does not have to provide the FDA with the evidence it relies on to substantiate safety before or after it markets its products; however, there is an exception for dietary supplements that contain a new dietary ingredient that is not present in the food supply as an article used for food in a form in which the food has not been chemically altered. At least 75 days before introducing such a dietary supplement into interstate commerce or delivering it for introduction into interstate commerce, the manufacturer or distributor must submit a notification to the FDA with the information on the basis of which the firm has concluded that the new dietary ingredient (NDI)-containing dietary supplement will reasonably be expected to be safe. In addition, the FDA's regulations require those who manufacture, package, or hold dietary supplements to follow current good manufacturing practices that help ensure the identity, purity, quality, strength, and composition of dietary supplements. The FDA generally does not approve dietary supplement claims or other labeling before use.

Under the FD&C Act, a firm is responsible for ensuring that the dietary supplements it manufactures or distributes are not adulterated, misbranded, or otherwise in violation of federal law. If a manufacturer or distributor makes a structure/function claim (a claim about effects on a structure or function of the human body), a claim of a benefit related to a classical nutrient deficiency disease, or a claim of general well-being in the labeling of a dietary supplement, the firm must have substantiation that the claim is truthful and not misleading. Facilities that manufacture, process, pack, or hold dietary supplements or dietary ingredients for consumption in the United States must register with the FDA, as required by the Public Health Security and Bioterrorism Preparedness and Response Act of 2002 and implementing regulations, before beginning such operations.

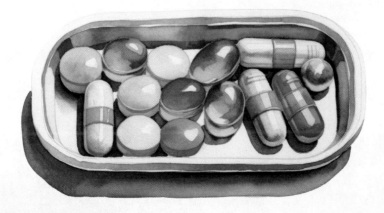

The FDA is responsible for enforcing the laws and regulations governing dietary supplements. To identify violations, the agency conducts inspections, monitors the marketplace, examines dietary supplements and dietary ingredients offered for import, and reviews NDI notifications and other regulatory submissions for dietary supplements, such as postmarket notifications of a structure/function claim or other claim made under section 403(r)(6) of the FD&C Act. It also investigates adverse event reports and complaints from consumers, healthcare professionals, other regulatory agencies, and industry.

When must a manufacturer or distributor notify the FDA about a dietary supplement it intends to market in the United States?

The Dietary Supplement Health and Education Act (DSHEA) requires that a manufacturer or distributor notify the FDA in advance and submit safety information if it intends to market a dietary supplement in the United States that contains a "new dietary ingredient," unless the new dietary ingredient is present in the food supply as an article used for food in a form in which the food has not been chemically altered. The notification must be submitted to the FDA at least 75 days before introducing the product into interstate commerce or delivering it for introduction into interstate commerce. Along with information about the new dietary ingredient and the dietary supplement in which it will be marketed, the notification must include the safety information on which the notifier has based its conclusion that the new dietary ingredient will be reasonably expected to be safe when used under the conditions recommended or suggested in the labeling of the dietary supplement.

What information must the manufacturer disclose on the label of a dietary supplement?

FDA regulations require dietary supplement labels to bear a product name and a statement that it is a "dietary supplement" or equivalent term replacing "dietary" with the name or type of dietary ingredient in the product (e.g., "iron supplement" or "herbal supplement"); the name and place of business of the manufacturer, packer, or distributor; nutrition labeling in the form of a Supplement Facts panel (except for some small volume products or those produced by eligible small businesses); a list of "other ingredients" not declared in the Supplement Facts panel; and the net quantity of contents. The Supplement Facts panel must list the serving size and number of servings per container, declare each dietary ingredient in the product, and except for dietary ingredients that are part of a proprietary blend, provide information on the amount of the dietary ingredient per serving. Depending on the type of ingredient, the amount per serving must be declared as a quantitative amount by weight, as a percentage of the daily value, or both. Finally, dietary supplement labels must provide a domestic address or domestic phone number for reporting serious adverse events to the manufacturer, packer, or distributor whose name and place of business are listed on the label.

Must all ingredients be declared on the label of a dietary supplement?

Yes, ingredients not listed on the Supplement Facts panel must be listed in the "other ingredients" list beneath. The types of ingredients listed there could include the sources of dietary ingredients, if not listed in the Supplement Facts panel (e.g., rose hips as the source of vitamin C), other food ingredients (e.g., water and sugar), food additives, and color additives. Gelatin, starch, stabilizers, preservatives, and flavors are additional examples of ingredients commonly declared in the "other ingredients" list.

Are dietary supplement serving sizes standardized or are there restrictions on the amount of a dietary ingredient that can be in one serving?

Other than the manufacturer's responsibility to meet the safety standards and labeling requirements for dietary supplements and to comply with current good manufacturing regulations, there are no laws or regulations that limit the serving size of a dietary supplement or the amount of a dietary ingredient that can be in a serving of a dietary supplement. This decision is made by the manufacturer and does not require FDA approval.

Where can I get information about a specific dietary supplement?

Because the FDA does not approve dietary supplements before they are marketed, the agency often does not know when new products come on the market. Therefore, it is not able to keep a complete list of all dietary supplements sold in the United States. If you want more detailed information about a specific dietary supplement than the label provides, it is recommended that you contact the manufacturer of the product directly. The name and address of the manufacturer or distributor can be found on the label of the dietary supplement.

Who has the responsibility for ensuring that a product meets the safety standards for dietary supplements?

Because the law prohibits the distribution and sale of adulterated dietary supplements, manufacturers and distributors have initial responsibility for ensuring that their dietary supplements meet the safety standards for dietary supplements. When manufacturers and distributors do not fulfill that responsibility and adulterated dietary supplements reach the market, the FDA has authority to enforce the law to protect consumers. In general, the FDA is limited to postmarket enforcement because, unlike drugs that must be proven safe and effective for their intended use before marketing, there are no provisions in the law for the FDA to approve dietary supplements for safety before they reach the consumer. However, manufacturers and distributors of dietary supplements must record, investigate, and forward to the FDA any reports they receive of serious adverse events associated with the use of their products. The FDA evaluates these reports and any other adverse event information reported by healthcare providers or consumers to identify early signals that a product may present safety risks to consumers. You can find more information on reporting adverse events associated with the use of dietary supplements at the FDA's "How to Report a Problem with Dietary Supplements."

How can consumers inform themselves about safety and other issues related to dietary supplements?

It is important to be well informed about health-related products before purchasing them. The FDA advises consumers to consult with a healthcare professional before deciding to take a dietary supplement. Consumers should also carefully read the label of any dietary supplement they are thinking of using. To help consumers in their search to be better informed, the FDA has prepared additional educational materials. Please visit its "Information for Consumers on Using Dietary Supplements."

What is the FDA's oversight responsibility for dietary supplements?

Because dietary supplements are under the umbrella of foods, the FDA's Center for Food Safety and Applied Nutrition (CFSAN) is primarily responsible for the agency's oversight of these products. The FDA's role in regulating dietary supplements includes (among other things) inspecting dietary supplement manufacturing establishments, reviewing new dietary ingredient (NDI) notifications and other regulatory submissions for dietary supplements, investigating complaints, monitoring the dietary supplement marketplace, examining dietary supplements and dietary ingredients offered for import to determine whether they meet U.S. requirements, and reviewing adverse event reports from firms, consumers, and healthcare providers to identify products that may be unsafe. However, by law, the FDA does not approve dietary supplements or their labeling, although certain types of claims sometimes used in dietary supplement labeling require premarket review and authorization (e.g., health claims).

Does the FDA routinely analyze the content of dietary supplements?

No. The FDA has limited resources to analyze the composition of food products, including dietary supplements, and, therefore, focuses its resources first on public health emergencies and products that may have caused injury or illness. Priority then goes to products suspected to be adulterated, fraudulent, or otherwise in violation of the law. The remaining resources are used to analyze product samples collected during inspections of manufacturing firms or pulled from store shelves as part of the FDA's routine monitoring of the marketplace. The FDA does not test dietary supplements before they are sold to consumers. Consumers may contact the dietary supplement manufacturer or a commercial laboratory for an analysis of a product's content.

Is it legal to market a dietary supplement product to treat, prevent, or cure a specific disease?

No. A product sold as a dietary supplement and represented explicitly or implicitly for treatment, prevention, or cure of a specific disease or class of diseases meets the definition of a drug and is subject to regulation as a drug.

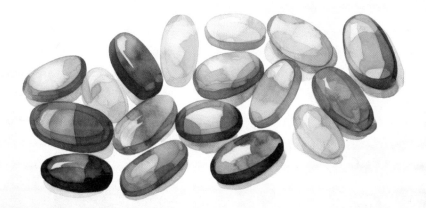

How are advertisements for dietary supplements regulated?

The Federal Trade Commission (FTC) regulates advertising, including infomercials, for dietary supplements. The FDA and FTC share responsibility for the oversight of dietary supplements and related promotion, with the FDA generally responsible for safety, quality, and labeling, and the FTC generally responsible for advertising. Both the FDA and FTC have the authority to take enforcement actions against dietary supplements and firms if they identify violations. In addition, the FDA considers advertising when evaluating the intended use of a product labeled as a dietary supplement. For more information on the FTC's role in regulating dietary supplement advertising, please visit the FTC website. Advertising and other promotional material sent through the mail are also subject to regulation by the U.S. Postal Inspection Service.

What kinds of claims can be made on dietary supplement labels?

Among the claims that can be used on dietary supplement labels are three categories of claims that are defined by the FD&C Act and FDA regulations: health claims (claims about the relationship between a dietary ingredient or other food substance and reduced risk of a disease or health-related condition), structure/function claims (claims about effects on a structure or function of the human body), and nutrient content claims (claims characterizing the level of a nutrient or other dietary ingredient in a dietary supplement). Different requirements apply to each of these claim types. For more information on the regulation of health claims, structure/function claims, and nutrient content claims, please see the FDA's "Label Claims for Conventional Foods and Dietary Supplements."

Two less common types of dietary supplement labeling claims defined by statute are claims of a benefit related to a classical nutrient deficiency disease (when accompanied by a statement disclosing the prevalence of the nutrient deficiency disease in the United States) and claims of general well-being from consumption of a nutrient or other dietary ingredient. These dietary supplement claims are subject to the same requirements as structure/function claims, including the disclaimer that must accompany the claim and the requirement for the manufacturer to have substantiation that the claim is truthful and non-misleading. Finally, dietary supplements, like conventional foods, may make other labeling claims that are not defined by statute or regulation (e.g., claims about taste or ingredient quality), as long as those claims are not false or misleading.

Who regulates the use of the term "organic" on dietary supplements under the National Organic Program?

The U.S. Department of Agriculture (USDA) regulates the use of the term "organic" under the National Organic Program (NOP). NOP is a federal regulatory program that develops and enforces consistent national standards for organically produced agricultural products sold in the United States.

Why do some dietary supplements have wording on the label that says: "This statement has not been evaluated by the Food and Drug Administration. This product is not intended to diagnose, treat, cure, or prevent any disease"?

This statement, known as a disclaimer, is required by law, 21 U.S.C. 343(r)(6)(C) and 21 CFR 101.93(b)–(d), when a manufacturer makes a structure/function claim or certain other claims in dietary supplement labeling. In general, structure/function claims describe the role of a nutrient or dietary ingredient intended to affect the structure or function of the body in humans or characterize the documented mechanism by which a nutrient or dietary ingredient acts to maintain such structure or function. The other dietary supplement labeling claims that require the disclaimer are claims of a benefit related to a classical nutrient deficiency disease and claims of general well-being from consumption of a dietary ingredient. These three types of claims are not approved by the FDA and do not require FDA evaluation before they are used in dietary supplement labeling. Accordingly, DSHEA requires that when a dietary supplement label or other labeling includes such a claim, the claim must be accompanied by a disclaimer informing consumers that the FDA has not evaluated the claim. The disclaimer must also state that the product is not intended to "diagnose, treat, cure, or prevent any disease" because only a drug can legally make such a claim.

[From: https://www.fda.gov/food/information-consumers-using-dietary
-supplements/questions-and-answers-dietary-supplements]

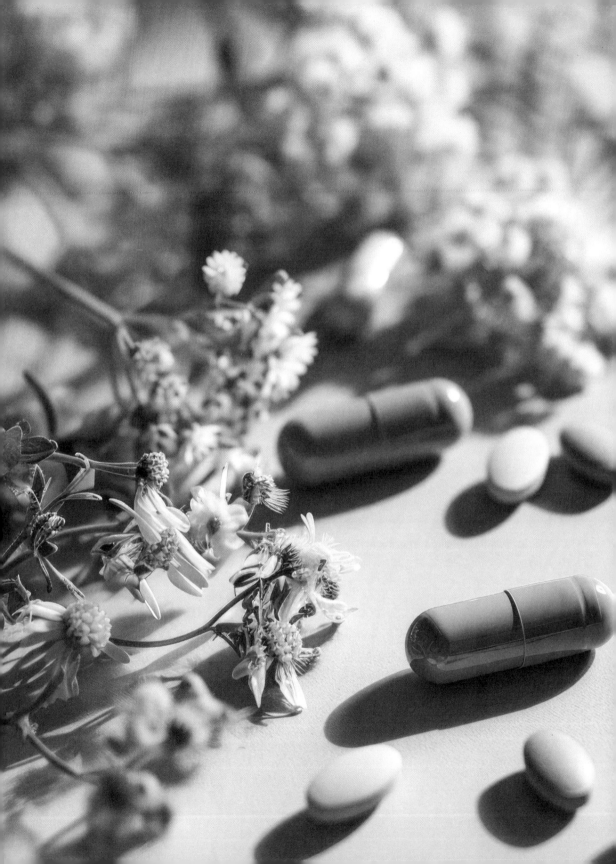

THREE

VITAMINS & SUPPLEMENTS
A to Z Reference Guide

VITAMIN A

Vitamin A, a crucial nutrient often overshadowed in nutritional discourse, offers an array of significant benefits indispensable for human health. This critical vitamin, abundantly found in various foods, contributes to numerous bodily functions and physiological processes.

The benefits of vitamin A begin with its profound impact on ocular health. This vitamin is integral to maintaining proper vision, particularly under conditions of low light. Deficiency in vitamin A can result in night blindness—a condition characterized by impaired vision in dim light.

The role of vitamin A extends to maintaining skin health. It fosters the generation of new cells, contributing to healthy, rejuvenated skin. Beyond its cosmetic appeal, vitamin A enhances the integrity of our skin and mucous membranes—the body's first line of defense against infectious pathogens. Consequently, vitamin A holds significant importance in both external aesthetic maintenance and internal health preservation.

Further, vitamin A is essential for immune system functionality. It bolsters the production and function of white blood cells, a critical component in the body's defense mechanism against illness and infection. Therefore, vitamin A serves as a vital ingredient in fortifying our body's immunity.

Lastly, the antioxidant properties of vitamin A are noteworthy. This vitamin combats the harmful effects of free radicals, which contribute to chronic illnesses and aging processes. By neutralizing these harmful particles, vitamin A aids in preventing heart disease, inflammation, and other associated health conditions.

VITAMIN B1 (THIAMINE)

Vitamin B1, also known as thiamine, is essential in the nutrient spectrum. It is predominantly found in whole grains, legumes, and certain meats. Thiamine is vital for our body's energy production, aiding in the conversion of nutrients into energy, ensuring our physiological systems function optimally.

Additionally, thiamine plays a significant role in maintaining a robust nervous system. Proper nerve communication relies on this vitamin, ensuring every part of our body receives timely and accurate messages. A deficiency in thiamine can lead to disruptions in this system.

While thiamine is indispensable, it's important to consume it in appropriate amounts. Excessive intake, although rare, can lead to imbalances, so adhering to recommended dietary amounts is advisable.

VITAMIN B2 (RIBOFLAVIN)

Introducing riboflavin, often referred to as vitamin B2. This nutrient is abundant in foods such as eggs, green vegetables, and dairy products. Riboflavin is instrumental in protecting our body's cells from potential damage.

Beyond its protective role, riboflavin is essential for maintaining eye health, ensuring clear and optimal vision. Moreover, it contributes to the health and vitality of our skin.

It's noteworthy that our bodies cannot store riboflavin for extended periods, necessitating regular intake. Balance is crucial, and it's always best to maintain consumption within the recommended daily intake.

VITAMIN B3 (NIACIN)

Niacin, commonly recognized as vitamin B3, has multiple health benefits. It's found in a variety of foods, including poultry, fish, legumes, and grains. One of niacin's primary roles is supporting brain function, contributing to cognitive clarity and concentration.

Niacin also plays an essential role in skin health, promoting a healthy complexion. It also aids our digestive system, ensuring efficient nutrient conversion into energy.

It's crucial to note that while niacin offers several benefits, excessive intake can lead to symptoms like facial flushing. It's recommended to acquire niacin primarily from natural food sources and adhere to dietary guidelines.

VITAMIN B5 (PANTOTHENIC ACID)

Vitamin B5, identified as pantothenic acid, offers numerous health advantages. Responsible for converting food into energy, it plays an integral role in ensuring our bodies remain energized.

B5 also supports the health of our hair, skin, and eyes. By promoting red blood cell production, it ensures these organs maintain their health. Moreover, B5 is involved in cholesterol production and the processing of other vitamins.

Maintaining a balance in B5 intake is important. Insufficient amounts can result in symptoms like fatigue, whereas overconsumption, although not commonly harmful, can occasionally cause digestive issues. Prioritizing balance and deriving nutrients from natural foods remains the optimal strategy.

VITAMIN B6

Vitamin B6, also known as pyridoxine, is a water-soluble vitamin that plays a vital role in various bodily functions. It is predominantly found in a variety of foods, including poultry, fish, potatoes, and non-citrus fruits.

The most notable benefit of vitamin B6 lies in its role in brain development and function. It aids in the production of neurotransmitters, the chemicals that facilitate communication between nerve cells. This makes it crucial for normal brain development and function, and in promoting mental health.

Vitamin B6 is also involved in protein metabolism, assisting in the breakdown and utilization of protein from our diet. This is crucial for the growth, repair, and functioning of our bodies.

Moreover, it plays a vital role in maintaining a healthy immune system. Vitamin B6 supports the production of antibodies, which are necessary to fight off many diseases.

On the other hand, while vitamin B6 is generally safe at the recommended daily intake levels, an excess can lead to harmful effects. These can include nerve damage that can cause tingling and numbness in the limbs and may also lead to difficulty walking. Therefore, it is critical to adhere to recommended doses and maintain a balanced diet to gain the benefits of vitamin B6 without risking overconsumption.

VITAMIN B12

Vitamin B12, also known as cobalamin, is an essential water-soluble vitamin. It is naturally present in a wide variety of animal foods and fortified in others, offering us a wealth of health benefits when consumed in adequate amounts.

A primary benefit of vitamin B12 lies in its fundamental role in red blood cell formation. Without sufficient vitamin B12, red blood cell production can be impaired, potentially leading to a specific type of anemia known as megaloblastic anemia, characterized by larger and fewer red blood cells.

Moreover, vitamin B12 is vital for maintaining a healthy nervous system. It contributes to the production of myelin, a substance that insulates nerve fibers and enhances nerve-impulse transmission. Deficiency in B12 can result in a range of neurological complications, including numbness, tingling, balance issues, and memory loss.

Further, this vitamin plays an essential role in energy production. It aids in converting the food we eat into glucose, which provides us with energy, making it a crucial nutrient for overall vitality.

Vitamin B12 also plays a significant role in maintaining heart health. It works to reduce levels of homocysteine, an amino acid linked to increased risk of heart disease when found in high amounts in the body.

Despite its numerous benefits, it's essential to note that excessive vitamin B12, while rare, can lead to potential side effects like dizziness, headache, anxiety, and nausea. Hence, it is always recommended to adhere to recommended dietary allowances.

VITAMIN C

Vitamin C, also known as ascorbic acid, is an essential nutrient known for its diverse range of health benefits. This vitamin, abundant in many fruits and vegetables, significantly contributes to our body's various physiological processes.

One of the primary benefits of vitamin C is its crucial role in enhancing immune function. This vitamin bolsters the production of white blood cells, fortifying our defense mechanism against infections. Additionally, its antioxidative properties shield these cells from harmful free radicals.

Vitamin C also plays a significant role in cardiovascular health. Regular intake may

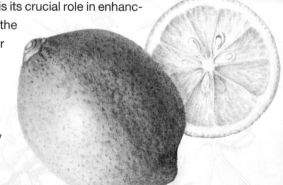

reduce the risk of heart disease, help prevent LDL cholesterol oxidation, and lower blood pressure, thereby promoting heart health.

Further, vitamin C enhances the body's absorption of iron, crucial for preventing conditions like iron-deficiency anemia. Its benefits also extend to skin health, promoting collagen production necessary for maintaining healthy skin, hair, nails, and connective tissues.

Additionally, vitamin C's potent antioxidative properties help combat oxidative stress, which is linked to chronic diseases such as cancer and heart disease. Lastly, adequate vitamin C intake is associated with a lower risk of cognitive decline, thereby playing an important role in cognitive health.

VITAMIN D

Recognized as the "sunshine vitamin," vitamin D is a unique nutrient our bodies can synthesize from sunlight. Yet, its role in health extends far beyond its unique production process, providing us with a spectrum of benefits essential for overall well-being.

First and foremost, vitamin D plays a critical role in bone health. It aids in the absorption of calcium and phosphorus, essential minerals for bone formation and strength. A deficiency in vitamin D can lead to soft bones in children (rickets) and fragile bones in adults (osteomalacia).

The benefits of vitamin D also reach our immune system. This vitamin contributes to the body's defense mechanisms by modulating the immune responses, strengthening our natural defenses against various diseases and infections.

Vitamin D is associated with the regulation of mood and warding off depression. There is growing evidence that adequate levels of vitamin D can help maintain a positive mood and reduce the risk of depression.

Notably, vitamin D also plays a role in cardiovascular health. Emerging research suggests that adequate vitamin D levels can help lower the risk of hypertension, heart disease, and stroke by maintaining optimal blood pressure levels and promoting heart muscle function.

Vitamin D has also been linked to a decreased risk of certain types of cancers, including breast and colon cancer. It is believed to inhibit cancer cell growth and promote cell differentiation, thereby playing a role in cancer prevention.

Lastly, vitamin D is essential for the proper functioning of the pancreas, which produces insulin. It is, therefore, implicated in the management and prevention of type 2 diabetes, with research showing that insufficient vitamin D levels may impair insulin secretion and glucose tolerance.

VITAMIN E

Delving into the realm of essential nutrients, vitamin E stands out for its distinct roles and health benefits. This fat-soluble vitamin, found plentifully in nuts, seeds, and leafy green vegetables, is instrumental in maintaining our well-being.

One of the pivotal roles of vitamin E resides in its antioxidative properties. By neutralizing harmful free radicals, vitamin E helps protect cells from oxidative stress, a key factor contributing to aging and various chronic diseases.

Vitamin E has a unique role in skin health. As a powerful antioxidant, it protects the skin from damage caused by free radicals and UV radiation. Furthermore, its anti-inflammatory properties can support skin healing, making it a widely recognized nutrient in skin care.

Additionally, vitamin E aids in maintaining a robust immune system. It enhances cellular defense and improves the body's ability to combat infections and diseases, reinforcing our immune response.

Moreover, vitamin E is known for its contribution to heart health. It aids in preventing the oxidation of LDL cholesterol—an important factor in the development of atherosclerosis. Thus, regular intake of vitamin E can contribute to the reduction of heart disease risk.

Emerging research also associates vitamin E with eye health. It's believed to reduce the risk of age-related macular degeneration and cataracts, two common causes of vision impairment and blindness in older adults.

Vitamin E has also been implicated in cognitive health. Studies suggest that adequate vitamin E intake could help slow cognitive decline and might play a role in Alzheimer's disease prevention.

VITAMIN K

Vitamin K, present in foods like leafy greens and fermented dairy, is primarily known for its role in blood clotting. It ensures that minor injuries don't lead to excessive bleeding and also aids in bone health. There are different forms of vitamin K, with K1 found in plants and K2 in animal sources and fermented foods. While it's necessary for many body functions, individuals on certain medications, especially blood thinners, should monitor their vitamin K intake to avoid potential interactions.

SUPPLEMENTS

BIOTIN

Biotin, another member of the B-vitamin family, plays a role in the metabolism of fats, carbohydrates, and proteins. It's present in foods like eggs, nuts, and whole grains and has gained popularity for its purported benefits for hair, skin, and nails. While biotin deficiencies are uncommon, excessive intake, especially from supplements, might interfere with certain lab test results.

CAFFEINE

Caffeine is a natural stimulant most commonly found in coffee, tea, and various energy drinks. It primarily affects the brain, warding off tiredness and improving concentration and focus. It serves as a reliable companion for individuals seeking to overcome morning grogginess or midday lethargy. Caffeine's capacity to improve physical performance has made it an essential component in the routines of athletes and fitness enthusiasts. Its metabolic and thermogenic effects also make it a valuable aid in weight management. Beyond its immediate impacts, caffeine consumption in moderate quantities has been associated with potential long-term health benefits, including a reduced risk of conditions such as Parkinson's disease and type 2 diabetes.

CALCIUM

Calcium is an essential mineral primarily known for its crucial role in building and maintaining strong bones and teeth. Rich sources include dairy products, leafy greens, and fortified foods. Beyond skeletal health, calcium aids in muscle function, nerve transmission, and blood clotting. While integral to our health, it's vital to maintain balance; excessive calcium can lead to kidney stones or negatively impact the absorption of other essential minerals.

CHOLINE

Choline, essential for numerous bodily functions, is paramount for brain development and liver health. Rich food sources include eggs, poultry, and fish. Apart from its primary

Coffea Arabica

roles, excessive choline intake can sometimes lead to side effects, like a fishy body odor or lowered blood pressure.

COENZYME Q10 (COQ10)

CoQ10, present naturally within our cells, plays a pivotal role in cellular energy production. Rich food sources include organ meats and whole grains. Furthermore, CoQ10 has been recognized for its antioxidant properties, helping combat oxidative stress. While typically well-tolerated, high supplemental doses can sometimes lead to digestive discomfort.

FOLATE

Folate, a B-vitamin variant, is central to DNA synthesis and repair processes. Highly present in leafy greens and fortified cereals, it's of particular importance during early pregnancy, helping prevent neural tube defects. Caution is advised with excessive intake, as it can sometimes mask vitamin B12 deficiency symptoms.

INOSITOL

Predominantly found in fruits, beans, and grains, inositol plays a vital role in maintaining cell membrane integrity. Additionally, it has shown potential in mood regulation and other neural functions. While generally safe, an overconsumption can occasionally cause gastrointestinal issues.

MAGNESIUM

Integral to many biochemical reactions, magnesium plays pivotal roles in muscle and nerve function, bone health, and energy production. Abundant sources encompass nuts, seeds, and certain green vegetables. Proper magnesium balance is paramount; while a deficiency can lead to several complications, an excess, particularly from supplements, might cause digestive disturbances.

MELATONIN

Produced in the pineal gland, melatonin is a hormone instrumental in regulating our sleep-wake cycle. While certain foods contain minute amounts, melatonin is frequently consumed as a supplement to aid sleep. It is generally safe for short-term use, but potential side effects, such as dizziness or grogginess, warrant caution.

Scale cereale

POTASSIUM

Potassium is an essential mineral and electrolyte that plays critical roles in maintaining proper muscle contractions, nerve functions, and fluid balance. Rich sources include bananas, beans, and potatoes. Adequate potassium intake is vital for heart health and proper cellular function. However, it's important to strike a balance; while a deficiency can lead to symptoms like fatigue and muscle cramps, excessive potassium levels can be harmful, particularly for those with kidney disorders.

QUERCETIN

Quercetin, a flavonoid, is primarily found in various fruits and vegetables, with onions and apples being particularly rich sources. It's renowned for its antioxidant properties and its potential anti-inflammatory effects. While dietary quercetin is generally safe, excessive intake from supplements may result in headaches or tingling sensations.

SELENIUM

Selenium is a trace mineral found in soil and certain foods, including Brazil nuts, fish, and grains. It's instrumental in DNA synthesis, protecting cells from damage, and thyroid hormone metabolism. Additionally, selenium plays a role in defending against oxidative stress and may support immune function. It's essential to consume selenium in moderation; while deficiencies can lead to specific health issues, excessive intake can result in symptoms like gastrointestinal problems or hair loss.

TAURINE

Taurine is an amino acid often found in energy drinks and certain meat and fish types. It plays vital roles in various body functions, including calcium signaling, lipid metabolism, and neurotransmission. Taurine has also shown potential in supporting cardiovascular health and the function of the central nervous system. While it's generally safe for most individuals, excessive consumption, particularly from supplements, may lead to potential side effects like nausea or headaches.

ZINC

Zinc, a trace mineral, is fundamental for immune system efficiency, protein synthesis, and DNA formation. Predominant in meats, dairy, and nuts, it's vital for cellular metabolism. Zinc is indispensable; however, overconsumption can interfere with the absorption of other minerals, such as copper, and lead to digestive issues.

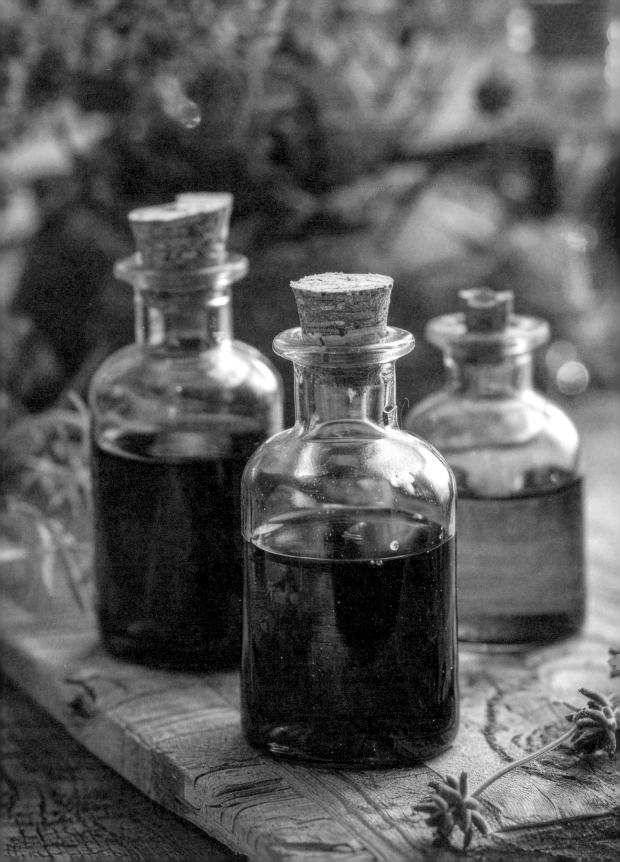

FOUR

COSMETIC HERBS
A to Z Reference Guide

Natural products have been utilized since antiquity to enhance human beauty. Whether for ornamentation, ritual and religious purposes, or simply personal enhancement, nearly every culture has recorded usage of plant extracts, earth dyes, and aromatic oils in unique and individual ways. In fact, the discovery and use of natural "cosmetics" and natural "medicines" might have more in common than we thought and may well have developed concurrently.

Coinciding with the development of synthetic drugs that followed the end of World War II, cosmetics underwent a similar transformation. As more and more of our natural pharmacopeia was replaced with synthetic drugs, so, too, were natural beauty aids discarded in favor of more "modern," high-tech synthetic products. Development was concentrated on synthetic cosmetics, and this trend has continued to the present day. However, in the 1960s, with the emphasis on more natural lifestyles, there came a surge in demand for a new group of perfumes, soaps, fragrances, oral care products, and other cosmetics that were free of synthetic components.

This interest led to the birth of new companies dedicated to the manufacture of cosmetics and other beauty aids free of the petrochemicals, artificial colors, and other adulterants that dominate mainstream cosmetic manufacturing.

A particular field in natural products dealing with the healing effects of essential oils is called aromatherapy. It was developed by the French perfumer and chemist René-Maurice Gattefossé, and French physician Jean Valnet later collaborated with the biochemist Marguerite Maury to develop a complete system of skin care and rejuvenation.

It is important to note that there are laws imposed on the manufacture of foods, drugs, and cosmetics that require certain preservatives be added to protect the consumer. Also, all labels must be written to conform with the Personal Care Products Council guidelines. Consequently, it may appear to a consumer who is purchasing a natural product that "on investigation of the ingredient label," there are synthetic-appearing items listed that give the impression of being synthetics, when in fact they are natural substances.

Some examples of these synthetic-sounding ingredients that are actually natural products include:

ACETIC ACID: A component of acetylated alcohol. It is an acid that is generally derived from vinegar. It is present in apples, grapes, oranges, peaches, pineapple, strawberries, and many other plants. It is used in skin care products as a vehicle for other ingredients because it causes no known allergic reactions and resembles the sterols normally found on human skin.

ACRYLIC ACID: This unsaturated liquid acid comes from red and green algae.

AZULENE: This is distilled from chamomile flowers or from yarrow.

BUTYLADIPATE: An emollient and pH adjusting agent derived from beets.

CAPRYLIC/CAPRIC GLYCERIDE: This oily liquid is derived from palm kernel or coconut oil.

CETYL ALCOHOL: Found in coconut, palm kernel, and other vegetable oils. It is a constituent of most plant waxes. It is a natural emollient.

COCAMIDOPROPYL BETAIN: Derived from the salts of coconut oil.

DECYL OLEATE: Derived from olive oil.

GLYCERYL OLEATE: A stabilizer and emollient derived from olive oil.

GLYCERYL STEARATE: An emulsifier derived from palm kernel or soy oil.

IMIDAZOLIDINYL UREA: Used to preserve cosmetics against bacterial contamination and to prolong shelf life.

ISOPROPYL ALCOHOL: Derived from petrochemicals—it is *not* a natural product.

LYSOZYME: A basic protein that is an effective bactericide.

PERHYDROSQUALENE: An emollient that comes from bran, olive, and wheat germ oils.

PHYTOSTEROL: Derived from soybeans, this is an emollient and emulsion stabilizer.

As you can see from these examples, reading labels can become an extremely confusing business. Substances that sound synthetic may, in fact, be natural products with standardized names. Additionally, Food and Drug Administration (FDA) requirements may demand that certain synthetic ingredients *must* be added to the product. The manufacturer must use the substance in order to conform to FDA requirements.

A good rule of thumb is to trust a manufacturer who emphasizes *cruelty-free* products. Such manufacturers have made an effort to avoid using any ingredients (natural or synthetic) where significant animal trials have taken place. Since synthetics are generally tested on animals while natural products often have been used for centuries by humans, these manufacturers tend to use natural ingredients, adding synthetics only when the law demands.

Other important labelling clues: organically grown botanicals, botanical ingredients free of irradiation, grown without pesticides, and containers that are biodegradable. Each of these attributes indicate that the manufacturer is committed to providing a quality, natural product.

The information provided in the previous list will aid in understanding ingredients on the label and help users better determine the true content of cosmetics. What follows is a list of natural ingredients contained in products used for hair, skin, teeth, eyes, feet, and body.

Always remember: simpler is better.

ALOE VERA
Used since the time of the ancient Egyptians to treat burns; it moistens and softens the skin. Soothes minor irritations of gum and mouth lining. Please be aware that the leaves need to be processed correctly so the irritants are sufficiently removed.

ANEMONE
Soothing; used to treat skin problems. It can help to reduce the appearance of hairline and deep wrinkles on the skin, while also deeply moisturizing and improving skin elasticity.

ANGELICA
Antiseptic, antibacterial, and bacteriostatic; used externally to treat infections and skin fungus, and to assist with wound healing. Helps to brighten skin and make it look more even and uniform. When applied topically, it works to calm and soothe the skin and heal problems such as eczema and breakouts.

ARGININE
Can enhance the appearance of skin by improving hydration and texture.

ARGAN OIL Has nourishing and hydrating properties; can help repair damaged hair, reduce frizz, and promote shine.

AVOCADO OIL Emollient and antibacterial. It is well-known that this ingredient protects the skin from drying winds and enhances hair, thanks to its moisturizing and antioxidant properties.

BALM As the name states, it soothes the skin. Provides a longer period of moisture and protection, which help to heal the skin.

BASIL Antiseptic; used as a skin toner and cleanser. Basil oil possesses anti-inflammatory properties that work well in preventing skin irritations, small wounds, and sores. The soothing effects of basil leaves aid in healing eczema.

BEESWAX Used in skin emulsions as a thickening agent and emollient; unbleached beeswax is better to use since it has much lower pH levels. Beeswax creates a protective barrier on skin's surface, guarding against environmental irritants and harsh weather. It's noncomedogenic, making it ideal for acne-prone and sensitive skin.

BEETS An emollient and pH adjusting agent; it is the source of the ingredient butyladipate. Helps fight acne and helps hydrate parched skin. Beet can also be used as a natural cheek and lip tint.

BELLADONNA At one time, it was used as a cosmetic dye and to dilate the pupils of the eyes; it is still used as a dye.

BENZOIN From the resin of the tree *Styrax benzoin*; antiseptic, deodorizing, and soothing to irritated skin. It is used as a natural preservative in many cream and ointment recipes. Used to help soothe dry skin. Mildly astringent, it can help with tone.

BERGAMOT From the peel of the green bitter orange, it is antiseptic and astringent, and has been used as an antiperspirant. Bergamot oil is added to black tea to make Earl Grey tea. Bergamot oil is used widely in many external skin and hair applications. It tans the skin and increases its sensitivity to light.

Caution should therefore be used when sunbathing. Is an effective spot treatment for acne due to its immunomodulatory, wound-healing, and anti-inflammatory properties.

BIRCH (Black) Very astringent; it is found in body and foot creams and toners, and in some natural dandruff preparations.

BLACKBERRY Astringent and tonic; used in skin preparations. Used to improve skin complexion and reduce the appearance of wrinkles. Also used in hair care to add shine and strengthen hair.

BLESSED THISTLE Astringent: used in skin care products to tone the skin. It is known for its astringent properties, which can shrink and tighten the top layers of skin. This helps reduce secretions, relieve irritation, and improve tissue firmness.

BLOODROOT Anti-plaque; also traditionally used as a natural red dye coloring. Also used to produce natural, orange, and pink dyes.

BOSWELLIN OIL is distilled from the resin; used in Egypt for corpse preservation. Its current use in natural products cosmetics is as an aid to treat wrinkles and raw or chapped skin, and as a fragrance factor. Helps to reduce inflammation and soothe the skin, while promoting skin firmness and reducing the appearance of wrinkles.

BURDOCK Used to slow the secretion of oil. Its anti-inflammatory and antibacterial properties can help improve various skin conditions, such as eczema, acne, and wrinkles.

CAJEPUT Antiseptic and antimicrobial; thought to be an external anodyne. This oil is mainly found in hair preparations dealing with scalp infection, dandruff, and/or hair loss. It is irritating to sensitive skin. Natural antiseptic that soothes and brightens skin, improving acne, scarring, and wrinkles for a youthful appearance.

CALENDULA (Marigold) Antiseptic and anti-inflammatory; oil and a blossom extract are used for skin conditions and to tone delicate skin. Is a natural anti-inflammatory and antimicrobial, good to use on sensitive or irritated skin to help calm and alleviate skin conditions such as redness, dryness, and minor irritations.

CAMPHOR Very strong external medicine employed to heal bruises, burns, and wounds. Its antifungal, antiseptic, and antibacterial properties can be beneficial for the skin. It can be used to treat skin conditions and fungal infections, as well as reduce inflammation and itchiness.

CARROT SEED OIL Contains carotene and stimulates cell renewal. It has been added to wrinkle creams and facial oils. Most often mixed with almond oil, it will dye the skin due to the carotene content. Carrot seed oil is a great source of antioxidants that can help shield the skin from free radical damage. Additionally, it has moisturizing properties that can help to hydrate the skin and reduce the appearance of fine lines and wrinkles.

CASTOR OIL Emollient; often used as a base and to bind ingredients together. Its healing properties can help soothe dry skin and protect against wrinkles. Additionally, it can speed up hair growth and be used to treat skin conditions such as eczema, dermatitis, and rosacea.

CEDARWOOD Antiseptic and astringent; used in haircare for dandruff and to eliminate greasy hair. Externally, it is used to treat a variety of skin conditions. Due to its manly fragrance, it is very popular as an additive to men's products. As it is soothing to the skin, it is found in aftershave lotions in particular. Can help soothe irritation, inflammation, redness, itchiness, and dryness.

CHAMOMILE An anti-inflammatory used in skin treatments. Useful against infections. When chamomile tea is mixed with lemon, it is an effective highlight rinse for light-colored hair. The ingredient azulene is usually distilled from chamomile. Chamomile can help soothe sensitive skin, promote wound healing, and reduce redness, hyperpigmentation, and acne.

CITRONELLA Possesses fungicidal, antibacterial, and insect repellent properties; used for skin fungus and infections. Citronella has been added to bath soaps and preparations. It can deodorize and refresh body odors, eliminate lice, slow the signs of aging, and improve skin's moisture absorption.

CLOVE Antiseptic and pain-relieving, it is used externally to treat warts, calluses, infected wounds, and insect stings. Men's cosmetics and fragrances seem to favor clove as an agreeable scent. Reduces sagging skin, fine lines, wrinkles, and pigmentation. Calms and soothes irritated skin.

COLTSFOOT High mucilage content; used for soothing skin. Helps reduce inflammation, conditions the skin, reduces oxidative stress, safeguards against microbial function, and gives the skin a more youthful appearance.

CUCUMBER Astringent, tonic, and refreshing, cucumber has been used for centuries to freshen and tone facial skin. Reduces puffiness and dark circles, and fights aging, while it hydrates, soothes, and nourishes the skin with vitamins, antioxidants, and nutrients.

CYPRESS The expressed distilled oil is astringent and deodorizing. It is also an insect repellent and, like clove, is favored as fragrance for men's cosmetic preparations. An astringent can help draw out excess oil from the skin, making it a great option for people with acne. It constricts the skin, which can reduce the appearance of prominent pores. Witch hazel is a well-known oil with astringent properties, but compared to it, cypress is gentler and kinder to the skin.

DEVIL'S CLAW Anti-inflammatory; used in skin products. When applied topically can help heal sores and skin lesions.

DOGWOOD The young branches are sometimes stripped of their bark and used to clean teeth.

ECHINACEA Helps treat sensitive or inflamed gums. An antioxidant-rich plant that provides incredible benefits for the skin, proven to boost collagen production, provide hydration, brighten the skin, and enhance skin's natural moisturizing factor. Additionally, it helps protect skin's outer layer, which helps to lock in moisture.

EUCALYPTUS It is very strong and can irritate the skin. Diluted in oil, it has been used as an insect repellent; stronger preparations are applied topically to herpes blisters.

EYEBRIGHT Used for its soothing properties. It can help reduce puffiness and redness around the eyes, making it a common ingredient in eye creams and serums.

FENNEL Extract of fennel seeds are used to formulate many natural toothpastes, as the seeds are beneficial for gums; it also helps heal mouth infections. It has a pleasing taste. Fennel is known for its antioxidant properties and is used to rejuvenate the skin.

FLAX Anti-inflammatory, demulcent, and emollient; the source of linseed. Flaxseeds contain omega-3 fatty acids that are beneficial for the skin's health. Flaxseed oil is used in skin care products to moisturize and nourish the skin.

FO-TI The Chinese drink a tea of this herb to prevent gray hair. It is also used in hair care products to strengthen and nourish hair.

GARLIC Strongly antiseptic and fungicidal, oil of garlic is used to treat warts as well as calluses and corns on the feet. Its antimicrobial properties make it useful in skin care products designed to combat acne and other skin issues.

GINGER Used for its invigorating and warming effects on the skin.

GINSENG *Panax ginseng* (Korean ginseng) is used to heal and soften skin. It's known for its energizing and revitalizing properties to promote a more youthful and radiant complexion.

GOLDENSEAL Antibacterial; it is used extensively in many female douche preparations. This herb is also found in many products for tooth and gum health and maintenance. Used for its antimicrobial and healing properties, goldenseal can be found in ointments and creams to aid in the healing of minor skin irritations.

GREEN TEA EXTRACT Packed with antioxidants and is used to protect the skin from free radicals and reduce signs of aging.

GROUNDSEL Used in herbal medicine to stop bleeding gums.

GUAR GUM Used as a thickening agent in various skin care and hair care products, such as lotions and shampoos.

HENNA Used as a hair dye since antiquity; imparts a reddish tint to the hair. It provides a natural way to dye hair and is also used for creating temporary body art.

HORSETAIL Taken internally, the silica content strengthens hair, nails, and teeth; externally it is used for skin conditions. Used in hair care products to strengthen hair and promote hair growth.

JASMINE Has a soothing effect on sensitive skin; utilized mainly as a fragrance for bath oils. Its pleasant fragrance is often used in perfumes and scented cosmetics. Its essential oil is also used for its skin-soothing properties.

JOJOBA OIL A versatile ingredient used in skin care and hair care products for its moisturizing and balancing properties.

JUNIPER BERRY Antibacterial, astringent, and toning; the oil is used in conjunction with other herbs to provide a refreshing facial steam bath. Used in skin care products for its astringent and detoxifying properties.

LADY'S MANTLE Used for skin conditions and for skin care in general. Skin care products for sensitive skin often contain this ingredient due to its skin-soothing and anti-inflammatory properties.

LAVENDER There are two distinctly separate lavenders, English and French; they have altogether different fragrances. Both scents are used in various cosmetic and bath preparations. Lavender oil is antibacterial and antiseptic. Some external skin care products include this for warts and eczema as well as athlete's foot. Lavender is widely used for its calming and aromatherapeutic qualities.

LEMON Astringent, antibacterial, and antiseptic; it is somewhat irritating, but has been found useful in the treatment of acne. It is included in many sun-tanning preparations as it enhances skin light sensitivity. It is used for its brightening and exfoliating properties.

LEMON BALM Used for sunburn relief and skin allergies, and as an insect repellent; it is very strong, so only highly diluted preparations are available. Some success treating herpes blisters has been reported. Products designed for sensitive skin often include lemon balm for its soothing and calming effects.

LEMONGRASS Deodorizing and refreshing; this oil has a delightful, totally unique fragrance and in bath oil can be very stimulating.

LICORICE Soothes minor irritations of the gum and mouth lining; used as a breath freshener. Used in skin care products to reduce redness and discoloration, and a popular choice in products for hyperpigmentation.

LINDEN Extracts from the blossoms are used to soothe irritated skin.

MADDER Used as a natural dye in cosmetics, particularly in lip and cheek products.

MAIDENHAIR FERN Used in hair care products for its strengthening and nourishing properties.

MARSHMALLOW The tea is useful as a rinse for oily hair and to add luster. Used in skin care products for its hydrating and soothing effects on the skin.

MUSTARD The oil expressed from the seeds is combined with a massage oil (to dilute the strength of the mustard oil, which can be quite irritating) and applied externally for the relief of muscle aches and pains due to injury or infirmity. Historically used in hair care products for its potential to stimulate hair growth and improve scalp health.

MYRRH One of the ancient Egyptian components of embalming agents, the oil is extracted from the resin of the plant. Today it is found in many natural preparations, such as skin care products that treat fungus infections and eczema, as well as wrinkles and rough skin, and in toothpastes and mouthwashes as an aid for bad breath and gum disease. Additionally, the exotic fragrance is a pleasing addition for those wishing a strong fragrance. Also used for its skin rejuvenation properties, particularly in antiaging products.

NEEM OIL Provides deep skin nourishment, reduces signs of aging, and effectively tackles acne.

NETTLE Astringent; used in hair products and facials. Nettle extract is used in hair care products for its reputed ability to promote hair growth and reduce hair loss.

OATMEAL Used for its soothing and moisturizing properties. Oatmeal baths and creams are popular for sensitive or irritated skin. Particularly recommended for eczema and psoriasis.

OLIVE OIL Used for its moisturizing and softening effects on the skin and hair. It can help reduce dryness and improve hair texture, making it a common ingredient in conditioners and hair treatments.

ORANGE BLOSSOM The oil is nonirritating and is used as a fragrance as well as for chapped skin and acne (mixed with avocado oil). It is found in many bath preparations. Used in cosmetics for its pleasant fragrance and skin-soothing properties.

ORANGE BLOSSOM WATER Astringent and refreshing; it is added to many facial preparations and is a component of an herbal facial steam formula. Used as a natural toner and skin freshener in skin care routines.

PANSY Used in skin care products for its anti-inflammatory properties and ability to soothe sensitive skin.

PAPAYA Used in cosmetics for its natural exfoliating properties and can help promote a brighter complexion.

PATCHOULI OIL Used in perfumes for its own odor as well as its ability to preserve the scent of other fragrances. Used for its exotic fragrance and can be found in perfumes, lotions, and oils.

PEPPERMINT Cooling and stimulating for the skin; also used as a breath freshener. Known for its cooling and invigorating properties, it helps promote scalp circulation, which can lead to increased hair growth and a refreshed feeling.

PRIMROSE OIL Used for its hydrating and soothing effects on the skin.

QUASSIA Commonly used for its ability to reduce inflammation and soothe the skin.

RESTHARROW Emollient; used for itching and eczema. Used for its skin-soothing properties and is often found in products for irritated skin.

ROSE Astringent; rose water soothes irritated skin. Rose essential oils are popular ingredients in cosmetics for their hydrating, soothing, and antiaging properties.

ROSEMARY Potential to promote hair growth and improve scalp health. It is believed to stimulate hair follicles, strengthen hair, and reduce dandruff.

SAGE Used in dandruff shampoo preparations and for gum disease, and for its astringent and purifying qualities, often used for oily skin.

SESAME OIL Emollient; used in skin care products and in sunscreens. Used for its moisturizing and nourishing properties. It's particularly beneficial for dry skin.

SHEA BUTTER Highly moisturizing ingredient used in cosmetics, especially in body creams and lip balms.

SLIPPERY ELM BARK Softens and lubricates the skin; non-greasy and therefore added to more subtle cosmetics as an emollient. Used in skin care products for its soothing and healing properties, especially for irritated or sensitive skin.

SQUIRTING CUCUMBER Ecballine, a compound derived from the fruits, is used in treating baldness as well as a cure against scalp diseases.

TEA TREE Antiseptic and antifungal, tea tree oil distilled from the leaves is used in salves, ointments, lotions, hair care products, and oral care products. It is renowned for its antimicrobial properties and is used for acne and blemish control.

THYME Used for its antimicrobial and scalp-cleansing effects, thyme can help combat dandruff and support a healthier scalp.

TURMERIC Used in cosmetics for its anti-inflammatory and brightening properties; can help to even out skin tone.

VITAMIN A Often in the form of retinol, it is used in antiaging cosmetics to promote skin renewal and reduce the appearance of wrinkles. Vitamin A is taken internally to strengthen skin and eye health.

VITAMIN C Used in cosmetics for its brightening and antioxidant properties, helping to even out skin tone and protect against free radicals. Vitamin C is an immune-enhancing agent that is taken for its assistance with general bodily health.

WALNUT Used to soothe the skin and reduce enlarged pores. Used as a natural exfoliant in cosmetics, particularly in scrubs and cleansers.

WILLOW BARK Natural exfoliating and clarifying properties. It helps remove excess oil, dead skin cells, and product buildup from the scalp, promoting cleaner and healthier hair.

WITCH HAZEL Astringent; used in liniments for body aches and pains; also, a common ingredient in face creams and lotions. Witch hazel is one of the more profound examples of a historical herb whose use endures to this day.

WORMWOOD Antiparasitic when taken internally, wormwood is a topical anesthetic for local irritations such as poison ivy and sunburn.

YARROW Heals wounds and cleans oily skin; along with chamomile, it is the source of the ingredient azulene. Used in cosmetics for its soothing and anti-inflammatory effects on the skin.

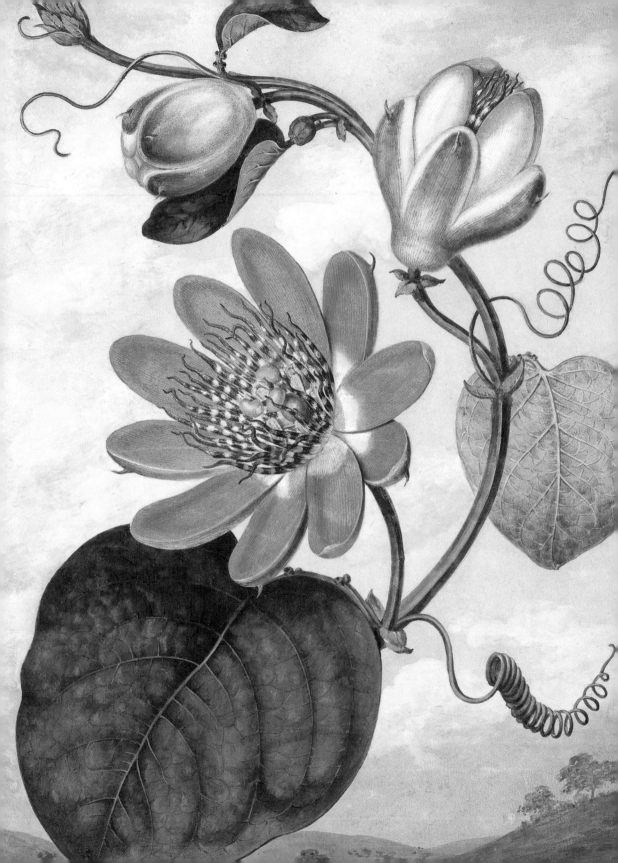

ACKNOWLEDGMENTS

Undertaking the production of any massive reference guide takes extreme effort as well as close attention to factual information. Synthesizing all data is a profoundly intense task.

The team that assisted in this task includes:

Kate Hartson, editor in chief, who assembled the working team and is responsible for the book being completed.

Sean McGowan, researcher and writer, who patiently and professionally researched, wrote updates, and integrated the working manuscript.

Blaire Taylor, researcher and writer, who painstakingly updated over 300 herbal entries with the latest scientific findings—a formidable job.

Night & Day Design, who have produced a stunning volume. We are grateful for their remarkable design featuring classic renderings of the botanical world.

Winged passionflower (*Passiflora alata*), 1799 by Sydenham Teak Edwards.

NO. XXII. BOTANICAL: ECONOMICAL USES OF PLANTS—*CONTINUED.*
V. MEDICINAL PLANTS.

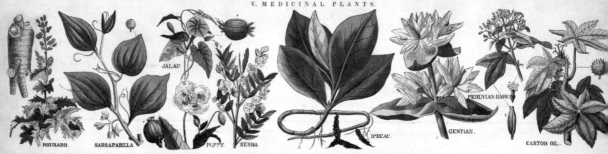

RHUBARB.   SARSAPARILLA   JALAP.   POPPY.   SENNA   IPECAC.   GENTIAN.   PERUVIAN BARK.   CASTOR OIL.

VI. PLANTS USED FOR BEVERAGES.

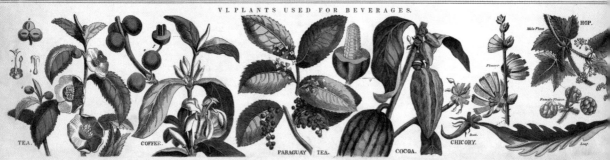

TEA.   COFFEE.   PARAGUAY TEA.   COCOA.   CHICORY.   Male Plant   HOP.   Flower   Female Flower.   Root.   Leaf

VII. PLANTS USED FOR MANUFACTURES.

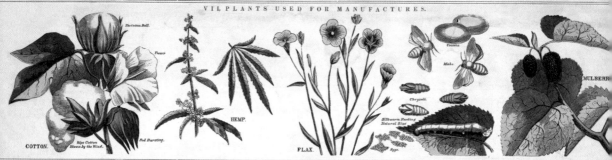

COTTON.   The Cotton Ball.   Flower   Ripe Cotton Blown by the Wind.   Pod Bursting.   HEMP.   FLAX.   Cocoon.   Moth.   Chrysalis.   Silkworm Feeding Natural Size   Eggs.   MULBERRY

VIII. MISCELLANEOUS.

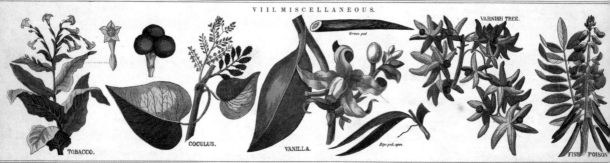

TOBACCO.   COCULUS.   VANILLA.   Green pod   Ripe pod, open.   VARNISH TREE.   FISH POISON

IX. PLANTS USED FOR COLORING.   X. SPICES.

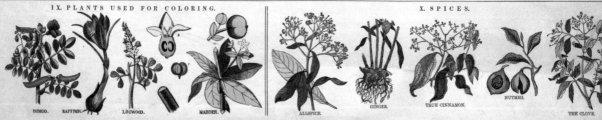

INDIGO.   SAFFRON.   LOGWOOD.   MADDER.   ALLSPICE   GINGER.   TRUE CINNAMON.   NUTMEG.   THE CLOVE.

GLOSSARY

ADAPTOGEN An agent that causes adaptive reactions; adaptogenic drugs appear to increase SNIR (state of nonspecifically increased resistance) in the human body, protecting against diverse stresses.

ADSORBENT A drug used to produce absorption of exudates or diseased tissues.

ALKALOID An alkaline principle of organic origin; any nitrogenous base, especially one of vegetable origin having a toxic effect.

ALTERATIVE An agent that tends to gradually alter a condition.

AMENORRHEA Absence of or suppression of menstruation.

AMINO ACID Amino acids are a large group of organic compounds characterized by the presence of both an amino and a carboxyl radical. They serve as the building blocks from which proteins are constructed and are the end products of protein digestion.

ANABOLIC Marked by or promoting the conversion of simple substances into more complex compounds; usually considered "constructive" metabolism.

ANALGESIC Medicine used to allay pain.

ANEMIA A disorder characterized by a decrease in hemoglobin in the blood to levels below the normal range.

ANESTHETIC Medicine used to produce anesthesia or unconsciousness.

ANODYNE Any medicine that allays pain.

ANTACID Medicines used to neutralize acid in the stomach and intestines.

ANTHELMINTIC (VERMIFUGE) Medicines capable of destroying or expelling worms that inhabit the intestinal canal.

ANTHOCYANINS A group of pigments that cause flowers and plants to be reddish purple in color.

ANTHRAQUINONE Glycoside that acts as a laxative.

ANTIOXIDANT An agent that diminishes the effects of harmful free-radical compounds.

ANTIPHLOGISTIC An agent that tends to relieve inflammation.

ANTIPYRETIC Medicine that reduces the bodily temperature in fevers.

ANTISCORBUTIC A remedy for or counteractant to scurvy.

ANTISEPTIC A substance that prevents infection; tending to inhibit the growth and reproduction of microorganisms.

ANTISPASMODIC Medicine that relieves nervous irritability and minor spasms.

APERIENT An extremely mild, weak laxative.

APHRODISIAC A substance used to increase sexual power or excitement.

AROMATIC An agent used chiefly to expel gas from the stomach and intestines. Also employed to make other medicines, less agreeable in taste and smell, more palatable, due to the fragrant smells and tastes of the aromatics.

ASTRINGENT Tightens and contracts skin and/or mucous membranes. Externally used as lotions and gargles, internally to check diarrhea.

AYURVEDIC MEDICINE The "science of the lifespan"; a system of healing developed and practiced in India.

BACTERIA Small, unicellular microorganisms.

BIOFLAVONOID Colored flavones found in many fruits; essential for absorption and metabolism of ascorbic acid; needed for maintenance of collagen and capillary walls.

BLOOD PRESSURE The pressure exerted by the blood on the walls of the arteries.

CALMATIVE Simply a calming agent, not necessarily a sedative.

CAPILLARY FRAGILITY Weakness of the capillaries (tiny blood vessels where blood and tissue cells exchange substances).

CARBOHYDRATE Group of organic compounds, including sugar, starch, cellulose, and gum.

CARCINOGENIC A substance that can induce cancer.

CARDIOTONIC A substance that tones the heart.

CARMINATIVE A substance that removes gases from the gastrointestinal tract.

CATARRH Inflammation of the air passages of the nose and trachea.

CATHARTIC Laxative and aperient—Mild promotion of evacuation of the bowels by action on alimentary canal. Purgative—Induces copious evacuation of the bowels, generally used to treat stubborn constipation in adults.

CATHETER Flexible, hollow tube that is inserted into a vessel of the body to instill or remove fluids.

CHI "Life-force," "inner energy," and other undefinable (to Westerners) health manifestations known to traditional Chinese medicine.

CHOLAGOGUE An agent that increases the flow of bile into the intestines.

CHOLESTEROL Fat-soluble steroid alcohol found in animals fats, oils, and egg yolk; continuously synthesized in the body, mainly in the liver.

COLLAGEN A protein that can be prepared from connective tissue and from which gelatin can be made.

CORDIAL A refreshing medicine that is held to revive the "spirits," being cheering, invigorating, and exhilarating.

CORTISONE A glucocorticoid (may also be prepared synthetically) often prescribed as an anti-inflammatory.

COUMARIN An anticoagulant.

CYTOTOXIN A substance that has a toxic effect on certain organs, tissues, and cells; produced by injection of foreign cells.

DECOCTION A preparation made by boiling a plant material in water.

DEMULCENT A medicine, used internally, that possesses soothing, mucilaginous properties, shielding surfaces and/or mucous membranes from irritating substances.

DEPURATIVE An agent that purifies or cleanses, generally: "depurate a wound" or "depurate a fluid."

DEXTRAN-SULFATE Created when dextran is boiled with chlorosulfonic acid; used in Japan to reduce blood clotting; may be antiviral.

DIAPHORETIC An agent that increases perspiration. Commonly used for relief of the common cold; administered hot, before bedtime.

DIURETIC Medicine that increases urination; often combined with demulcents.

DOCTRINE OF SIGNATURES An ancient medical theory that "like cures like."

DYSPEPSIA Uncomfortable digestion.

EMETIC A medicine that provokes vomiting.

EMMENAGOGUE A substance with medicinal properties designed to assist and promote menstrual discharge.

EMOLLIENT Generally, of oily or mucilaginous nature; used externally for its softening, supple, or soothing qualities.

ENEMA An injection of solution into the rectum and colon for cleansing or therapeutic purposes.

ESTROGENIC A substance causing estrus.

EXPECTORANT Medicine that promotes the discharge of matter from the lungs, whether it be mucus, pus, or any other morbid accumulation.

FEBRIFUGE Any medicine that mitigates or dispels fever.

FOLLICLE STIMULATING HORMONE (FSH) Secreted by anterior pituitary gland; stimulates growth and maturation of Graafian follicles in the ovary and promotes spermatogenesis in the male.

GALACTAGOGUE A substance that increases the flow of milk.

GAMMA GLOBULIN Protein found in blood; concentration related to ability to resist infection.

GLUTATHIONE A substance that takes up and gives off hydrogen; important in cellular respiration.

GLYCOPROTEIN A compound in which a protein is joined with a carbohydrate nonprotein.

GLYCOSIDE Carbohydrate that yields a sugar and non-sugar on hydrolysis.

HDL High-density lipoprotein; protein that may stabilize low-density lipoprotein; also important in transporting cholesterol and other lipids.

HEMOSTATIC Medicine that arrests hemorrhages.

HEPATIC An agent that promotes the action of the liver and the flow of bile.

HISTAMINE A compound found in all cells where tissue is damaged; associated with allergies and other inflammatory reactions.

HYDRAGOGUE Purgative; causing watery evacuations.

HYDROCORTISONE A cortisone derivative used in the treatment of rheumatoid arthritis.

HYPERTENSIVE An agent that increases blood pressure.

HYPNOTIC An agent producing sleep.

HYPOGLYCEMIA Low blood sugar.

HYPOTENSIVE An agent that causes low blood pressure.

IMMUNOSTIMULANT An agent that stimulates immune responses.

INFUSION A preparation made by steeping a plant material in hot water.

INTERFERON An antiviral glycoprotein.

LAXATIVE An agent that increases the peristaltic motion of the bowels, without purging or producing a fluid discharge. *Never to be used when pregnant.*

LDL Low-density lipoprotein; protein containing more cholesterol and triglycerides than protein.

LITHOTROPIC An agent that dissolves stones in the urinary organs.

MENORRHAGIA Weakness due to heavy menstrual bleeding.

NARCOTIC An agent that induces a hypnotic stupor.

NEPHRITIC An agent useful in kidney complaints.

NERVINE An agent that has a soothing influence and quiets the nerves without numbing them.

PANACEA A "cure-all."

PECTORAL A medicine adapted to cure or relieve complaints of the breast and lungs.

PHOTOTOXIC Making the skin more susceptible to damage by ultraviolet light.

POLYSACCHARIDE A complex carbohydrate.

PROPHYLAXIS Medicine that prevents the development of disease.

PURGATIVE An agent that induces copious evacuation of the bowels. Generally used only for stubborn cases, such as chronic constipation among adults. *Never to be used when pregnant.*

REFRIGERANT Cooling.

RELAXANT Relaxing muscle fiber and alleviating spasm; allaying nervous irritation due to excitement, strain, or fatigue.

RUBEFACIENT An agent that when applied exernally produces redness of the skin, by virtue of drawing the blood and fluids toward the skin's surface; helpful in treatment of boils and blisters.

SAPONIN A complex glycoside that forms a soapy lather in water.

SEDATIVE An agent that allays irritability or nerve action and induces a state of calmness.

SOPORIFIC Causing sleep.

STIMULANT An agent that temporarily increases activity of cardiac, bronchial, gastric, cerebral, intestinal, nervous, motor, vasomotor, respiratory, or secretory organs.

STOMACHIC A stimulant to the stomach.

SUDORIFIC An agent that causes copious perspiration.

TANNIN An astringent phenolic plant constituent.

THROMBOSIS A clot in the bloodstream that blocks the blood vessel.

TONIC Medicine that leads to a feeling of vigor or well-being.

VERMICIDE Medicine that kills intestinal worms.

VERMIFUGE *See* ANTHELMINTIC.

VOLATILE OIL (ESSENTIAL OIL) A mixture of hydrocarbons that are less soluble in water than alcohol or fat.

VULNERARY Useful for healing wounds.

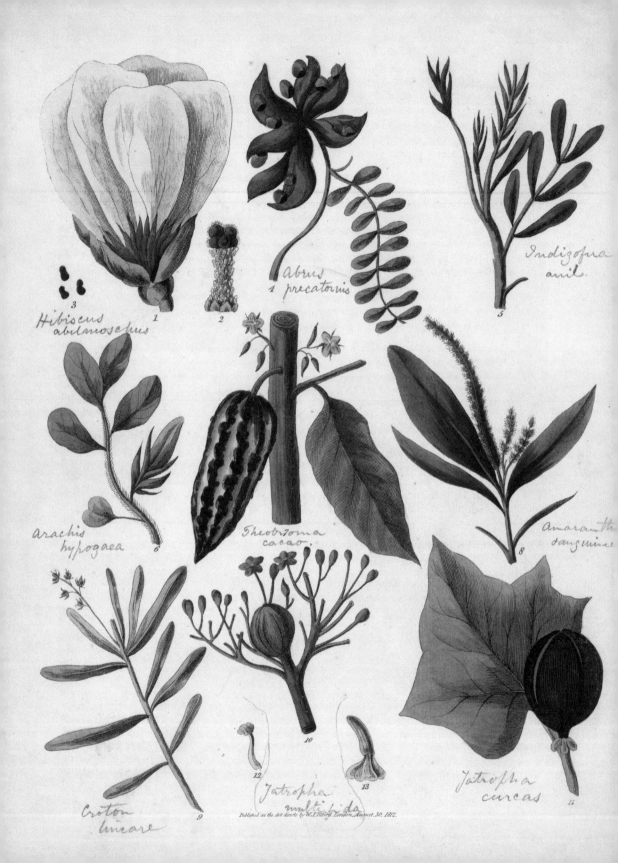

3

Hibiscus
abelmoschus

1

2

Abrus
1 *precatorius*

Indigofra
anil.

5

Arachis
hypogaea   5

Theobroma
cacao.

Amaranth
sanguine   8

12

10

13

Croton
lineare   9

Jatropha
multifida

Jatropha
curcas   11

Published as the Act directs by W.J. Tilling. London. August. 30. 1812.

REFERENCES

GENERAL REFERENCES

Bernier, G.A. *Great Moments in Pharmacy*. Detroit, MI: Northwood Institute Press, 1966.

Carper, J. *The Food Pharmacy: Dramatic New Evidence That Food Is Your Best Medicine*. New York, NY: Bantam Books, 1988.

Chung Shan Medical College. *Kanpo no rinsho oy* (The Clinical Applications of Chinese Herbal Formulas). Tokyo, Japan: Dental and Pharmaceutical Press, 1976.

Fluck, Hans. *Medicinal Plants*. Berkshire, England: W. Foulsham & Co., Ltd, 1988.

Holmes, P. *The Energetics of Western Herbs: Integrating Western and Oriental Herbal Traditions*. Boulder, CO: Artemis, 1989.

Hsu, H., et al., eds. *Oriental Materia Medica: A Concise Guide*. Long Beach, CA: Oriental Healing Arts Institute, 1986.

Hsu, H. *Taiwan ti chu chang chungyao yuao tsai tu chie* (An Illustrated Guide to the Medicinal Plants of Taiwan). Taipei: Chinese National Health Administration, Committee on Chinese Herbal Medicine, 19n.

Kiangsu New Medical College. *Chung yao ta tsu tien* (Dictionary of Chinese Herbal Drugs). Shanghai, Science and Technology Press, 1978; Hong Kong, Commercial Press Ltd., 1978.

Kidd, P.M., and W. Huber. *Living with the AIDS Virus: A Strategy for Long-Term Survival*. HK Biomedical Inc., 1990.

Lawrence, George H.M. *Taxonomy of Vascular Plants*. New York, NY: Macmillian Company, 1969.

Lust, John. *The Herb Book*. New York, NY: Bantam Books, 1974.

Marderosian, A.D., and L.E. Liberti. *Natural Product Medicine: A Scientific Guide to Foods, Drugs, Cosmetics*. Philadelphia, PA: George F. Stickley Co., 1988.

Mills, Simon Y. *The Dictionary of Modern Herbalism*. New York, NY: Thorsons Publishing Group, 1985.

Millspaugh, Charles F. *American Medicinal Plants*. New York, NY: Dover Publications, Inc., 1974 (originally published in two volumes in 1892).

Mowrey, D.B. *The Scientific Validation of Herbal Medicine*. New York, NY: McGraw Hill, 1986.

National Academy of Science. *Herbal Pharmacology in the People's Republic of China: A Trip Report of the American Herbal Pharmacology Delegation*. Washington, DC: National Academy of Science, 1975.

Ratafia, M., and T. Purinton. The untapped market in plant derived drugs. *Medical Marketing and Media,* 58–68, June 1988.

Spalding, B.J. Modern drugs from folk remedies. *Chemical Week,* 52–53, February 27, 1985.

Takagi, K., et al. *Wakan yakubutsugaku* (The Pharmacology of Medicinal Herbs in East Asia). Tokyo, Japan: Nanzando, 1982.

Tyler, V.E., L.R. Brady, and J.E. Robbers. *Pharmacognosy* (9th ed.). Philadelphia, PA: Lea & Febiger, 1988.

Uphof, J.C.T. *Dictionary of Economic Plants*. Stuttgart, Germany: J. Cramer Verlag, 1968.

Vogel, V.J. *American Indian Medicine*. Norman, OK: University of Oklahoma, 1970.

Weiner, M.A. *Earth Medicine, Earth Foods: Plant Remedies, Drugs and Natural Foods of the North American Indian*. New York, NY: Ballantine Books, 1990.

Weiner, M.A. *The Herbal Bible*. Mill Valley, CA: Quantum Books, 1992.

Weiner, M.A. *Maximum Immunity*. Boston, MA: Houghton-Mifflin, 1986.

Weiner, M.A. *Secrets of Fijian Medicine*. Mill Valley, CA: Quantum Books, 1983.

Weiner, Michael and Janet. *Weiner's Herbal*. Mill Valley, CA: Quantum Books, 1990.

Weiss, R.F. *Herbal Medicine*. Beaconsfield, England: Beaconsfield Publishers Ltd, 1988.

Wood, G.B., and F. Bache. *United States Dispensary* (20th ed.). Philadelphia, PA: Lippincott Co., 1918.

RECENT SCIENTIFIC REFERENCES FOR SPECIFIC PLANTS

AGRIMONY

Swanston-Flatt, S.K., Day, C., Balley, C.J., and Flatt, P.R. Traditional plant treatments for diabetes. Studies in normal and streptozotopin diabetic mice. *Diabetologia*, 33(8): 162–164, 1990.

ALOE VERA

Brown, J.S., and Marcy, S.A. The use of botanicals for health purposes by members of a prepaid health plan. *Research in Nursing and Health*, 14(5): 339–350, 1991.

Davis, R.H., et al. Wound healing: Oral and topical activity of Aloe vera. *Journal of the American Podiatric Medical Association*, 79(11): 559–562, 1989.

Davis, R.H., Parker, W.L., and Murdoch, D.P. Aloe vera as a biologically active vehicle for hydrocortisone acetate. *Journal of the American Podiatric Medical Association*, 81(1): 1–9, 1991.

Davis, R.H., Parker, W.L., Sampson, R.T., and Murdoch, D.P. The isolation of an active inhibitory system from an extract of aloe vera. *Journal of the American Podiatric Medical Association*, 81 (5): 258–261, 1991.

Fulton, J.E., Jr. The stimulation of postdermabrasion wound healing with stabilizing aloe vera gel-polyethylene oxide dressing. *Journal of Dermatologic Surgery and Oncology*, 167(5): 460–467, 1990.

Hunter, D. and Frumkin, A. Adverse reactions to vitamin E and aloe vera preparation after dermabrasion and chemical peel. *Cutis*, 47(3), 193–196, 1991.

McCauley, R.L, Heggers, J.P., and Robson, M.C. *Postgraduate Medicine*, 88(8): 67–68, 73–77, 1990.

Schmidt, J.M., and Greenspoon, J.S. Aloe vera dermal wound gel is associated with a delay in wound healing. *Obstetrics and Gynecology*, 78(1): 115–117, 1991.

Thompson, J.E. Topical use of aloe vera derived allantoin gel in otolaryngology [letter]. *Ear, Nose, and Throat Journal*, 70(1): 56, 1991.

Thompson, J.E. Topical use of aloe vera derived allantoin gel in otolaryngology [letter]. *Ear, Nose, and Throat Journal*, 70(2): 119, 1991.

ANEMONE

Martin, M.L., San Roman, L., and Dominquez, A. In vitro activity of protaenominin, an antifungal agent. *Planta Medica*, 56(1): 66–69, 1990.

Martin, M.L, et al. Pharmacologic effects of lactones isolated from Pulsatilla alpina subsp. apiifolia. *Journal of Ethnopharmacology*, 24(Z-3): 185–191, 1988.

Zhang, X.Q., Liu, A.R., and Xu, L.X. Determination of ranunculin in Pulsatilla chinensis and synthetic ranunculin by reversed phase HPLC. *Yao Hsueh Hsueh Pao*, 25(12): 932–935, 1990.

ANGELICA

Inamori, Y, et al. Antibacterial activity of two chalcones, xanthoangelol and 4-hydroxyderricin, isolated from the root of Angelica keiskei. *Chemical and Pharmacological Bulletin*, 39(6): 1604–1605, 1991.

Keji, C. Certain progress in the treatment of coronary heart disease with traditional medicinal plants in China. *American Journal of Chinese Medicine*, 9(3):193–196, 1981.

Mei, Q.B., Tao, J.Y., and Cui, B. Advances in the pharmacological studies of radix Angelica sinensis (Oliv) Diels (Chinese Danggui). *Chinese Medical Journal*, 104(9): 776–7871, 1991.

Murakami, S., et al. Inhibition of gastric H+, K(+)-ATPase by chalcone derivatives, xanthoangelol and 4-hydroxyderricin, from Angelica keiskel Koidzumi. *Journal of Pharmacy and Pharmacology*, 42(10), 723–726, 1990.

Okuyama, T., et al. Antitumor promotion by principles obtained from Angelica keiskei. *Planta Medica*, 57(3): 242–246, 1991.

Usuki, S. Blended effects of herbal components of tokishakuyakusan on somatomedin C/insulin-like growth factor 1 level in rat corpus luteum. *American Journal of Chinese Medicine*, 19(1): 61–64, 1991.

Usuki, S. Effects of herbal components of tokishakuyakusan on progesterone secretion by corpus luteum in vitro. *American Journal of Chinese Medicine*, 19(1): 57–60, 1991.

Wang, L.R., Li, H.Y., and Xie, C.K. Reverse-phase HPLC determination of coumarins in the traditional Chinese drug bal-zhi (Angelica dahurica forma bai-zhi). *Pharmaceutica Sinica*, ZS(Z): 131–136, 1990.

Wang, Y.P. Progress of pharmacological research on angelica polysaccharide. *Chinese Journal of Modern Developments in Traditional Medicine*, 11(1): 61–63, 1991.

Yan, Z., Niu, Z., Pan, N., Xu, G., and Yang, X. Analysis of essential oils in roots and fruits of Angelica in Northeast China. *Journal of Chinese Materia Medica*, 15(7): 419–421, 447, 1990.

Yu, S., et al. Research on the processing of Angelica based on the analysis of water soluble constituents. *Journal of Chinese Materia Medica*, 16(3): 148–149, 190, 1991.

Zhuang, X.X. Protective effect of Angelica injection on arrhythmia during myocardial ischemia reperfusion in rat. *Chinese Journal of Modern Developments in Traditional Medicine*, 11(6): 360–361, 326, 1991.

ANISE

el-Shobaki, F.A., Saleh, Z.A., and Saleh, N. The effect of some beverage extracts on intestinal iron absorption. *Journal of Nutritional Sciences*, 29(4): 264–269, 1990.

Moharram, A.M., Abdel-Mallek, A.Y., and Abdel-Hafez, A.I. Mycoflora of anise and fennel seeds in Egypt. *Journal of Basic Microbiology*, 29(7): 427–435, 1989.

Spencer, D.G., Jr., Yaden, S., and Lal, H. Behavioral and physiological detection of classically conditioned blood pressure reduction. *Psychopharmacology Berlin*, 95(1): 25–28, 1988.

van Toorenenbergen, A.W., Huijakes-Heins, M.J., Leijnse, B., and Dieges, P.H. Immunoblot analysis of IgE-binding antigens in spices. *International Archives of Allergy and Applied Immunology*, 86(1): 117–120, 1988.

ARROWROOT

Rolston, D.D., Matthew, P., and Mathan, V.I. Food-based solutions are a viable alternative to glucose-electrolyte solutions for oral hydration in acute diarrhoea—studies in a rat model of secretory diarrhoea. *Transactions of the Royal Society of Tropical Medicine and Hygiene*, 84(1): 156–159, 1990.

ARTICHOKE

Benveniste, I., Lesot, A., Hasenfratz, M.P., Kochs, G., and Durst, F. Multiple forms of NADPH-cytochrome P450 reductase in higher plants. *Biochemical and Biophysical Research Communications*, 177(1): 105–112, 1991.

Bosque, M.A., Schumacher, M., Domingo, J.L, and Uobet, J.M. Concentrations of lead and cadmium in edible vegetables from Tarragona Province, Spain. *Science of the Total Environment*, 95: 61–67, 1990.

Gabriac, B., Werc-Reichart, D., Teutsch, H., and Durst, F. Purification and immunocharacterization of a plant cytochrome P450: the cinnamic acid 4-hydroxylase. *Archives of Biochemistry and Biophysics*, 288(1): 302–309, 1991.

Gross, K.C., and Acosta, P.B. Fruits and vegetables are a source of galactose: Implications in planning the diets of patients with galactosaemia. *Journal of Inherited Metabolic Diseases*, 14(2): 253–258, 1991.

Merelah, K.A., Bunner, D.L, Ragland, D.R., and Creasla, D.A. Protection against microcystin-LR-induced hepatotoxicity by Silymarin: biochemistry, histopathology, and lethality. *Pharmaceutical Research*, 8(2): 273–271, 1991.

Tavazza, M., Lucioli, A., Ancora, G., and Benvenuto, E. DNA cloning of artichoke mottled crinkle virus RNA and localization and sequencing of the goat protein gene. *Plant Molecular Biology*, 13(6): 685–692, 1989.

ASHWAGANDHA

Al-Hindawi, M.K., Al-Deen, J.H., Nabi, M.H., and Ismail, M.A. Anti-inflammatory activity of some Iraqi plants using intact rats. *Journal of Ethnopharmacology*, 26(2): 163–168, 1989.

Asthana, R., and Raina, M.K. Pharmacology of *Withania somnifera* (linn) dunal—a review. *Indian Drugs*, 26(5): 199–205, 1989.

Atal, C.K., and Schwarting, A.E. Investigation of amino acids in the berries of *Withania somnifera* Dunal, *Current Science*, 29: 22, 1960.

Begum, V.H., and Sadique, J. Effect of *Withania somnifera* on glycosaminoglycan synthesis in carrageenin-induced air pouch granuloma. *Biochemical Medicine and Metabolic Biology*, 38(3): 2n-277, 1987.

Begum, V.H., and Sadique, J. Long-term effect of herbal drug *Withania somnifera* on adjuvant induced arthritis in rats. *Indian Journal of Experimental Biology*, 26(11): 871–882, 1988.

Bhattacharya, S.K., Goel, R.K., Kaur, R., and Ghosal, S. Antistress activity of sitonindosides VII and VIII, new acylsterylglucosides from *Withania somnifera*. *Phytotherapy Research*, 1(1): 32–37, 1987.

Brekhman, I.I. Panax ginseng. *Med. Sci Serv*, 4: 17–26, 1967.

Brekhman, I.I., and Dardymov, I.V. New substances of plant origin which increase non-specific resistance. *Annual Review of Pharmacology and Toxicology*, 9: 419–430, 1969.

Chandra, V., Singh, A., and Kapoor, LD. Studies on alkaloidbearing plants. I. *Withania somnifera* dunal. *Indian Drugs Pharm. Ind.,* September–October, 1, 1970.

Elsakka, M., Grigorescu, E., Stanescu, U., and Domeanu, V. New data referring to chemistry in *Withania somnifera* species. *Revista Medico-Chirurgicala a Sodetatii de Media Si Naturalisti Din Iasi*, 94(2): 385–387, 1990.

Elsakka, M., Pavelescu, M., and Grigorescu, E. *Withania somnifera,* a plant with a great therapeutic future. *Revista Medico-Chirurgicala a Sodetatii de Medid Si Naturalisti Din Iasi*, 93(2): 349–350, 1989.

Ghosal, S., et al. Immunomodulatory and CNS effects of sitoindosides IX and X, two new glycowithanolides from *Withania somnifera*. *Phytotherapy Research*, 3(5): 201–206, 1989.

Kapoor, L.D. *CRC Handbook of Ayurvedic Medicinal Plants*. Boca Raton, FL: CRC Press, 1990.

Kulkarni, R.R., et al. Treatment of osteoarthritis with a herbomineral formulation: a double-blind, placebo-controlled, cross-over study. *Journal of Ethnopharmacology*, 33(1-2): 91–95, 1991.

Kupchan, S.M., et al. *Journal of the American Chemistry Society*, 87: 5805, 1965.

Kuppurajan, K., et al. Effect of Ashwagandha (*Withania somnifera* dunal) on the process of ageing in human volunteers.

Singh, N. et al. Prevention of urethan-induced lung adenomas by *Withania somnifera* (L.) dunal in albino mice. *International Journal of Crude Drug Research*, 24(2): 90–100, 1986.

Singh, N., et al. *Withania somnifera* (Ashwagandha), a rejuvenating herbal drug which enhances survival during stress (an adaptogen). *International Journal of Crude Drug Research*, 20(1): 29–35, 1982.

ASTRAGALUS

Chang, C.Y., Hou, Y.D., and Xu, F.M. Effect of *Astragalus membranaceus* on enhancement of mouse natural killer cell activity. *Chung-kuo I Hsueh K'o Hsueh Yuan Hsueh Pao*, 4(4): 231–234, 1983.

Chu, D.T., et al. Immunotherapy with Chinese medicinal herbs. II. Reversal of cyclophosphamide-induced immune suppression by administration of fractionated *Astragalus membranaceous* in vivo. *Journal of Clinical and Laboratory Immunology*, 25:125–129, 1988.

Chu, D.T., Wong, W.L., and Mavligit, G.M. Immunotherapy with Chinese medicinal herbs I. Immune restoration of local xenogeneic graft-versus-host reaction in cancer patients by fractionated *Astragalus membranaceous* in vitro.

Journal of Clinical and Laboratory Immunology, 25(3):119–123, 1988.

Hou, Y., Ma, G.L., Wu, S.H., U, Y.Y., and U, H.T. Effect of radix astragali seu hedysari on the interferon system. *Chin Med*, 94(1): 35–40, 1981.

Li, Y.Y., Liu, X.Y., Shi, L.Y., Li, Y.X., and Hou, Y.D. Induction characteristic of lymphoblastoid interferon. *Chung-kuo I Hsueh K'o Hsueh Yuan Hsueh Pao*, 2: 250–252, 1980.

Peng, J., Wu, S., Zhang, L., Hou, Y., and Colby, B. Inhibitory effects of interferon and its combination with antiviral drugs on adenovirus multiplication. *Chung-kuo I Hsueh K'o Hsueh Yuan Hsueh Pao*, 6(2): 116–119, 1984.

BARBERRY

Amann, M., Nagakura, N., and Zank, M.H. Purification and properties of (S)-tetrahydrorotoberberine oxidase from suspension-cultured cells of *Berberis wilsoniae. European Journal of Biochemistry*, 175(1): 17–25, 1988.

Dong, H. Effects of storage time on the berberine content in *Berberis amurensis* Rupr. *Chinese Materia Medica*, 12(9): 19–20, 62, 1987.

Gupta, R.S., and Dixit, V.P. Testicular cell population dynamics following palmitine hydroxide treatment in male dogs. *Journal of Ethnopharmacology*, 25(2): 151–157, 1989.

Morales, M.A., et al. Effects of 7-0-demethylisothalicberine, a bisbenzylisoquinoline alkaloid of *Berberis chilensis* on electrical activity of frog cardiac pacemaker cells. *General Pharmacology*, 20(5): 621–625, 1989.

BEARBERRY

Borkowski, B. Diuretic action of several flavone drugs. *Planta Medica*, 8: 95–104, 1960.

Graham, R.C.B., and Noble, R.L. Comparison of in vitro activity of various species of lithospermum and other plants to inactive gonadotrophin. *Endocrinology*, 56: 239, 1955.

Jahodar, L., Jilek, P., Patkova, M., and Dvorakova, V. Antimicrobial action of arbutin and the extract from the leaves of *arctostaphylos uva-ursi* in vitro. *Cesk Farm*, 34(5): 174–178, 1985.

Kubo, M., Ito, M., Nakata, H., and Matsuda, H. Pharmacological studies on leaf of Arctostaphylos uva-ursi (L) Spreng. I. Combined effect of 50% methanol extract from Arctostaphylos uva-ursi. *Journal of the Pharmacological Society of Japan*, 110(1): 59–67, 1990.

Leslie, G.B. A pharmacometric evaluation of nine bio-strath herbal remedies. *Medita*, 8(10): 3–19, 1978.

Matsuda, H., Nakata, H., Tanaka, T., and Kubo, M. Pharmacological studies on leaf of Arctostaphylos uva-ursi (L) Spreng. II. Combined effect of arbutin and prednisolone or dexamethazone on immuno-inflammation. *Journal of the Pharmacological Society of Japan*, 110(1): 68–76, 1990.

Matsuda, H., Tanaka, T., and Kubo, M. Pharmacological studies on leaf of Arctostaphylos uva-ursi (L) Spreng. III. Combined effect of arbutin and indomethacin on immuno-inflammation. *Journal of the Pharmacological Society of Japan*, (4-5): 253–254, 1991.

May, G., and Willuhn, G. Antiviral activity of aqueous extracts from medicinal plants in tissue cultures. *Arzneim-Forsch*, 28(1): 1–7, 1978.

Namba, T., Tsunezuka, M., Bae, K.H., and Hattori, M. Studies on dental caries prevention by traditional Chinese medicines Part I. Screening of crude drugs for antibacterial action against streptococcus mutans. *Shoyakugaku Zasshi*, 35(4): 295–302, 1981.

Namba, T., et al. Studies on dental caries prevention by traditional Chinese medicines (Part IV) Screening of crude drugs for antiplaque action and effects of artemisia capillaris spikes on adherence of streptococcus mutans to smooth surfaces and synthesis of glucan. *Shoyakugaku Zasshi*, 38(3): 253–263, 1984.

Racz, G., Fazakas, B., and Rac-Kotllla, E. Trichomonacidal and anthelmintic activity in Roumanian folkloric plants. (Abstract). *Planta Medica*, 39: 257A, 1980.

Schaufelberger, D., and Hostettmann, K. On the molluscicidal activity of tannin containing plants. *Planta Medica*, 48(2): 105–107, 1983.

Swanson-Flatt, S.K., Day, C., Bailey, C.J., and Flatt, P.R. Evaluation of traditional plant treatments for diabetes: studies in streptozotocin diabetic mice. *Acta Diabetologica Latina*, 26(1): 51–55, 1989.

Ueki, H., Kalbara, M., Sakagawa, M., and Hayashi, S. Antitumor activity of plant constituents. I. *Yakugaku Zasshi*, 81: 1641–1644, 1961.

BEE POLLEN

Iarosh, A.A., Macheret, E.L, Iarosh, A.A., and Zapadniuk, B.V. Changes in the immunological reactivity of patients with disseminated sclerosis treated by prednisolone and the preparation Proper-Myll. *Vrachebnoe Delo*, Feb(2): 83086, 1990.

Koshte, V.L., Kagen, S.L., and Aalberse, R.C. Cross-reactivity of IgE antibodies to caddia fly with arthropoda and mollusca. *Journal of Allergy and Clinical Immunology*, 84(2): 174–183, 1989.

Koslik, S. Possible utilization of the favorable effects of bee pollen in patients with chronic renal insufficiency. *Vnitrni Lakarstvi*, 33(8): 633–640, 1987.

Lin, F.L., Vaughan, T.R., Vandewalker, M.L., and Weber, R.W. Hypereosinophilia, neurologic, and gastrointestinal symptoms after bee-pollen ingestion. *Journal of Allergy and Clinical Immunology*, 83(4): 793–796, 1989.

Liu, X., and Li, L. Morphological observation of effect of bee pollen on intercellular lipofuscin in NIH mice. *Journal of Chinese Materia Medica*, 15(9): 561–563, 578, 1990.

Ludianskii, E.A. The use of apiotherapy and radon baths in treating syringomyelia. *Zhurnal Nevropatologii i Paikhiartrii Imani*, 91(3): 102–103, 1991.

Pham-Dalegua, M.H., Etievant, P., and Masson, C. Molecular parameters involved in bee-plant relationships: a biological and chemical approach. *Biochimie*, 69(607): 661–670, 1987.

Profet, M. The function of allergy: immunological defense against toxins. *Quarterly Review of Biology*, 66(1): 23–62, 1991.

Qian, B., Zang, X., and Liu, X. Effects of bee pollen on lipid peroxides and immune response in aging and malnourished mice. *Journal of Chinese Materia Medica*, 15(5): 301–303, 319, 1990.

Sabbah, A., Le Dauphin, C., and Haulin, M.G. Comparative study of ELISA and RIA technics for the detection of specific IpG4. *Allergie et Immunologie*, 20(6): 232–235, 1988.

Wai, J., Cao, S., Liang, N., and Du, Y. Chemical components of bee's pollen from buckwheat (agopyrum esculentum Moench). *Journal of Chinese Materia Medica*, 15(5): 293–295, 318, 1990.

Wojcicki, J., et al. Effect of pollen extract on the development of experimental atherosclerosis in rabbits. *Atherosclerosis*, 62: 39–45, 1986.

BELLADONNA

Fukui, A., Nakashima, Y., and Kimura, K. Anesthetic management of a patient with Sjogren's syndrome associated with an allergic reaction to various antiphlogistics and sedatives. *Japanese Journal of Anesthesiology*, 40(4): 627–631, 1991.

Kushnir, S., et al. Nucleo-cytoplasmic incompatibility in hybrid plants possessing an Atropa genome and a Nicotinaa plastome. *Molecular and Genera Genetica*, 225(2): 225–230, 1991.

Liu, W.Z. Construction and application of atropine flowthrough sensor in flow injection analysis. *Pharmaceutica Sinica*, 25(6): 451–456, 1990.

Terashchenko, A.V., et al. The conservative treatment of children with vesico-urateral reflux. *Uroligiia i Nefrologiia*, Mar-Apr(2): 24–28, 1991.

BILBERRY

Bonati, A. How and why should we standardize phytopharmaceutical drugs for clinical validation? *Journal of Ethnopharmacology*, 32(1-3): 195–197, 1991.

Cristoni, A., and Magistretti, M.J. Antiulcer and healing activity of *Vaccinium myrtillus* anthocyanosides. *Farmaco, Edizione Pratica*, 42(2): 29–43, 1987.

Fokina, G.I., Frolova, T.V., Roikhel, V.M., and Pogodina, V.V. Experimental phytotherapy of tick-borne encephalitis. *Voprosy Virusologil*, 36(1): 18–21, 1991.

Magistrettl, M.J., Conti, M., and Cristoni, A. Antiulcer activity of an anthocyanidin from *Vaccinium myrtillus*. *ArzneimeittelForschung*, 38(5): 686–690, 1988.

Morazzoni, P., Livig, S., Scilingo, A., and Malandrino, S. *Vaccinium myrtillus* anthocyanosides pharmacokinetics in rats. *Arzneimeittel-Forschung*, 41 (2): 128–131, 1991.

Saija, A., et al. Effect of *Vaccinium myrtillus* anthocyanins on trilodothyronine transport into brain in the rat. *Pharmacological Research*, 22(Suppl 3): 59–60, 1990.

BLOODROOT

Eisenberg, A.D., Young, D.A., Fan-Hsu, J., and Spitz, L.M. Interactions of sanguinarine and zinc on oral streptococci and Actinomyces species. *Caries Research*, 25(3): 185–190, 1991.

Harper, D.S., Mueller, L.J., Fine, J.B., Gordon, J., and Laster, L.L. Clinical efficacy of a dentifrice and oral rinse containing sanguinaria extract and zinc chloride during 6 months of use. *Journal of Periodontology*, 61(6): 352–358, 1990.

Harper, D.S., Mueller, L.J., Fine, J.B., Gordon, J., and Laster, L.L. Effect of 6 months use of a dentrifice and oral rinse containing sanguinaria extract and zinc chloride upon the microflora of the dental plaque and oral soft tissues. *Journal of Periodontology*, 61(6): 359–363, 1990.

Kuftinec, M.M., Mueller-Joseph, L.J., and Kpozyk, R.A. Sanguinaria toothpaste and oral rinse regimen clinical efficacy in short- and long-term trials. *Journal of Clinical Dentistry*, 1 (3): 59–66, 1989.

Walker, C. Effects of sanguinarine and Sanguinaria extract and microbiota associated with the oral cavity. *Journal of the Canadian Dental Association*, 56(7 Suppl): 13–30, 1990.

Walker, C. New perspectives on Sanguinaria clinicals: individual toothpaste and oral rinse testing. *Journal of the Canadian Dental Association*, 56 (7 Suppl): 19–30, 1990.

BONESET

Beier, R.C., and Norman, J.O. The toxic factor in white snakeroot: identity, analysis and prevention. *Veterinary and Human Toxicology*, 32(Suppl): 81–89, 1990.

Beier, R.C., Norman, J.O., Irvin, T.R., and Witzel, D.A. Microsomal activation of constituents of white snakeroot (Eupatorium rugosum Houtt) to form toxic products. *American Journal of Veterinary Research*, 19(1): 583–585, 1987.

Chan, M.Y., Zhao, X.L., and Ogle, C.W. A comparative study on the hepatic toxicity and metabolism of *Crotaleria assemica* and *Eupatorium* species. *American Journal of Chinese Medicine*, 17(3-4): 165–170, 1989.

Elema, E.T., Schripaema, J., and Malingra, T.M. Flavones and flavonol glycosides from *Eupatorium cannabrinum* L. *Pharmaceutisch Weekbled*, 11(5): 161–164, 1989.

Hendrika, H., Hulzing, H.J., and Bruins, A.P. Ammonium positive-ion and hydroxide negative-ion chemical ionization gas chromatography-mass spectrometry for the identification of pyrrolizidine alkaloids in *Eupatorium rotundifolium* L var. ovatum. *Journal of Chromatography*, 128(2): 352–356, 1989.

Hirschmann, G.S., and Ferro, E. Indigo from *Eupatorium* leaves. *Journal of Ethnopharmacology*, 26(1): 93–94, 1989.

Lexa, A., et al. Choleretic and hepatoprotective properties of *Eupatorium cannabinum* in the rat. *Planta Medica*, 55(2): 127–132, 1989.

Woerdenbag, H.J., et al. Induction of DNA damage in Ehrlich ascites tumor cells by exposure to eupatoriopicrin. *Biochemical Pharmacology*, 39(11); 2279–2293, 1969.

Woerdenbag, H.J., Lemstra, W., Malingre, T.M., and Konings, A.W. Enhanced cytostatic activity of the sesquiterpene lactone eupatoriopicrin by glutathione depletion. *British Journal of Cancer*, 59(1): 69–75, 1989.

Zhao, X.L, Chan, M.Y., Kumana, C.R., and Ogle, C.W. A comparative study on the pyrrolizidine alkaloid content and the pattern of hepatic pyrrolic metabolite accumulation in mice given extracts of Eupatorium plant species, *Crotaleria assemica* and an Indian herbal mixture. *American Journal of Chinese Medicine*, 15(1-2), 59–67, 1987.

Zhao, X.L., Chan, M.Y., and Ogle, C.W. The identification of pyrrolizidine alkaloid-containing plants–a study on 20 herbs of the Compositae family. *American Journal of Chinese Medicine*, 17(1-2); 71–79, 1989.

BOSWELLIN

11th European Congress of Rheumatology, Vol. 5/8-2. Supplement issue, 1987.

Atal, C.K., et al. Salai guggal a new nonsteroidal anti-inflammatory agent and its probable mode of action. Recent Advances in Mediators of Inflammation and Anti-inflammatory Agents, Symposium, Nov. 2–4, 1984.

Atal, C.K., Sharma, M.L, Kaul, A., Khajuria, and Singh, G.B. Effect of "Salai guggal"-a new non-steroidal anti-inflammatory drug on leucocyte migration. XV Annual Conference of IPS.

Bhargava, G.G., Negi, J.S., and Ghua, S.R.D. Studies on the chemical components of salai gum. *Indian Forester*, 104: 174–181, 1978.

Council of Scientific and Industrial Research. Recent advances in mediators of inflammatory agents R.R.I. Symposium, 1984.

Gupta, V.N., Yadav, D.S., Jain, M.P., and Atal, C.K. Chemistry and pharmacology of gum resin of *Boswellia serrata* (salai guggal). *Indian Drugs*, 24(5): 221–231, 1987.

Kar, A. & Menon, M.K. Analgesic effect of the gum resin of *Boswellia serrata* Roxb. *Life Sciences*, 8(1): 1023–1028, 1969.

Kulkarni, R.R., et al. Treatment of osteoarthritis with a herbomineral formulation: a double-blind, placebo-controlled, cross-over study. *Journal of Ethnopharmacology*, 33(1-2): 91–95, 1991.

Menon, M.K., and Kar, A. Analgesic and psychopharmacological effects of the gum resin of *Boswellia serrata*. *Planta Medica*, 19: 332–341, 1971.

Pardhy, R.S., and Bhattacharya, S.C. Tetracyclic triterpene acids from the resin of *Boswellia serrata* Roxb. *Indian Journal of Chemistry*, 16(B): 174–175, 1978.

Pardhy, R.S., and Bhattacharya, S.C. Boswellic acid, acetyl-boswellic acid and 11-keta-boswellic acid four pentacyclic triterpene acids from the resin of *Boswellia serrata* Roxb. *Indian Journal of Chemistry*, 16(B): 176–178, 1978.

Reddy, G.K., Chandrakasan, G., and Dhar, S.C. Studies on the metabolism of glycosaminoglycalis under the influence of new herbal anti-inflammatory agents. *Biochemical Pharmacology*, 38(2): 3527–3534, 1989.

Safayhi, H., Mack, T., and Ammon, H.P.T. Protection by boswellic acids against galactosamine/endotoxin-induced hepatitis in mice. *Biochemical Pharmacology*, 41(10): 1537–1537, 1991.

Singh, G.B., and Atal, C.K. Pharmacology of an extract of salai guggul *ex-Boswellia serrata,* a new nonsteroidal anti-inflammatory agent. *Agents Actions*, 18: 407–412, 1986.

Zutshi, U., Rao, P.G., Kaur, S., Singh, G.B., and Atal, C.K. Mechanism of cholesterol lowering effect of Salai guggal *ex-Boswelli serrat* XII Annual Conference of IPS.

BUCKTHORN

Goel, R.K., Des Gupta, G., Ram, S.N., and Panday, V.B. Antiulcerogenic and anti-inflammatory effects of emodin, isolated from *Rhamnus triquerta* wall. *Indian Journal of Experimental Biology*, 29(3): 80–83, 1991.

Goel, R.K., Panday, V.B., Dwivedi, S.P., and Rao, Y.U. Anti-inflammatory and anti-ulcer effects of kaempferol, a flavone, isolated from *Rhamnus procumbens*. *Indian Journal of Experimental Biology*, 26(2): 121–124, 1988.

Gundidza, M., and Sibanda, M. Antimicrobial activities of *Ziziphus abyssinica* and *Berchemia discolor*. *Central African Journal of Medicine*, 37(3): 80–83, 1991.

Ito, Y., Oka, H, and Lee, Y.W. Improved high-speed countercurrent chromatograph with three multilayer coils connected in series. II. Separation of various biological samples with a semi-preparative column. *Journal of Chromatography*, 198(1): 169–179, 1991.

Jiao, P.Y., and Fang, J.N. Studies in isolation, purification and structure of NLCA of *Rhamnus heterophyllus*. *Pharmaceutica Sinica*, 21(5): 353–356, 1989.

Kostrikova, E.V. Experimental study of wound-healing effect of the preparation "Askol" (artificial sea buckthorn oil). *Ortopediia Travmatologita i Protezirovanie*, fan(l): 32–36, 1989.

Martinez de Villarreal, L, et al. Effects of toxin T-511 from the Karwinskia humboldtiana (buckthorn) plant upon mouse embryos explanted at 11 days. *Toxicon*, 28(1): 119–152, 1990.

Nunes, P.H., Marinho, L.C., Nunes, M.L, and Scares, E.D. Antipyretic activity of an aqueous extract of *Zizyphus joazeiro* Mart. *Brazilian Journal of Medical and Biological Research*, 20(5): 599–601, 1987.

Terencio, M.C., Sanz, M.J., and Paya, M. A hypotensive procyanidin-glycoside from *Rhamnus lydoides* ssp. lycioides. *Journal of Ethnopharmacology*, 30(2): 205–214, 1990.

Turner, N.J., and Habda, R.J. Contemporary use of bark for medicine by two Salishan native elders of southeast Vancouver Island, Canada. *Journal of Ethnopharmacology*, 29(1): 59, 1990.

van den Dikkenberg, M.I., and Holtkamp, B.M. Alder buckthorn poisoning in horses. *Tridschrift voor Diergenesskunda*, 112(6): 310–311, 1987.

Zhang, T.Y., Lee, Y.W., Fang, O.C., Xiao, R., and Ito, Y. Preliminary applications of cross-axis synchronous flow-through coil planted centrifuge for large-scale preparative counter-current chromatography. *Journal of Chromatography*, 151: 185–193, 1988.

BUPLEURUM

Amagaya, S., et al. Effects of Shosaikoto, an Oriental herbal medicinal mixture, on age-induced amnesia in rats. *Journal of Ethnopharmacology*, 28: 349–356, 1990.

Amagaya, S., and Ogihara Y. Effects of Shosaikoto, an Oriental herbal medicinal mixture, on restraint-stressed mice. *Journal of Ethnopharmacology*, 28: 357, 1990.

BURDOCK

Proctor, V.A., and Cunningham, F.E. The chemistry of lysozyme and its use as a food preservative and pharmaceutical. *Critical Review Food Science Nutrition*, 25(1): 359–395, 1988.

Smarda, J. Viroids: molecular infectious agents. *Acta Virologica*, 31(6): 505–521, 1987.

Swanston-Flatt, S.K., et al. Glycaemic effects of traditional European plant treatments for diabetes. Studies in normal and streptozotocin diabetic mice. *Diabetes Research*, 10(2): 69–73, 1989.

BUTCHER'S BROOM

Cahn, J., Herold, M., and Sanault, B. Antiphiogistic and anti-inflammatory activity of F 191. Int. Symp. Non-Steroidal Anti-Inflammatory Drugs, Milano, 1964.

Cappelli, R., Nicora, M., and Di Perri, T. Use of extract of *Ruscus aculeatus* in venous disease in the lower limbs. *Drugs Under Experimental and Clinical Research*, 11(1): 277–293, 1988.

Capra, C. Studio farmacologico e tossicologico di componenti del *Ruscus aculeatus* L. *Fitoterapia,* 43: 99, 1972.

Caujolle, F., Meriel, P., and Stanilas, E. Sur Jes propriétés pharmacologiques de *Ruscus aculeatus* L. *Ann. Pharm. Franc.*, 11: 109, 1953.

Chabanon, R. Expérimentation du proctolog dans les hémorroides et les fissures anales. *Gaz. Mtd de France*, 83: 3013, 1976.

Marcelon, G., Verbeuren, T.J., Lauressergues, H., and Vanhoutte, P.M. Effect of *Ruscus aculeatus* on isolated canine cutaneous veins. *Gen. Pharmac.*, 14: 103, 1983.

Moscarella, C. Contribution a l'etude pharmacologique du *Ruscus aculeatus* L (Fragon épineux). Thése de Pharmacie, Toulouse, 1953.

Weindorf, N., and Schultz-Ehrenburg, U. Controlled study of increasing venous tone in primary varicose veins by oral administration of *Ruscus aculeatus* and trimethylhespiridinchalcone. *Zeitschrift fur Haukrankhsiten*, 52(1): 28–38, 1987.

CASCARA SAGRADA

Borkje, B., Pederson, R., Lund, G.M., Enehaug, J.S., and Berstad, A. Effectiveness and acceptability of three bowel cleansing regimens. *Scandinavian Journal of Gastroenterology*, 26(2): 162–166, 1991.

de Witte, P., and Lemli, L. The metabolism of anthranoid laxatives. *Hepatogastroenterology*, 37 (6): 601–605, 1990.

Phillip, J., Schubert, G.E., Thiel, A, and Wolters, U. Preparation for colonoscopy using Golytely—a sure method? Comparative histological and clinical study between lavage and saline laxatives. *Medizinische Klinik*, 85(7): 115–120, 1990.

CAYENNE

Basha, K.M., et al. Capsaicin: A therapeutic option for painful diabetic neuropathy. *Henry Ford Hospital Medical Journal*, 39(2): 138–140, 1991.

De, A.K.Y., and Ghosh, J.J. Short- and long-term effects of capsaicin on the pulmonary antioxidant enzyme system in rats. *Phytotherapy Research*, 3(5), 1989.

Govindarajan, V.S., and Sathyanarayana, M.N. Capsicum-production, technology, chemistry and quality. Part V. Impact on physiology, pharmacology, nutrition, and metabolism; structure, pungency, pain, and desensitization sequences. *Critical Review Food Science Nutrition*, 29(6): 135–171, 1991.

Jancso, N., Jancso-Gabor, A., and Szolcanyi, J. Direct evidence for neurogenic inflammation and its prevention by denervation and by pretreatment with capsaicin. *Br. Journal Pharmacol.*, 31:138, 1967.

Marabii, S., Ciabatti, P.G., Polli, G., Fusco, B.M., and Geppetti, P. Beneficial effects of intranasal applications of capsaicin in patients with vasomotor rhinitis. *European Archives of OtoRhino-laryngology*, 218(4): 181–184, 1991.

Rayner, H.C., Atkins, R.C., and Westerman, R.A. Relief of local stump pain by capsaicin cream. *Lancet*, 1276–1277, 1989.

Teel, R.W. Effects of capsaicin on rat liver S9-mediated metabolism and DNA binding of aflatoxin. *Nutrition and Cancer*, 15(1): 27–32, 1991.

CHAMOMILE

Fokina, G.I., Frolova, T.V., Roikhel, V.M., and Pogodina, V.V. Experimental phytotherapy of tick-borne encephalitis. *Voprosy Virusologii*, 36(1): 18–21, 1991.

Glowania, H.J., Raulin, C., and Swoboda, M. Effect of chamomile on wound healing–a clinical double-blind study. *Zeitschrift fur Hautkrankheiten*, 62(17): 1262, 1267–1271, 1987.

Maiche, A.G., Grohn, P., and Maki-Hokkonen, H. Effect of chamomile cream and almond ointment on acute radiation skin reaction. *Acta Oncologica*, 30(3): 395–398, 1991.

Subiza, J., et al. Anaphylactic reaction after the ingestion of chamomile tea: a study of cross-reactivity with other composite pollens. *Journal of Allergy and Clinical Immunology*, 81(3): 353–359, 1989.

Subiza, J., et al. Allergic conjunctivitis to chamomile tea. *Annals of Allergy*, 55(2): 127–132, 1990.

CHASTEBERRY

Belie, I., Bergant-Dolar, J., Stucin, D., and Stucin, M.A. Biologically active substance from *Vitex agnus-castus*. *Vestnick Sloven Kemi Drutva*, 5: 63, 1958.

Goerler, K., Dehlke, D., and Soicke, H. Iridoid derivatives from *Vitex agnus castus*. *Planta Medica*, 50(6): 530–531, 1985.

Gomaa, C.S., El-Moghazy, M.A., Halim, F.A., and El-Sayyad, A.E. Flavonoids and iridoids from *Vitex agnus castus*. *Planta Medica*, 33: 277, 1978.

Haller, J. Animal experimentation with the Lipschutz technic on the activity of a phytohormone

on gonadotrophin function. *Geburtschilfe Frauenheilkund*, 18: 1347, 1958.

Hansel, R., and Winde, E. Constituents of the verbenaceae. 2. Agnuside, a new glycoside from *vitex agnus castus. Arzneimittel-Forschung*, 9: 180–190, 1959.

Jochle, W. Menses-inducing drugs. Their role in antique, medieval and renaissance gynaecology and birth control. *Contraception*, 10: 425, 1974.

Perrot, E., and Paris, R.R. *Les plantes medicinales, Part I.* Presses Universitaires De France, Paris, 1971.

Stewart, A. *Vitex agnus castus* in premenstrual tension. Available from Gerard House Ltd., Bournemouth, England, 1987.

Wollenweber, E., and Mann, K. Flavonols from the fruits of *Vitex agnus castus. Planta Medica*, 48: 126–127, 1983.

CHINESE CUCUMBER

Chao, Z., and Liu, J. Chemical constituents of the pericarp of *Tricosanthes rosthornii* Harms. *Journal of Chinese Materia Medica*, 16(2): 97–99, 127, 1991.

Ferrari, P., et al. Toxicity and activity of purified trichosanthin. 5(7): 865–870, 1991.

Lee-Huang, S., et al. TAP 29: An antihuman immunodeficiency virus protein from *Trichosanthes kirilowii* that is nontoxic to intact cells. *Proceedings of the National Academy of Sciences of the United States of America*, 88(15): 6570–6574, 1991.

McGrath, M.S., et al. GLQ 223: An Inhibitor of human immunodeficiency virus replication in acutely and chemically infected cells of lymphocyte and mononuclear phagocyte lineage. *Proceedings of the National Academy of Science*, 86: 2844–2848, April 1989.

Schnittman, S.M., et al. The reservoir for HIV-1 in human peripheral blood is a T cell that maintains expression of C D4. *Science*, 245: 305–308, 1989.

Wang, Q.C., et al. Tricosanthin-monoclonal antibody conjugate specifically cytotoxic to human hepatoma cells in vitro. *Cancer Research*, 51(3): 3353–3355, 1991.

CINCHONA

Abdulraharnn, S., et al. High-performance liquid chromatographic-mass spectrometric assay of high-value compounds for pharmaceutical use from plant cell tissue culture: Cinchona alkaloids. *Journal of Chromatography*, 562(1-2): 719–721, 1991.

Kirk, K., et al. Enhanced choline and Rb+ transport in human erythrocytes infected with the malaria parasite *Plasmodium falciparum. Biochemical Journal*, 278(Pt 2): 521–525, 1991.

Sabchareon, A., et al. Red cell and plasma concentrations of combined quinine-quinidine and quinine in falciparum malaria. *Annals of Tropical Pediatrics*, 11(4): 315–324, 1991.

CINNAMON

Buch, J.G., Dikshit, R.K., and Mansuri, S. Effect of certain volatile oils on ejaculated human spermatozoa. *Indian Journal of Medical Research*, 87(4): 361–363, 1988.

Conner, D.E., and Beuchat, L.R. Effects of essential oils from plants on growth of food spoilage yeasts. *Journal of Food Science*, 49(2): 429–434, 1984.

Fitzpatrick, F.K. Plant substances active against mycobacterium tuberculosis. *Antibiotic Chemotherapy*, 4: 528, 1954.

Gupta, M. Essential oils: A new source of bee repellents. *Chem India (London)*, 5: 161–163, 1987.

Morozumi, S. A new antifungal agent in cinnamon. *Shinkin To Shinkinsho*, 19: 172–180, 1978.

Namba, T., et al. Studies on development of immunomodulating drugs (11) effect of Ayurvedic medicines on blastogenesis of lymphocytes from mice. *Shoyakugaku Zasshi*, 43(3): 250–255, 1989.

Noding, A., Stoa, K.F., and Nordal, A. Investigation of the estrogenic effect of extracts of Ceylon cinnamon. *Norsk Farm Selskap*, 12: 68–73, 1950.

Raharivelomanana, P.J., Terrom, G.P., Bianchini, J.P., and Coulanges, P. Study of the antimicrobial action of various oil extracts from madagascan plants. 11. The aluraceae. *Arch Institute Pasteur Madagascar*, 56(1): 261–271, 1989.

Sivaswamy, S.W., Balachandran, B., Balanehru, S., and Sivaramakrlshnan, V.W. *Indian Journal of Experimental Biology*, 29(8): 730–737, 1991.

Sugaya, A., Tsuda, T., Sugaya, E., Usami, M., and Takamura, K. Local anaesthetic action of the Chinese medicine saikokeishi-to. *Planta Medica*, 37: 274–276, 1979.

Sugaya, E., et al. Inhibitory effect of a mixture of herbal drugs (TJ-960, SK) on pentylenetetrazol-induced convulsions in E1 mice. *Epilepsy Research*, 2(5): 337–339, 1988.

Ungsurungsie, M., Paovalo, C., and Noonai, A. Mutagenicity of extracts from Ceylon Cinnamon in the rec assay. *Food and Chemical Toxicology*, 22(2): 109–112, 1984.

CITRUS

Clegg, R.J., Middleton, B., Bell, G.D., and White, D.A. Inhibition of hepatic cholesterol synthesis by monoterpenes administered in vivo. *Biochemical Pharmacology*, 29: 2125–2127, 1980.

Elegbede, J., Elson, C., Tanner, M., Qureshi, A., and Gould, M. Regression of rat primary mammary tumors following dietary d-limonene. *Journal of the National Cancer Institute*, 323–325, 1986.

Elson, C., Maltzman, T., Boston, J., Tanner, M., and Gould, M. Anti-carcinogenic activity of d-limonene during the initiation and promotion/progression stages of DMBA-induced rat mammary carcinogenesis. *Carcinogenesis*, 9: 331–332, 1988.

Evans, D., Miller, D., Jacobsen, K., and Bush, P. Modulation of immune responses in mice by d-limonene. *Journal of Toxicological and Environmental Health*, 20: 51–66, 1987.

Igimi, J., Hisatsugu, T., and Nishimura, M. The use of d-limonene preparation as a dissolving agent of gallstones. *American Journal of Digestive Disorders*, 21: 926, 1976.

Maltzman, T., Tanner, M., Elson, C., and Gould, M. Anticarcinogenic activity of specific orange peel oil monoterpenes. *Federation Proceedings*, 45: 970, 1986.

Wattenberg, L. Inhibition of neoplasia by minor dietary components. *Cancer Research*, 43(supplement): 2448–2453, 1983.

CLOVE

Al-Khayat, M.A., and Blank, G. Phenolic spice components sporostatic to *Bacillus subtilis. Journal of Food Safety*, 50(4): 971–980, 1985.

Buch, J.G., Dikshit, R.K., and Mansuri, S.M. Spermicidal effects of certain volatile oils on human spermatozoa in vitro. *Journal of Andrology*, 6(2): Abstr-M41, 1985.

Buch, J.G., Dikshit, R.K., and Mansuri, S.M. Effect of certain volatile oils on ejaculated human spermatozoa. *Indian Journal of Medical Research*, 87(4): 361–363, 1988.

Burapanont, P., Siriwongpairat, P., and Leartskulpiriya, M. Preparation and evaluation of cough pills. *Undergraduate Special Project Report 1984:* 30pp, 1984.

Caceres, A., Giron, L.M., Alvarado, S.R., and Torres, M.F. Screening of antimicrobial activity of plants popularly used in Guatemala for the treatment of dermatomucosal diseases. *Journal of Ethnopharmacology*, 20(3): 223–237, 1987.

Conner, D.E., and Beuchat, L.R. Effects of essential oils from plants on growth of food spoilage yeasts. *Journal of Food Safety*, 49(2): 429–434, 1984.

Dabral, P.K., and Sharma, R.K. Evaluation of the role of rumalaya and geriforte in chronic arthritis: A preliminary study. *Probe*, 22(2): 120–127, 1983.

Dhawan, B.N., Patnaik, G.K., Rastogi, R.P., Singh, K.K., and Tandon, J.S. Screening of Indian plants for biological activity, VI. *Indian Journal of Experimental Biology*, 15: 208, 1977.

Giron, L.M., Aguilar, G.A., Caceres, A., Arroyo, G.L. Anticandidal activity of plants used for the treatment of vaginitis in Guatemala and clinical trial of *Solanum nigrescens* preparation. *Journal of Ethnopharmacology*, 22(3): 307–313, 1988.

Guerin, J.C., and Reveillere, H.P. Antifungal activity of plant extracts used in therapy. II. Study of 40 plant extracts against 9 fungi species. *Ann. Pharm. Fr.*, 43(1): 77–81, 1985.

Gupta, M. Essential oils: A new source of bee repellents. *Chem. Ind. (London)*, 5: 161–163, 1987.

Iwasaki, M., Ishikawa, C., Maesuura, Y., Ohhashi, E., and Harada, R. Antioxidants of allspice and clove. *Sagami foshi Daigaku* Kiyo, 48: 1–6, 1984.

Janssen, A.M., Chin, N.L., Scheffer, J.J.C., and Baerheim-Svendsen, A. Screening for antimicrobial activity of some essential oils by the agar overlay technique. *Phann. Weekbl (Sd. Ed.)*, 8(6): 289–292, 1986.

Janzen, D.H., Juster, H.B., and Bell, E.A. Toxicity of secondary compounds to the seed-eating larvae of the bruchid beetle *Callosobruchus maculatus*. *Phytochemistry*, 16: 223–227, 1977.

Kramer, R.E. Antioxidants in clove. *Journal of the American Oil Chemists' Society*, 62(1): 111–113, 1985.

Maruzzella, J.C., Scrandis, O., Scrandis, J.B., and Grabon, G. Action of odoriferous organic chemicals and essential oils on wood-destroying fungi. *Plant Dis. Rept*, 44: 789, 1960.

Namba, T., Tsunezuka, M., Bae, K.H., and Hattori, M. Studies on dental caries prevention by traditional Chinese medicines Part I. Screening of crude drugs for antibacterial action against *Streptococcus mutans*. *Shoyakugaku Zasshi*, 35(4): 295–302, 1981.

Namba, T., et al. Studies on dental caries prevention by traditional Chinese medicines (Part IV) screening of crude drugs for antiplaque action and effects of *Artemisia capillaris* spikes on adherence of *Streptococcus mutans* to smooth surfaces and synthesis of glucan. *Shoyakugaku Zasshi*, 38(3): 253–263, 1984.

Nes, I.F., Skjelkvale, R., Olsvik, O., and Berdai, B.P. The effect of natural spices and oleoresins on *Lactobacillus plantarum* and *Staphylococcus aureus*. *Microb. Assoc. Interact Food Proc. Int Iums-ICFMH Sym. 12th 1983 1984*: 435–440, 1984.

Reiter, M., and Brandt, W. Relaxant effects on tracheal and ileal smooth muscles of the guinea pig. *Arzneim-Forsch*, 35(1): 408–414, 1985.

Saito, Y., Kimura, Y., and Sakamoto, T. The antioxidant effects of petroleum ether soluble and insoluble fractions from spices. *Eiyo To Shokuryo Vryo*, 29: 505–510, 1976.

Salem, F.S. Evaluation of clove oil and some of its derivatives as trichomonacidal agents. *Journal Drug Res (Egypt)*, 12: 115–119, 1980.

Seetharam, K.A., and Pasricha, J.S. Condiments and contact dermatitis of the finger-tips. *Indian Journal Dermatol. Venereal Leprol*, 53(6): 325–328, 1987.

Shukia, B., Khanna, N.K., and Godhwani, J.L Effect of brahmi rasayan on the central nervous system. *Journal of Ethnopharmacology*, 21(1): 65–74, 1987.

Singh, B.G., and Agrawal, S.C. Efficacy of odoriferous organic compounds on the growth of keratinophilic fungi. *Current Science*, 57(14): 807–809, 1988.

Soytong, K., Rakvidhvasastra, V., Sommartya, T. Effect of some medicinal plants on growth of fungi and potential in plant disease control. Abstr. 11th Conference of Science and Technology, Thailand. Kasetsart University, Bangkok, Thailand. 24-26 October, 1985: 361, 1985.

Srivastava, K.C., and Justesen, U. Inhibition of platelet aggregation and reduced formation of thromboxane and lipoxygenase products in platelets by oil of cloves. *Prostaglandins Leukotrienes Med.,* 29(1): 11–18, 1987.

Stager, R. New studies on the effect of plant odors of ants. *Mitt Schwetz. Antomol. Ges.,* 15: 567, 1933.

Takechi, M., and Tanaka, Y. Purification and characterization of antiviral substance from the bud of *Syzygium aromatica. Planta Medica,* 42: 69–74, 1981.

To-A-Nun, C., Sommart, T., and Rakvidhyasastra, V. Effect of some medicinal plants and spices on growth of aspergillus. Abstr. 11th Conference of Science and Technology, Thailand. Kasetsart University, Bangkok, Thailand. 24-26 October: 364–365, 1985.

Tu, H.Y. Pharmaceuticals for peptic ulcer. *Patent-Japan Kokai Tokkyo Koho-79 76,* 815: 1979.

Ungsurungsie, M., Suthlenkul, O., and Paovalo, C. Mutagenicity screening of popular Thai spices. Food *Chem. Toxicol.,* 20: 527–530, 1982.

Urata, M. Antitrichophyton agents containing natural phytoncides. *Patent-Japan Kokai Tokyo Koho-63 30,* 324: 1988.

Wagner, H., Wierer, M., and Bauer, R. Screening of essential oils and phenolic compounds for in vitro-inhibition of prostaglandin biosynthesis. *Planta Medica,* 6: 1986.

Watanabe, F., Nozaka, T., Tadaki, S.I., and Morimoto, I. Desmutagenicity of clove extracts on TRP-P-2-induced mutagenesis in salmonella typhimurium TA 98. *Shoyakugaku Zasshi,* 43(4): 324–330, 1989. .

Wesley-Hadzija, B., and Bohing, P. Influences of some essential oils on the central nervous system of fish. *Ann. Pharm. Fr.,* 14: 283, 1956.

CLOVER (RED)

Cassady, J.M., et al. Use of a mammalian cell culture benzo(a)pyrene metabolism assay for the detection of potential anticarcinogens from natural products: inhibition of metabolism by biochanin A., an isoflavone from *Trifolium pratense L. Cancer Research,* 48(22): 6257–6261, 1988.

Chae, Y.H., et al. Effects of synthetic and naturally occurring flavonoids on benzo(a)pyrene metabolism by hepatic microsomes prepared from rats treated with cytochrome P-450 inducers. *Cancer Letters,* 60(1): 15–24, 1991.

COLTSFOOT

Fu, J.X. Measurement of MEFV in 66 cases of asthma in the convalescent stage and after treatment with Chinese herbs. *Chinese Journal of Modern Developments in Traditional Medicine,* 9(11): 658–659, 644, 1989.

Li, Y.P., and Wang, Y.M. Evaluation of tussilagone: a cardiovascular-respiratory stimulant isolated from Chinese herbal medicine. *General Pharmacology,* 19(2): 261–263, 1988.

Wang, C. Chemical studies of flower buds of *Tussilago farfara* L. *Yao Hsueh Pao,* 24(12): 913–916, 1989.

ECHINACEA

Anonymous. *Journal of the National Cancer Institute,* 81(2): 162–164, 1989.

Bauer, R., Jurcic, K., Puhlmann, J., and Wagner, H. Immunological in vivo examinations of echinacea extracts. *Arzneim-Forsch,* 38(2): 276–281, 1988.

Coeugniet, E.G., and Elek, E. Immunomodulation with *Viscum album* and *Echinacea purpurea* extracts. *Onkologie,* 10(3): 27–33, 1987.

Hartwell, J.L Plants used against cancer. A survey. *Lloydia,* 32: 247–296, 1969; 33: 97–194; 288–392, 1970.

Hewett, A.C. *Echinacea purpurea, Echinacea angustifolia, echafolta. Dental Rev.,* 20: 1218–1230, 1906.

Kabellk, J. The echinacea: Possibly an important medicinal plant? *Ziva,* 13(1): 4–5, 1965.

Lersch, C., et al. Stimulation of the immune response in outpatients with hepatocellular carcinomas by low doses of cyclophosphamide (LDCY), *Echinacea purpurea* extracts (Echinacin) and thymostimulin. *Archiv fur Geschwulstfor schung,* 60(5): 379–383, 1990.

Luettlg, B., et al. Macrophage activation by the polysaccharide arabinogalactan isolated from plant cell cultures of *Echinacea purpurea. Journal of the National Cancer Institute,* 81(9): 669–675, 1989.

Roesler, J., et al. Application of purified polysaccharides from cell cultures of the plant *Echinacea purpurea* to mice mediates protection against systemic infections with Listeria monocytogenes and *Candida albicans. International Journal of Immunopharmacology,* 19(1): 27–37, 1991.

Schumacher, A., and Friedberg, K.D. The effect of *Echinacea angustifolia* on nonspecific cellular immunity in the mouse. *Atzneim-Forschung,* 41(2): 141–147, 1991.

Stimpel, M., Proksch, A., Wagner, H., and Lohmann-Matthes, M.L Macrophage activation and induction of macrophage cytotoxicity by purified polysaccharide fractions from the plant *Echinacea purpurea. Infimmun,* 46(3): 845–849, 1984.

Tragni, et al. Anti-inflammatory activity of *Echinacea angustifolia* fractions separated on the basis of molecular weight *Pharmacological Research Communications,* Suppl 5: 87–90, 1988.

Tubaro, A., et al. Anti-inflammatory activity of a polysaccharidic fraction of *Echinacea angustifolia. Journal of Pharmacy and Pharmacology,* 39(7): 567–569, 1987.

Voaden, D.J., and Jacobson, M. Tumor inhibitors. 3. Identification and synthesis of an oncolytic hydrocarbon from American coneflower roots. *I Med Chem,* 15: 619, 19n.

Wacker, A., and Hilbig, W. Virus inhibition by *Echinacea purpurea. Planta Medica,* 33: 89, 1978.

Wagner, H., et al. Immunologically active polysaccharides from tissue cultures of *Echinacea purpurea.* Proc 34th Annual Congress on Medicinal Plant Research-Hamburg, Sept 22-27, 1986.

Wagner, H., Zenk, M.H., and Ott, H. Polysaccharides derived from echinacea plants as immunostimulants. Patent-Ger Offen-3, 541,945 : l0pp, 1988.

EPHEDRA

Arch, J. R. S., Ainsworth, A. T., and Cawthorne, M. A. Thermogenic and anorectic effects of ephedrine and congener in mice and rats. *life Sci.,* 30: 1817, 1982.

Astrup, A., et al. Enhanced thermogenic responsiveness during chronic ephedrine treatment in man. *Am. J. Clin. Nutr.,* 42: 83, 1985.

Dulloo, A.G., and Miller, D.S. Obesity: a disorder of the sympathetic nervous system. *World Rev. Nutr. Diet,* 50: 1, 1987.

Dulloo, A.G., and Miller, D.S. Reversal in obesity in the genetically obese fa/fa Zucker rat with an ephedrine/methylzanthine (caffeine) thermogenic mixture. *Journal of Nutrition,* 117: 383–389, 1987.

Jeculer, E., and Schultz, Y. New evidence for a thermogenic defect in human obesity. *Int J. Obesity,* 9 (Suppl 2): 1, 1985.

Kalix, P. The pharmacology of psychoactive alkaloids from ephedra and catha. *Journal of Ethnopharmacology,* 32(1-3): 201–208, 1991.

Katzeff, H.L, et al. Metabolic studies in human obesity during overnutrition and undernutrition: Thermogenic and hormonal responses to norepinephrine. *Metabolism,* 35: 166, 1988.

Lansberg, L, Saville, M.E., and Young J.B. Sympathoadrenal system and regulation of thermogenesis. *Am. J. Physio.,* 247: 181, 1984.

Morgan, J.B., York, D.A., Wasliewska, A., et al. A study of the thermogenic responses to a meal and to a sympathomimetic drug (ephedrine) in relation to energy balance in man. *Br. J. Nutr.,* 47: 21, 1982.

Pasquali, R., Cesari, M.P., Melchionda, N., Stefanini, C., Raitano, A., and Labo, G. Does ephedrine promote weight loss in low-energy-adapted obese women? *International Journal of Obesity,* 11: 163–168, 1987.

Roth, R.P., et al. Nasal decongestant activity of pseudoephedrine. *Annals of OTOL,* 86, 1977.

EUCALYPTUS

Cal, Z., U, X., and Xu, X. Determination of eucalyptole in eucalyptus oil by gas chromatography. *Journal of Chinese Materia Medica,* 15(5): 298–299, 319, 1990.

Hong, C.Z., and Shellock, F.G. Effects of a topically applied counterirritant (Eucalyptamint) on cutaneous blood flow and on skin and muscle temperatures. A placebo-controlled study. *American Journal of Physical Medicine and Rehabilitation,* 70(1): 29–33, 1991.

Swanston-Flatt, S.K., Day, C., Balley, C.J., and Flatt, P.R. Traditional plant treatments for diabetes. Studies in normal and streptozotopin diabetic mice. *Diabetaolgoia*, 33(8): 162–164, 1990.

Takasalki, M., et al. Inhibitors of skin-tumor promotion. VIII. Inhibitory effects of euglobals and their related compounds on Epstein-Barr virus activation. *Chemical and Pharmaceutical Bulletin*, 38(10): 2737–2739, 1990.

FENNEL

Abdul-Ghani, A.S., and Amin, R. The vascular action of aqueous extracts of *Foeniculum vulgare* leaves. *Journal of Ethnopharmacology*, 24(2-3): 213–218, 1988.

FENUGREEK

Madar, Z., Abel, R., Samiah, S., and Arad, J. Glucose-lowering effect of fenugreek in non-insulin dependent diabetics. *European Journal of Clinical Nutrition*, 42(1): 51–54, 1988.

Sambalah, K., and Srinivasan, K. Influence of spices and spice principles on hepatic mixed function oxygenase system in rats. *Indian Journal of Biochemistry and Biophysics*, 26(4): 254–258, 1989.

Sauvaire, Y., et al. Implication of steroid saponins and sapogenins in the hypocholesterolemic effect of fenugreek. *Lipids*, 26(3). 191–197, 1991.

Sharma, R.D., Raghuram, T.C., and Rao, N.S. Effect of fenugreek seeds on blood glucose and serum lipids in type I diabetes. *European Journal of Clinical Nutrition*, 44(4): 301–306, 1990.

FEVERFEW

Hayes, N.A., and Foreman, J.C. The activity of compounds extracted from feverfew on histamine release from rat mast cells. *Journal of Pharmacy and Pharmacology*, 39(6): 466–470, 1987.

Hobbs, C. The modern rediscovery of feverfew. *HerbalGram*, 20: 36, 1989.

Hobbs, C. Feverfew. *HerbalGram*, 20: 27–35, 1989.

Johnson, E.S., et al. Efficacy of feverfew as prophylactic treatment of migraine. *British Medical Journal*, 291: 569, 1985.

Johnson, E.S., et al. Investigation of possible genotoxic effects of feverfew in migraine patients. *Human Toxicology*, 6: 533, 1987.

Loesche, W., et al. Effects of an extract of feverfew *(Tanacetum parthenium)* on arachiodonic acid metabolism in human blood platelets. *Biomedica Biochimica Acta*, 47(10- 11): S241–243, 1988.

Murphy, J.J., Heptinstall, S., and Mitchell, J.R. Randomized double-blind placebo-controlled trial of feverfew in migraine prevention. *Lancet*, 2(8604): 189–192, 1988.

Voyno-Yasenetskaya, T.A., et al. Effects of an extract of feverfew on endothelial cell integrity and on cAMP in rabbit perfused aorta. *J. Pharm. Pharmacol*, 40: 501–501, 1988.

FO-TI

Chung Shan Medical College. *Kanpo no rinsho oyo* (The Clinical Applications of Chinese Herbal Formulas). Tokyo: Dental and Pharmaceutical Press, 1976.

Hsu, H. *Chung yao tsai chih yen chiu* (Study of Chinese Medicinal Plants). Taipei: Modern Drug Press, 1980.

Huang, H.C., Chu, S.H., and Chao, P.O. Vasorelaxants from Chinese herbs, emodin and scoparoine, possess immunosuppressive properties. *European Journal of Pharmacology*, 198(2-3): 211–213, 1991.

Kam, J.K. Mutagenic activity of Ho Shao Wu *(Polygonum Multiflorum* thunb). *American Journal of Chinese Medicine*, 9(3): 213–215, 1981.

Muddathir, A.K., et al. Anthelmintic properties of *Polygonum glabrum. Journal of Pharmacy and Pharmacology*, 39(4): 296–300, 1987.

Singh, B., Pandey, V.B., Joshi, V.K., and Gambhir, S.S. Anti-inflammatory studies on *Polygonum glabrum. Journal of Ethnopharmacology*, 19(3): 255–267, 1987.

FOXGLOVE

Marullax, P.O. Digitalis: Is there a future for this classical ethnopharmacological remedy? *Journal of Ethnopharmacology*, 32(1-3): 111–115, 1991.

GARLIC

Amla, V., Verma, S.L, Shanna, T.R., Guptu, O.P., and Atal, C.K. Clinical study of *Allium cepa* Linn in patients of bronchial asthma. *Ind. J. Pharmacol.*, 13: 63, 1980.

Barone, F., and Tansey, M. Isolation, purification, identification, synthesis, and kinetics of activity of the anticandidal component of *Allium sativum,* and a hypothesis for its mode of action. *Mycologia*, 69: 793–825, 1977.

Belman, S. Inhibition of soybean lipoxygenase by onion and garlic oil constituents. *Proc. Am. Assoc. Cancer Res.*, 26: 131, 1985.

Belman, S. Onion and garlic oils and tumour promotion. *Carcinogenesis*, 4: 1063–1065, 1983.

Bilyk, A., Cooper, P., and Sapers, G. Varietal differences in distribution of quercetin and kaempferol in onion *(Allium cepa)* tissue. *Journal of Agricultural Food Chemistry*, 32: 274–285, 1984.

Bordia, A., and Verma, S. Effect of garlic feeding on regression of experimental atherosclerosis in rabbits. *Artery*, 7: 428–436, 1980.

Bordia, A., et al. The effect of active principle of garlic and onion on blood lipids and experimental atherosclerosis in rabbits and their comparison with clofibrate. *Journal of the Association of Physicians of India*, 25: 509–521, 1977.

Chi, M. Effects of garlic products in lipid metabolism in cholesterol-fed rats. *Proceedings of the Society for Experimental Biology and Medicine*, 171: 174–178, 1982.

Dabas, Y., Rao, V., Saxena, O., and Sharma, V. Efficacy of therapy against infectious genital tract disorders in bovine. *Indian Journal of Animal Science*, 53: 81–89, 1983.

Fenwich, G., and Hanley, A. The genus Allium-Part 2. CRC. *Critical Reviews in Food Science and Nutrition*, 22: 273–341, 1985.

Srivastiva. K.C. Effect of onion and ginger consumption on platelet thromboxane production in humans. *Prostaglandins, Leukotrienes and Essential Fatty Acids*, 35:183–185, 1989.

Subrahmanyan, V., Sreenivasamurthy, V., and Krishnamurthy, S.M. The effect of garlic on certain intestinal bacteria. *Food Science*, 7: 223–230, 1958.

Vanderhoek, J.Y., Makheia, A.N., and Balley, J.M. Inhibition of fatty acid oxygenases by onion and garlic oils: Evidence for the mechanism by which these oils inhibit platelet aggregation. *Biochemical Pharmacology*, 29: 3169–3173, 1980.

Wagner, H., Wierer, M., and Fessler, B. Effects of garlic constituents on arachidonate metabolism. *Planta Medica*, 53, 1987.

Yamada, Y., and Azuma, K. Evaluation of the in vitro antifungal activity of allicin. *Antimicrobial Agents and Chemotherapy*, 11: 743–749, 1977.

GINKGO

Barth, S.A., Inselmann, G., Engemann, R., and Heidennann, H.T. Influences of *Ginkgo biloba* on cyclosporin A induced lipid peroxidation in human liver microsomes in comparison to vitamin E, glutathione and N-acetylcysteine.

Braquet, P., and Hosford, D. Ethnopharmacology and the development of natural PAF antagonists as therapeutic agents. *Journal of Ethnopharmacology*, 32(1-3): 135–139, 1991.

Chung, K. F., et al. Effect of a ginkgolide mixture (BN 52063) in antagonizing skin and platelet responses to platelet activating factor in man. *Lancet*, January 31, 1987.

Massoni, G., Piovella, C., and Fratti, L. Effects microcirculatoires de la *Ginkgo biloba* chez les personnes agées. *Gioren. Geront*, 20: 444, 1972.

Peter, H. Vasoactivity of *Ginkgo biloba* preparation. 4th Conf. Hung. Ther. Invert. Pharmacol. Soc. Pharmacol. Hung. (Edited by Dumbovitch, B.), 177, 1968.

Ral, G.S., Shovlin, C., and Wesnes, K.A. A double-blind, placebo controlled study of *Ginkgo biloba* extract ("tanakan") in elderly outpatients with mild to moderate memory impairment. *Current Medical Research and Opinion*, 12(6): 350–355, 1991.

Sikora, R., et al. *Ginkgo biloba* extract in the therapy of erectile dysfunction. *Journal of Urology*, 141: 188A, 1989.

Warot, D., et al. Comparative effects of *Ginkgo biloba* extracts on psychomotor performances and memory in healthy subjects. *Therapie*, 46(1): 33–36, 1991.

GINSENGS

The drug that builds Russians. *New Scientist*, August 21, 1980.

Bohn, B., Nebe, C.T., and Birr, C. Flow-cytometric studies with *Eleutherococcus senticosus* extracts as an immunomodulatory agent. *Arzneimittel-Forschung*, 37(10): 1193–1196, 1987.

Darling, E. Do ginsenosides influence performance? *Notabene Medici*, 10(5): 241–246, 1980.

Domashenko, O.N., and Sotnik, I.P. Evaluation of the cationic-lysomal test in patients with pneumonia against a background of therapy. *Laboratornoe Delo*, (5): 15–17, 1989.

Elden, H.R. Ginsenosides: new uses for an old root. *Drug and Cosmetic Industry*, pp. 36–40, April 1990.

Forgo, I., and Schimert, G. The duration of effect of the standardized Ginseng extract G115® in healthy competitive athletes. *Notabene Medici*, 15(9): 636–640, 1985.

Forgo, I. On the question of influencing the performance of sportsmen. *Aerztliche Praxis*, 33(44): 1784–1786, 1981.

Itoh, T., Zang, Y. F., Murai, S., and Saito, H. Effects of *Panax ginseng* on the vertical and horizontal motor activities and on brain monoamine-related substances in mice. *Planta Medica*, 55: 429, 1989.

Kim, H., Jang, C., and Lee, M. Antinarcotic effects of the standardized ginseng extract G115® on morphine. *Planta Medica*, 56: 158, 1990.

McCaleb, R. Ginseng conference report. *Herbalgram*, No. 16, pp. 8–12, Spring 1988.

Takaku, T., Kameda, K., Matsuura, Y., Seklya, K., and Okuda, H. Studies on insulin-like substances in Korean red ginseng. *Planta Medica*, 56: 27, 1990.

GOLDENSEAL

Boyd, L.J. The pharmacology of the homeopathic drugs. *J. Amer Inst Homeopathy*, 21: 312–323, 1920.

D'Amico, M.L Investigation of the presence of substances having antibiotic action in higher plants. *Fitoterapia*, 21: 77, 1950.

Hay, G., and Willuhn, G. Antiviral activity of aqueous extracts from medicinal plants in tissue cultures. *Drug Res,* 28(1): 1–7, 1978.

GOTU KOLA

Arpala, M.R., et al. Effects of *Centella asiatica* extract on mucopolysaccharide metabolism in subjects with varicose veins. *International Journal of Clinical Pharmacology Research*, 10(4): 229–233, 1990.

Baltina, L.A., et al. Synthesis and antiphlogistic activity of protected glycopeptides of glycyrrhizic acid. *Pharm. Chem.* 226: 460–462, 1989.

Belcaro, G.V., Grimaldi, R., and Guidi, G. Improvement of capillary permeability in patients with venous hypertension after treatment with TTFCA. *Angiology*, 41 (7): 588, 1990.

Belcaro, G.V., Rulo, A., and Grimaldi, R. Capillary filtration and ankle edema in patients with venous hypertension treated with TTFCA. *Angiology*, 41(1): 12–18, 1990.

Finney, R.S.H., Somers, C.F., and Wilkinson, J.H. Pharmacological properties of glycyrrhetinic acid—a new anti-inflammatory drug. *Pharm. Pharmacol.*, 10: 687, 1958.

Fujita, H., Sakurai, T., Yoshida, M., and Toyoshima, S. Anti-inflammatory effects of glycyrrhizinic acid. *Oyo Yakuri*, 19: 481–484, 1980.

Gijon, J.R., and Murcia, C.R. Estudio farmacologico comparativo de la actividad anti-inflammatoria local del acido glicirretinico con la de la cortisona. *An. Real Acad. Fann.*, 26: 5, 1960.

Grimaldi, R., et al. Pharmacokinetics of the total triterpenic fraction of *Centella asiatica* after single and multiple administration to healthy volunteers. A new assay for asiatic acid. *Journal of Ethnopharmacology*, 28(2): 235–241, 1990.

Maquart, F.X., et al. Stimulation of collagen synthesis in fibroblast cultures by a triterpene extracted from *Centella asiatica. Connective Tissue Research*, 24(2): 107–120, 1990.

Montecchio, G.P., et al. Centella Asiatica Triterpenic Fraction (CATTF) reduces the number of circulating endothelial cells in subjects with postphlebitic syndrome. *Hannatologica*, 76(3): 256–259, 1991.

Pointel, J.P., et al. Titrated extract of *Centella asiatica* (TECA) in the treatment of venous insufficiency of the lower limbs. *Angiology*, 38(1 Pt 1): 46–50, 1987.

Sugishita, E., Amagaya, S., and Ogihara, Y. Studies on the combination of glycyrrhizae radix in shakuyakukanzo-to. *Pharmacobio Dyn,* 7: 427–435, 1984.

GREEN TEA

Ali, M., Afzal, M., Gubler, C.J., and Burka, J.F. A potent thromboxane formation inhibitor in green tea leaves. *Prostaglandins Leukotrienes and Essential Fatty Acids*, 40(4): 281–283, 1990.

Anonymous. Tea-totaling mice gain cancer protection. *Science News*, August 31, 1991, p. 133.

Bokuchava, M., Skoveleva, N.I., and Sanderson, G.W. The biochemistry and technology of tea manufacture. *CRC Critical Reviews in Food Science and Nutrition*, 12(4): 303–370, 1980.

Conney, A.H. Induction of microsomal enzymes by foreign chemicals and carcinogenesis by polycyclic aromatic hydrocarbons. G.H.A. Clowes Memorial Lecture. *Cancer Research*, 42: 4875–4917, 1982.

Cooke, R. Studies: Green tea may prevent cancer. *Newsday*, August 27, 1991.

Demirer, T., Icli, F., Uzunallmoglu, O., and Kucuk, O. Diet and stomach cancer incidence. A case-control study in Turkey. *Cancer*, 65(10): 2344–2348, 1990.

Ding, L.A. Inhibition effect of epicatechin on phenobarbitol-induced proliferation precancerous liver cells. *Chinese Journal of Pathology*, 19(4): 261–263, 1990.

Guo, B.Y., and Wan, H.B. Rapid determination of caffeine in green tea by gas-liquid chromatography with nitrogen-phosphorous-selective detection. *Journal of Chromatography*, 505(2):435–437, 1990.

Hara, Y., et al. Antitumor action of the green tea extract. Proc. Annual Meeting Japanese Society Cancer Research: 993, 1984.

Hattori, M., et al. Effect of tea polyphenols on glucan synthesis by glucosyltransferase from *Streptococcus mutans*. *Chemical and Pharmaceutical Bulletin*, 38(3): 717–720, 1990.

Higashi, A., et al. A case-control study of ulcerative colitis. *Japanese Journal of Hygiene*, 45(6): 1035–1043, 1991.

Huang, M.T., et al. Inhibition of the mutagenicity of bay-region diol-epoxides of polycyclic aromatic hydrocarbons by tannic acid, hydroxylated anthaquinones and hydroxylated cinnamic acid derivatives. *Carcinogenesis*, 6: 237–242, 1985.

Imanishi, H., et al. Tea tannin components modify the induction of sister-chromatic exchanges and chromosome aberrations in mutagen-treated cultured mammalian cells and mice. *Mutation Research*, 259(1): 79–87, 1991.

Kaiser, H.E. Cancer-promoting effects of phenols in tea. *Cancer*, 20: 614, 1967.

Kubota, K., et al. Effect of green tea on iron absorption in elderly patients with iron deficiency anemia. *Japanese Journal of Geriatrics*, 27(5): 1990.

Kursanov, A.L., et al. Biological effects of tea tannins. *Biokhim Chain. Proizvod*, 6, 1950, p. 170.

Lee, H.H., et al. Epidemiologic characteristics and multiple risk factors of stomach cancer in Taiwan. *Anticancer Research*, 10(4):875–881, 1990.

Li, Y., Yan, R.Q., Qin, G.Z., Qin, L.L., and Duan, X.X. Reliability of a short-term test for hepatocarcinogenesis induced by aflatoxin BI. *IARC Scientific Publications*, (105): 431–433, 1991.

Liu, X.L. Genotoxicity of fried fish extract, MelQ and inhibition by green tea antioxidant. *Chinese Journal of Oncology*, 12(3): 170–173, 1990.

Mgaloblishvili, E.K., Therapeutic effects of the green tea infusion. *Izdatelstvo Medgiz*, Batumi, 23, 1967.

Mgaloblishvili, E.K., and Tsutsunava, A.I. Healthful properties of the green tea infusion. *Bulletin USSR Research Institute Tea Subtrop. Cult.*, 1(26): 64, 1971.

Morton, J. Further association of plant tannins and human cancer. *Q.J. Crude Drug Research*, 12: 1829, 1972.

Nomura, A.M., Kolonel, L.N., Hankin, J.H., and Yoshizawa, C.N. Dietary factors in cancer of the lower urinary tract. *International Journal of Cancer*, 48(2): 199–205, 1991.

Oguni, I., Nasu, K., and Nomua, T. Epidemiological and physiological studies on the antitumor activity of the fresh green tea leaf. *Proceedings of the International Conference on Tea Quality and Human Health*, Nov. 4-9, 1987. Hanzhou, China Abstracts, p. 120.

Ruch, R.J., Cheng, S., and Klaunig, J.E. Prevention of cytotoxity and inhibition of intercellular communication by antioxidant catechins isolated from Chinese green tea. *Carcinogens*, 10(6): 1003–1008, 1989.

Sagesaka-Mitane, Y., Miwa, M., and Okada, S. Platelet aggregation inhibitors in hot water extract of green tea. *Chemical and Pharmaceutical Bulletin*, 38(3): 1990.

Stagg, G.V., and Millin, D.J. The nutritional and therapeutic value of tea. *Journal Sd. Food Agric.*, 26: 1439, 1975.

Taramoto, K., et al. Neutron activation analysis of manganese contents in ordinary hospital meals. *Osaka City Medical Journal*, 36(1): 53–59, 1990.

Tewes, F.J., Koo, L.C., Meisgen, T.J., and Rylander, R. Lung cancer risk and mutagenicity of tea. *Environmental Research*, 52(1): 23–33, 1990.

Wang, H., and Wu, Y. Inhibitory effect of Chinese tea on N-nitrosation in vitro and in vivo. *IARC Scientific Publications,* (105): 546–549, 1991.

Wang, W., and Chen, W.W. Antioxidative activity studies on the meaning of same original of herbal drug and food. *Chinese Journal of Modern Developments in Traditional Medicine*, 11 (3): 159–161, 1991.

Wang, Z.Y., Agarwal, R., Bickers, D.R., and Mukhtar, H. Protection against ultraviolet B radiation-induced photocarcinogenesis in hairless mice by green tea polyphenols. *Carcinogens*, 12(8): 1527–1530, 1991.

Wang, Z.Y., et al. Antimutagenic activity of green tea polyphenols. *Mutation Research*, 223: 273–285, 1989.

Wang, Z.Y., Khan, W.A., Bickers, D.R., and Mukhtar, H. Protection against polycyclic aromatic hydrocarbon-induced skin tumor initiation in mice by green tea polyphenols. *Carcinogens*, 10(2): 411–415, 1989.

Wang, Z.Y., Mukul, D., Bickers, D.R., and Mukhtar, H. Interaction of epicatechins derived from green tea with rat hepatic cytochrome P-450. *Drug Metabolism and Disposition*, 16(1): 98–103, 1988.

Yamaguchi, Y., Hayashi, M., Yamazoe, H., and Kunitomo, M. Preventive effects of green tea extract on lipid abnormalities in serum, liver and aorta of mice fed an atherogenic diet. *Nippon Yakurigaku Zasshi*, 97(6): 329–337, 1991.

Yan, Y.S. Effect of Chinese green tea extracts on the human gastric carcinoma cell in vitro. *Chinese Journal of Preventive Medicine*, 24(2): 80–82, 1990.

Zhao, B.L., Li, X.J., He, R.G., Cheng, S.J., and Xin, W.J. Scavenging effect of extracts of green tea and natural antioxidants on active oxygen radicals. *Cell Biophysics*, 14(2): 175–185, 1989.

GUARANA

Bydlowski, S.P., Yunker, R.L., and Subbiah, M.T. A novel property of an aqueous guarana extract *(Paullinia cupana):* inhibition of platelet aggregation in vitro and in vivo. *Brazilian Journal of Medical and Biological Research*, 21 (3): 535–538, 1988.

GUAR GUM

Miettinen, T.A., and Tarpila, S. Serum lipids and cholesterol metabolism during guar gum and plantago ovata and high fibre treatments. *Clinical Chimica Acta*, 183(3): 253–262, 1989.

Tonstad, S. Dietary supplementation in the treatment of hyperlipidemia. *Tidsskrift for den Norske Laegegorening*, 111(28): 3398–4000, 1991.

GUGGAL

Agarwal, R.C., et al. Clinical trial of gugulipid: A new hypolipidemic agent of plant origin in primary hyperlipidemia. *Indian Journal of Medical Research*: 626, 1986.

Bombardelli, E., et al. *Commiphora mukul* extracts: A reinvestigation on chemical constituents and biological activity. Unpublished Manuscript, Presented at the 32nd Annual Meeting of the American Society of Pharmacognosy, Chicago, Illinois, July 1991.

Bordia, A., and Chuttani, S.K. Effect of gum guggulu on fibrinolysis and platelet adhesiveness in coronary heart disease. *Indian Journal of Medical Research*, 70: 992–996, 1979.

Bordia, A., and Bansal, H.C. Essential oil of garlic in prevention of atherosclerosis. *Lancet*, 2: 1491, 1973.

Bordia, A., et al. Effect of the essential oil (active principle) of garlic on serum cholesterol, plasma fibrinogen, whole blood, coagulation time and fibrinolytic activity in alimentary lipaemia. *Journal Assoc. Phys. India*, 22: 267, 1974.

Chopra, R.N., Chopra, I.C., Handa, K.L, and Kapur, L.D. *Indigenous Drugs of India* (2nd. ed.). Calcutta, India: Academic Publishers, 1958, reprint 1982.

Chopra, R.N., Chopra, J.C., and Verma, B.S. *Supplement to glossary of Indian medicinal plants.* New Delhi, India: Publication and Information Directorate (CSIR), 1969.

Conant, R. Gum guggul: a protective herb from India. *Let's Live*: 68, 1991.

Das, D., Sharma, R.C., and Arora, R.B. Antihyperlipidaemic activity of fraction A of *Commiphora mukul* in monkeys. *Indian Journal Pharm.*, 5: 283, 1973.

DellaLoggia, R., Sosa, S., Tubaro, A., and Bombardelli, E. Anti-inflammatory activity of

Commiphora mukul extracts. Unpublished Manuscript, Presented at the 32nd Annual Meeting of the American Society of Pharmacognosy, Chicago, Illinois, July 1991.

Dev, S. A modern look at an age-old Ayurvedlc drug—guggulu. *Science* Age: 13, 1987.

Dhar, M.L., Dhar, M.M., Dhawan, B.N., Mehrotra, B.N., and Ray, C. Screening of Indian plants for biological activity. *Indian Journal of Experimental Biology*, 6: 232, 1968.

Dwarakanath, C., and Satyavati, G.V. Research in some of the concepts of Ayurveda and application of modern chemistry and experimental pharmacology therefore. *Ayurveda Pradeepika*, 1: 69, 1970.

Gujral, M.L., Sareen, K., Tangri, K.K., Amma, M.K.P., and Roy, A.K. Anti-arthritic and anti-inflammatory activity of gum guggal *(Balsamodendron mukul* Hook). *Indian Journal Physiol. Pharmacol.*, 4: 267, 1960.

Jain, R.C., Vyas, C.R., and Mahatma, O.P. Hypoglycemic action of onions and garlic, *Lancet*, 2: 1491, 1973.

Khanna, D.S., Agarwal, O.P., Gupta, S.K., and Arora, R.B. A biochemical approach to antiatherosclerotic action of *Commiphora mukul:* an Indian indigenous drug in Indian domestic pigs *(Sus scrofa)*. *Indian Journal of Medical Research*, 57: 900, 1969.

Malhotra, S.C., Ahuja, M.M.S., and Sundaram, K.R. Long-term clinical studies on the hypolipidaemic effect of *Commiphora mukul* (Guggulu) and Clofibrate. *Indian Journal of Medical Research*, 65(3): 390–395, 1977.

Menon, M.K., and Kar, A. Analgesic and psychopharmacological effects of the gum resin of *Boswellia serrata*. *Planta Medica*, 19: 333, 1971.

Mester, L., Mester, M., and Nityanand, S. Inhibition of platelet aggregation by "Guggulu" steroids. *Hippokrates Verlag GmbH*, 37: 367–369, 1979.

Nadkarni, A.K. *Dr. K.M. Nadkarni's Indian Materia Medica* (revised ed.). Bombay, India: Popular Book, 1954.

Sastry, V.V.S. Experimental and clinical studies on the effect of the oleogum resin of *Commiphora mukul* Engl. on thrombotic phenomena associated with hyperlipaemia, Thesis, Banaras Hindu University, Varanasi, 1967.

Satyavati, G.V. Effect of an indigenous drug on disorders of lipid metabolism with special reference to atherosclerosis and obesity (medaroga). Thesis, Banaras Hindu University, Varanasi, 1966.

Satyavati, G.V. Pathogenesis of atherosclerosis: an analogy between ancient and modern concepts.

Satyavati, G.V., Dwarakanath, C., and Tripathi, S.N. Experimental studies on the hypocholesterolemic effect of *Commiphora mukul* Engl. (Guggul). *Indian Journal of Medical Research*, 57(10): 1950–1962, 1969.

Shankar, R. Herbal hope for the heart. *Sci. Exp. of Ind. Exp.*: 3, 1988.

Tripathi, S.N., Shastri, V.V.S., and Satyavati, G.V. (Achayra) Experimental and clinical studies on the effect of Guggulu (*Commiphora mukul*) in hyperlipaernia and thrombosis. *Journal of Indian Medical Research*, 2: 10, 1968.

Tripathi, Y.B., Malhotra, O.P., and Tripathi, S.N. Thyroid stimulating action of z-guggulsterone obtained from *Commiphora mukul. Planta Medica*: 22–24, 1984.

HAWTHORN

Ammon, H.P.R., and Handel, M. Cratageus, toxicology and pharmacology, Part I. Toxicology. *Planta Medica*, 43: 105–120, 1981.

Ammon, H.P.R., and Handel, M. Cratageus, toxicology and pharmacology, Part II. Pharmacodynarnics. *Planta Medica*, 43: 313–322, 1981.

Ammon, H.P.R., and Handel, M. Cratageus, toxicology and pharmacology, Part III. Pharmacodynamics and pharmacokinetics. *Planta Medica,* 43: 209–239, 1981.

He, G. Effect of the prevention and treatment of atherosclerosis of a mixture of hawthorn and motherwort. *Journal of Modern Development in Traditional Medicine*, 10(6): 361, 326, 1990.

Hobbs, C., and Foster, S. Hawthorn, a literature review. *HerbalGram*, 22: 19–33, 1990.

Meier, B. Plant vs. synthetic medicines. *Schweiz Apothek-Zeit*, 19: 1989.

Occhluto, F., et al. Study comparing the cardiovascular activity of shoots, leaves and flowers of *C. laevigata* L. II. Effect of extracts and pure isolated active principles on the isolated rabbit heart. *Plantes Med. Phytoher*, 20: 52–63, 1986.

Zeylstra, H. Cratageus. *New Herbal Practitioner*, 9: 53–61, 1983.

HENNA

Sharma, V.K. Tuberculostatic activity of henna *(Lawsonia inermis Linn). Tubercle*, 71(4): 293–295, 1990.

HORSE CHESTNUT

Kunz, K., Schaffler, K., Biber, A, and Wauschkuhn, C.H. Bioavailability of beta-aescin after oral administration of two preparations containing aesculus extract to healthy volunteers.

Lehtole, T., and Huhtikengas, A. Radioimmunoassay of aescine, a mixture of triterpene glycosides. *Journal of Immunoassay*, 11(1): 17–30, 1990.

Magliulo, E., Carco, F.P., Gorini, S., and Barigazzi, G.M. Ricerche in vivo ed in vitro sull'azione antiflogistica dell'escina. *Arch. Sc. Med.*, 125: 207, 1968.

Manca, P., and Passarelli, E. Aspetti farmacologici dell'escina principio attivo dell'aesculus hyppocastanum. *Clin. Terap.*, 32: 297, 1965.

Senatore, F., Mscisz, A., Mrugasiewicz, K., and Gorecki, P. Steroidal constituents and anti-inflammatory activity of the horse chestnut bark. *Bollettino-Societa Italiano Biolgia Sperimentale*, 65(2): 137–141, 1989.

Siering, H. Die permeabilitat von zellmembranen, fur Ionen unter dem einfluss von Aescin. *Aizneim. Forsch*, 12: 376, 1962.

IPECAC

Hodgkinson, D.W., Jellett, L.B., and Ashby, R.H. A review of the management of oral drug overdose in the Accident and Emergency Department of the Royal Brisbane Hospital. *Archives of Emergency Medicine*, 8(1): 8–16, 1991.

Kornberg, A.E., and Dolgin, J. Pediatric ingestions: charcoal alone versus ipecac and charcoal. *Annals of Emergency Medicine*, 20(6): 648–651, 1991.

Tennebein, M., Wiseman, N., and Yatscoff, R.W. Gastronomy and whole bowel irritation in iron poisoning. *Pediatric Emergency Care*, 7(5): 286–288, 1991.

JUNIPER

Swanston-Flatt, S.K., Day, C., Bailey, C.J., and Flatt, P.R. Traditional plant treatments for diabetes.

Studies in normal and streptozotopin diabetic mice. *Diabetologia*, 33(8): 162–164, 1990.

KAVA

Cheng, D., et al. Identification by methane chemical ionization gas chromatography/mass spectrometry of the products obtained by steam distillation and aqueous acid extraction of commercial *Piper methysticum. Biomedical and Environmental Mass Spectrometry*, 17(5): 371–376, 1988.

Duffield, A.M., et al. Identification of some human urinary metabolites of the intoxicating beverage kava. *Journal of Chromatography*, 475: 273–281, 1989.

Duffield, P.H., Jamieson, D.D., and Duffield, A.M. Effect of aqueous and lipid-soluble extracts of kava on the conditioned avoidance response in rats. *Archives Internationales de Pharmacodynamie et de Therapie*, 301: 81–90, 1989.

Jamieson, D.D., Duffield, P.H., Cheng, D., and Duffield, A.M. Comparison of the central nervous system activity of the aqueous and lipid extract of kava. *Archives Internationales de Pharmacodynamie et de Therapie*, 301: 66–80, 1989.

Ruze, P. Kava-induced dermopathy: a niacin deficiency? *Lancet*, 335(8703): 1442–1445, 1990.

LAVENDER

Gamez, M.J., Jimenez, J., Navarro, C., and Zarzuelo, A. Study of the essential oil of *Lavandula dentata* L. *Pharmazie*, 45(1): 69–70, 1990.

Gamez, M.J., et al. Hypoglycemic activity in various species of the genus Lavandula. Part 1: *Lavandula stoechas* L. and *Lavandula multifida* L. *Pharmazie*, 42(10): 706–707, 1987.

Gamez, M.J., et al. Hypoglycemic activity in various species of the genus Lavandula. Part 2: *Lavandula dentata* and *Lavandula latifolia. Pharmazie*, 43(6): 441–442, 1988.

Shubine, L.P., Siurin, S.A., and Savchenko,V.M. Inhalations of essential oils in the combined treatment of patients with chronic bronchitis. *Vrachebnoe Delo*, (5): 66–67, 1990.

LEMONGRASS

da Silva, V.A., et al. Neurobehavioral study of the effect of beta-myrcene on rodents. *Brazilian*

Journal of Medical and Biological Research, 24(8): 827–831,1991.

Elson, C.E., et al. Impact of lemongrass oil, an essential oil, on serum cholesterol. Lipids, 24(8): 677–679, 1989.

Kauderer, B., Zamith, H., Paumgartten, F.J., and Spelt, G. Evaluation of the mutagenicity of beta-myrcene in mammalian cells in vitro. Environmental and Molecular Mutagenesis, 18(1): 28–34,1991.

Lorenzetti, B.B., et al. Myrcene mimics the peripheral analgesic activity of lemongrass tea. Journal of Ethnopharmacology, 34(1): 43–48, 1991.

Onawunmi, G.O. In vitro studies on the antibacterial activity of phenoxyethanol in combination with lemongrass oil. Pharmazie, 43(1): 42–44, 1988.

Rao, V.S., Menezes, A.M., and Viana, G.S. Effect of myrcene on nociception in mice. Journal of Pharmacy and Pharmacology, 42(12): 877–878, 1990.

LICORICE

Abe, N., Ebina, T., and Ishida, N. Interferon induction by glycyrrhizin and glycyrrhetinic acid in mice. Microbiology and Immunology, 26: 535, 1982.

Agarwal, R., Wang, Z.Y., and Mukhtar, H. Inhibition of mouse skin tumor-initiating activity of DMBA by chronic oral feeding of glycyrrhizin in drinking water. Nutrition and Cancer, 15(3-4): 187–193, 1991.

Baba, M., and Shigeta, S. Antiviral activity of glycyrrhizin against varicella-zoster virus in vitro. Antiviral Research, 7: 99–107, 1987.

Baker, M.E., and Fanestil, D.D. Licorice, computer-based analyses of dehydrogenase sequences, and the regulation of steroid and prostaglandin action. Molecular and Cellular Endocrinology, 78(1-2): 99-102, 1991.

Baltina, L.A., et al. Synthesis and antiphlogistic activity of protected glycopeptides of glycyrrhizic acid. Pharm. Chem. J., 226: 460–462, 1989.

Borst, J.G.G., Ten Holt, S.P., de Vries, L.A., and Molhuysen, J.A. Synergistic action of liquorice and cortisone in Addison's and Simmonds's disease. Lancet, 1: 657–668, 1953.

Finney, R.S.H., Somers, C.F., and Wilkinson, J.H. Pharmacological properties of glycyrrhetinic acid—a new anti-inflammatory drug. J. Pharm. Pharmacol., 10: 687, 1958.

Fujisawa, K., Watanabe, Y., and Kimura, K. Therapeutic approach to chronic active hepatitis with glycyrrhizin. Asian Medical Journal, 23: 745–756, 1981.

Fujita, H., Sakurai, T., Yoshida, M., and Toyoshima, S. Anti-inflammatory effects of glycyrrhizinic acid. Oyo Yakuri, 19: 481–484, 1980.

Gijon, J.R., and Murcia, C.R. Estudio farmacologico comparativo de la actividad anti-inflammatoria local del acido glicirretinico con la de la cortisona. An. Real Acad. Farm., 26: 5, 1960.

Hatano, T., et al. Phenolic constituents of licorice. IV. Correlation of phenolic constituents and licorice specimens from various sources and inhibitory effects of licorice extracts on xanthine oxidase and monoamine oxidase. Journal of the Pharmaceutical Society of Japan, 111(6): 311–321, 1991.

Kiso, Y., Tohkin, M., and Hikino, H. Assay method for antihepatotoxic activity using carbon tetrachloride induced cytotoxicity in primary cultured hepatocytes. Planta Medica, 49: 222–225,1983.

Kitagawa, K., Nishino, H., and Iwashima, A. Inhibition of the specific binding of 12-0-tetradecacanoylphorbol-13-acetate to mouse epidermal membrane fractions by glycyrrhetic acid. Oncology, 43: 127–130,1986.

Kraus, S.D. The anti-oestrogenic action of glycyrrhetic acid. Experimental Medicine and Surgery, 27: 411–420, 1969.

Segal, R., Pisanty, S., Wormser, R., Azaz, E., and Sela, M.N. Anticarcinogenic activity of liquorice and glycyrrhizin I: Inhibition of in vitro plaque formation by Streptococcus mutans. Journal of Pharmaceutical Sciences, 74: 79–81, 1985.

Sugishita, E., Amagaya, S., and Ogihara, Y. Studies on the combination of glycyrrhizae radix in shakuyakukanzo-to. Pharmacobio Dyn, 7: 427–435,1984.

Tanaka, S., Kuwai,Y., and Tabata, M. Isolation of monoamine oxidase inhibitors from Glycyrrhiza uralensis roots and the structure-activity relationship. Planta Medica: 5–7, 1987.

Teelucksingh, S., et al. Potentiation of hydrocortisone activity in skin by glycyrrhetinic acid. Lancet, 335: 1060–1063, 1990.

LOBELIA

Sopranzi, N., De Feo, G., Mazzanti, G., and Braghiroli, L. The biological and electrophysiological parameters in the rat chronically treated with *Lobelia inflata L. Clinica Terapeutica*, 137(4): 265–268, 1991.

MARIGOLD

Chemli, R., et al. *Calendula officinalis L* impact of saponins on toxicity, hemolytic effect, and anti-inflammatory activity. *Journal de Pharmacie de Belgique*, 45(1): 12–16, 1990.

Elias, R., et al. Antimutagenic activity of some saponins isolated from *Calendula officinalis L, C. arvensis L.* and *Hedera helix L. Mutagenesis*, 5(4): 327–331, 1990.

Krivenki, V.V., Potebnia, G.P., and Loiko, V.V. Experience in treating digestive organ diseases with medicinal plants. *Vrachebnoe Delo*, (3): 76–78, 1989.

Szakiel, A., and Kasprzyk, Z. Distribution of oleanolic acid glycosides in vacuoles and cell walls isolated from protoplasts and cells of *Calendula officinalis* leaves. *Steroids*, 53(3-5): 501–511, 1989.

MARSHMALLOW

Schultz, H., and Albroscheit, G. High-performance liquid chromatographic characterization of some medical plant extracts used in cosmetic formulas. *Journal of Chromatography*, 442: 353–361, 1988.

MATE

Acheson, K.J., Zahorska-Markiewicz, B., Pittet, P., Anantharaman, K., and Jéquler, E. Caffeine and coffee: Their influence on metabolic rate and substrate utilization in normal weight and obese individuals. *American Journal of Clinical Nutrition*, 33: 989–997, 1980.

Anonymous. *Nutrition Today*, 24(6): 4, Nov.-Dec. 1989.

Astrup, A., Toubro, S., Cannon, S., Hein, P., Breum, L., and Madsen, J. Caffeine: A double-blind, placebo-controlled study of its thermogenic, metabolic, and cardiovascular effects in healthy volunteers. *American Journal of Clinical Nutrition*, 51: 759–767, 1990.

Bonaa, K., Arnesen, E., Thelle, D.S., and Forder O.H. Coffee and cholesterol: Is it all in the brewing? The Tromso study. *British Medical Journal*, 297: 1103–1104, 1988.

Bukowiecki, L.J., Lupien, J., Folléa, N., and Jahjah, L. Effects of sucrose, caffeine, and cola beverages on obesity, cold resistance, and adipose tissue cellularity. *American Journal of Physiology*, 244: R500–507, 1983.

Cheraskin, E., Ringsdorf, W.M., Setyaadmadja, A.T.S.H., and Barrett, R.A. Effect of caffeine versus placebo supplementation on blood-glucose concentration. *Lancet*, 2: 1299–1300, 1967.

Dulloo, A.G., Geissler, G.A., Horton, T., Collins, A., and Miller, D.S. Normal caffeine consumption: Influence on thermogenic and daily energy expenditure in lean and postobese human volunteers. *American Journal of Clinical Nutrition*, 49: 44–50, 1989.

Fredholm, B.B. Gastrointestinal and metabolic effects of methylxanthines. In Dews, P. B., ed., *The Methylxanthine Beverages and Foods: Chemistry, Consumption, and Health Effects*. New York, NY: A.R. Liss Press, 1984, pp. 331–354.

Jung, R.T., Shetty, P.S., James, W.P.T., Barrand, M.A., and Callingham, B.A. Caffeine: Its effect on catecholamines and metabolism in lean and obese subjects. *Clin. Sci.*, 60: 527–535, 1981.

Malchow-Moller, A., Larsen, S., Hey, H., Stokholm, K.H., Juhl, E., and Quaade, F. Ephedrine as an anorectic: The story of the "Elsinore pill." *International Journal of Obesity*, 5: 183–187, 1981.

Whitsett, T.L, Manion, C.V., and Christensen, H.D. Cardiovascular effects of coffee and caffeine. *American Journal of Cardiology*, 53: 918–922, 1984.

MATHAKE

Collier, W.A., and Van De Plji, L. The antibiotic action plants, especially the higher plants, with results from Indonesian plants. *Chron Nat*, 105: 8, 1949.

Haddon, A.C. Reports of the Cambridge anthropological expedition to Torres Straits. Cambridge University Press, Cambridge England Book 6: 107, 1908.

Huxtable, R.J. Herbs along the western Mexican-American border. *Proc West Pharmacol Soc*, 26: 185–191, 1983.

Quisumbing, E. Medicinal plants of the Philippines. JMC Press, Inc. Quezon City, Philippines, 1978.

Tiwari, A.K., Gode, J.D., and Dubey, G.P. Effect of *Terminalia arjuna* on lipid profiles of rabbits fed hypercholesterolemic diet. *International Journal of Crude Drug* Research, 28(1): 43–47, 1990.

MILK THISTLE

Campos, R., Garrido, A., Guerra, R., and Valenzuela, A. Silybin dihemisuccinate protects against glutathione depletion and lipid peroxidation induced by acetaminophen on rat liver. *Planta Medica*, 55: 417–419, 1989.

Chander, R., Kapoor, N.K., and Dhawan, B.N. Hepatoprotective activity of silymarin against hepatic damage in *Mastomys natalensis* infected with *Plasmodium berghei. Indian Journal of Medical Research*, 90: 1989.

Ferenci, P, et al. Randomized controlled trial of silymarin treatment in patients with cirrhosis of the liver. *Journal of Hepatology*, 9(1): 105–113, 1989.

Kalmar, L., et al. Silibinin (Legalon-70) enhances the motility of human neutrophils immobilized by formyl-tripeptide, calcium ionophore, lymphokine and by normal human serum. *Agents and Actions*, 29(3-4): 239–246, 1990.

Mereish, K.A., Bunner, D.L., Regland, D.R., and Creasla, D.A. Protection against microcystin-LR-induced hepatotoxicity by silymarin: biochemistry, histopathology, and lethality. *Pharmaceutical Research*, 8(2): 273–277, 1991.

Valenzuela, A, Aspillaga, M., Vial, S., and Guerra, R. Selectivity of silymarin on the increase of the glutathione content in different tissues of the rat. *Planta Medica*, 55(5): 420–422, 1989.

MOTHERWORT

He, G. Effect of the prevention and treatment of atherosclerosis of a mixture of hawthorn and motherwort. *Journal of Modern Development in Traditional Medicine*, 10(6): 361, 326, 1990.

Kuant, P.G., Zou, X.F., Shang, F.Y., and Lang, S.Y. Motherwort and cerebral ischemia. *Journal of Traditional Chinese Medicine*, 8(1): 37–40, 1988.

Nagasaw, H., et al. Effects of motherwort (*Leonurus sibiricus* L.) on preneoplastic and neoplastic mammary gland growth in multiparous GR/A mice. *Anticancer Research*, 10(4): 1019–1023, 1990.

Zou, Q.Z., et al. Effect of motherwort on blood hyperviscosity. *American Journal of Chinese Medicine*, 17(1-2): 65–70, 1969.

OAK (WHITE)

Basden, K.W., and Dalvi, R.R. Determination of total phenolics on acorns from different species of oak

trees in conjunction with acorn poisoning in cattle. *Veterinary and Human Toxicology*, 29(1): 305–306, 1987.

Ipsen, H., and Hansen, O.C. The NH2-terminal amino acid sequence of the immunochemically partial identical major allergens of Alder (*Alnus glutinosa*) Aln g I, Birch (*Betula verrucosa*) Bet v I, hornbeam (*Carpinus betulus*) car b I and Oak (*Quercus alba*) Que a I pollen. *Molecular Immunology*, 28(1): 1279–1288, 1991.

Loria, R.C., Wilson, P., and Wedner, H.J. Identification of potential allergens in white oak (*Quercus alba*) pollen by immunoblotting. *Journal of Allergy and Clinical Immunology*, 81(1): 9–18, 1989.

PARSLEY

Christomanos, A.A. The pharmacology of apiol and some of its allies. *Naunyn-Schmiederbergs Arch Exp Pathol Pharmakol*, 123: 252–258, 1927.

Joachimoglu, G. Apiolum viride as an abortifacient. *Dtsch Med Wochenschr*, 52: 2079–2080, 1926.

Meyer, K., Kohler, A., Kauss, H. Biosynthesis of ferulic acid esters of plant cell wall polysaccharides in endomembranes from parsley cells. *FEBS Letters*, 290(1-2): 209–212, 1991.

Schmitt, D., Pakusch, A.E., and Matern, U. Molecular cloning, induction, and taxonomic distribution of caffeoyl-CoA 3-0-methyltransferase, an enzyme involved in disease resistance. *Journal of Biological Chemistry*, 266(26): 17416–17423, 1991.

PASSIONFLOWER

Li Q.M., et al. Mass spectral characterization of C-gycosidic flavonoids isolated from a medicinal plant (*Passiflora incarnata*). *Journal of Chromatography*, 562(1-2), 435–446, 1991.

PAU D'ARCO

Austin, F.G. Schistosoma mansoni chemoprophylaxis with dietary lapachol. *American Journal of Tropical Medicine and Hygiene*, 23(3): 412–415, 1974.

Avirutnant, W. and Pongpan, A. The antimicrobial activity of some Thai flowers and plants. *Mahidol Univ. J. Pharm. Sd.*, 10(3): 81–86, 1983.

Barros, G.S.G., Matos, F.J.A., Vieira, J.E.V., Sousa, M.P., and Medeiros, M.C. Pharmacological screening of some Brazilian plants. *J. Pharm Pharmacol*, 22: 116, 1970.

Da Consolacao, F., Linardi, M., De Oliveira, M.M., and Sampaio, M.R.P. A lapachol derivative active against mouse lymphocytic leukemia P-388. *J Med Chem*, 18: 1159, 1975.

Di Carlo, F.J., Haynes, L.J., Sliver, N.J., and Phillips, G.E. Reticuloendothelial system stimulants of botanical origin. *J. Reticuloendothelial Soc.*, 1: 224, 1964.

Dominguez, X.A., and Alcorn, J.B. Screening of medicinal plants used by Huastec Mayans of northeastern Mexico. *Journal of Ethnopharmacology*, 13(2): 139–156, 1985.

Ferreira De Santana, C., Goncalves De Lima, O., D'Albuquerque, I.L, Lacerda, A.L., and Martins, D.G. The antitumor and toxic properties of substances extracted from the wood of *Tabebuia avellanedae*. *Rev Inst Antibiot Univ Fed Pemambuco Recife*, 81: 89–94, 1968.

Forgacs, P., Jacquemin, H., Moretti, C., Provost, I., and Touche, A. Phytochemical and biological activity studies on 18 plants from French Guyana. *Plant Med. Phytother*, 17(1): 22–32, 1983.

Heal, R.E., Rogers, E.F., Wallace, R.T., and Starnes, O. A survey of plants of insecticidal activity. *Lloydia*, 13: 89–162, 1950.

Kingston, D.G.I., and Rao, M.M. Isolation structure elucidation and synthesis of two new cytotoxic napthoquinones from *Tabebuia cassinoides*. *Planta Medica*, 39: 230–231, 1980.

Oga, S., and Sekino, T. Toxicity and anti-inflammatory activity of *Tabebuia avellanedae* extracts. *Rev. Fae. Farm Bioqium Univ. Sau Paulo*, 7(1): 47–53, 1969.

Oguniana, E.O., and Ramstad, E. Investigations into the antibacterial activities of local plants. *Planta Medica*, 27: 354, 1975.

Rao, M.M., and Kingston, D.G.I. Plant anticancer agent XII. Isolation and structure elucidation of new cytotoxic quinones from *Tabebuia cassinoides*. *J. Nat Prod.*, 45: 600–604, 1982.

Spencer, C.F., et al. Survey of plants for antimalarial activity. *Lloydia*, 10: 145–174, 1947.

Wagner, H., Kreher, B., and Jurcic, K. Immunological investigations of naphthaquinone containing plant extracts, isolated quinones and other cytostatic compounds in cellular immunosystems. *Planta Medica*, 6; 1986.

PENNYROYAL

Gordon, W.P., et al. The metabolism of the abortifacient terpene, (R)-(+)-pulegone, to a proximate toxin, menthofuran. *Drug Metabolism and Disposition: The Biological Fate of Chemicals*, 15(5): 589–594, 1987.

PERIWINKLE (TROPICAL)

De Bruyn, et al. Modification of *Catharanthus roseus* alkaloids: a lactone derived from 17-deacetylvinblastine. *Planta Medica*, 55(4): 364–365, 1989.

Facchini, P.J., Neumann, A.W., and DiCosmo, F. Adhesion of suspension-cultured *Catharanthus roseus* cells to surfaces: effect of pH, ionic strength, and cation valency. *Biomaterials*, 10(5): 318–324, 1989.

Naaraniahti, T., et al. Electrochemical detection of indole alkaloids of *Catharanthus roseus* in high-performance liquid chromatography. *Analyst*, 114(10): 1229–1231, 1989.

Naaraniahti, T., et al. Isolation of Catharanthus alkaloids by solid-phase extraction and semipreparative HPLC. *Journal of Chromatographic Science*, 28(4): 173–174, 1990.

PINEAPPLE

Batkin, S., Taussig, S., and Szekerczes, J. Modulation of pulmonary metastasis (Lewis lung carcinoma) by bromelain, an extract of the pineapple stem (*Ananas comosus*) [letter]. *Cancer Investigation*, 6(2): 241–242, 1988.

Rowan, A.D., Buttle, D.J., and Barrett, A.J. The cysteine proteinases of the pineapple plant. *Biochemical Journal*, 266(3): 869–875, 1990.

Rowan, A.D., et al. Debridement of experimental full-thickness skin burns of rats with enzyme fractions derived from pineapple stem. *Burns*, 16(4): 243–246, 1990.

Noble, R.L. The discovery of the vinca alkaloids—chemotherapeutic agents against cancer. *Biochemistry and Cell Biology*, 68(12): 1344–1351, 1990.

Taussig, S.J., and Batkin, S. Bromelain, the enzyme complex of pineapple (*Ananas comosus*) and its clinical application. An update. *Journal of Ethnopharmacology*, 22(2): 191–203, 1988.

POMEGRANATE

Ferrara, L., et al. Identification of the root of *Punica granatum* in galenic preparations using TLC. *Bollettino-Societa Italiana Biolgia Sperimentale*, 65(5): 385–390, 1989.

Segura, J.J., Morales-Ramos, L.H., Verde-Star, J., and Guerra, D. Growth inhibition of *Entamoeba histolytica* and *E. invadens* produced by pomegranate root (*Punica granatum L.*). *Arhivos de Investigacion Medica*, 21(3): 235–239, 1990.

PSYLLIUM

Anderson, J.W., et al. Cholesterol-lowering effects of psyllium hydrophilic mucilloid for hypercholesterolemic men. *Archives of Internal Medicine*, 148(2): 292–296, 1988.

Bell, L.P., Hectorne, K.J., Reynolds, H., Balm, T.K., and Hunninghake, D.B. Cholesterol-lowering effects of psyllium hydrophilic mucilloid. Adjunct therapy to a prudent diet for patients with mild to moderate hypercholesterolemia.

Bell, L.P., Hectorne, K.J., Reynolds, H., and Hunninghake, D.B. Cholesterol-lowering effects of soluble-fiber cereals as part of a prudent diet for patients with mild to moderate hypercholesterolemia. *American Journal of Clinical Nutrition*, 52(6): 1020–1026, 1990.

Davidson, L.J., Belknap, D.C., and Flournoy, D.J. Flow characteristics of enteral feeding with psyllium hydrophilic mucilloid added. *Heart and Lung*, 20(4): 404–408, 1991.

Friedman, E., Lightdale, C., and Winawer, S. Effects of psyllium fiber and short-chain organic acids derived from fiber breakdown on colonic epithelial cells from high-risk patients. *Cancer Letters*, 43(1-2): 121–124, 1988.

Hallert, C., Kaldma, M., and Petersson, B.G. Ispaghula husk may relieve gastrointestinal symptoms in ulcerative colitis in remission. *Scandinavian Journal of Gastroenterology*, 26(7): 747–750, 1991.

Haskell, W.L., et al. Role of water-soluble dietary fiber in the management of elevated plasma cholesterol in healthy subjects. *American Journal of Cardiology*, 69(5): 433–439, 1992.

Heather, D.J., Howell, L., Montana, M., Howell, M., and Hill, R. Effect of a bulk-forming cathartic on diarrhea in tube-fed patients. *Heart and Lung*, 20(4): 409–413, 1991.

James, J.M., Cooke, S.K., Barnett, A., and Sampson, H.A. Anaphylactic reactions to a psyllium-containing cereal. *Journal of Allergy and Clinical Immunology*, 88(3 Pt. 1): 402–408, 1991.

Levin, E.G., et al. Comparison of psyllium hydrophilic mucilloid and cellulose as adjuncts to a prudent diet in the treatment of mild to moderate hypercholesterolemia. *Archives of Internal Medicine*, 150(9): 1822–1827, 1990.

Lipsky, H., Gloger, M., and Frishman, W.H. Dietary fiber for reducing blood cholesterol. *Journal of Clinical Pharmacology*, 30(8): 699–703, 1990.

Miettinen, T.A., and Tarpila, S. Serum lipids and cholesterol metabolism during guar gum and plantago ovata and high fibre treatments. *Clinical Chimica Acta*, 183(3): 253–262, 1989.

Misra, S.P., Thorat, V.K., Sachdev, G.K., and Anand, B.S. Long-term treatment of irritable bowel syndrome: results of a randomized controlled trial. *Quarterly Journal of Medicine*, 73(270): 931–939, 1989.

Neal, G.W., and Balm, T.K. Synergistic effects of psyllium in the dietary treatment of hypercholesterolemia. *Southern Medical Journal*, 83(10): 1131–1137, 1990.

Pape, D. Improvement in blood lipids and lipoproteins by simple nutritional modification, exemplified by a high-fiber modified so-called "heart diet" of a West German clinic: the therapeutic gain due to expanding and high fiber foods. *Vasa. Supplementum*, 33: 247–249, 1991.

Pastors, J.G., Blaisdell, P.W., Balm, T.K., Asplin, C.M., and Pohl, S.L. Psyllium fiber reduces rise in postprandial glucose and insulin concentrations in patients with non-insulin-dependent diabetes. *American Journal of Clinical Nutrition*, 53(6): 1431–1435, 1991.

Stewart, R.B., Hale, W.E., Moore, M.T., May, F.E., and Marks, R.G. Effect of psyllium hydrophilic mucilloid on serum cholesterol in the elderly. *Digestive Diseases and Sciences*, 36(3): 329–334, 1991.

Sussman, G.L., and Dorian, W. Psyllium anaphylaxis. *Allergy Proceedings*, 11(5): 241–242, 1990.

Turley, D.D., Daggy, B.P., and Dietschy, J.M. Cholesterol-lowering action of psyllium mucilloid in the hamster: sites and possible mechanism of action. *Metabolism: Clinical and Experimental*, 40(10): 1063–1073, 1991.

Wolever, T.M., et al. Effect of method of administration of psyllium on glycemic response and carbohydrate digestibility. *Journal of the American College of Nutrition*, 10(4): 364–371, 1991.

RASPBERRY (RED)

Alonso, R., Cadavid, I., and Calleja, J.M. A preliminary study of hypoglycemic activity of *Rubus fruticosus*. *Planta Medica Suppl.*, 40: 102–106, 1980.

Bamford, D.S., Percival, R.C., and Tothill, A.U. Raspberry leaf tea: a new aspect to an old problem. *British Journal of Pharmacology*, 40: 1970.

Burn, J.H., and Withell, E.R. A principle in raspberry leaves which relaxes uterine muscle. *Lancet*, 2: 1941.

Kim, M.S., Lee, N.G., Lee, J.H., Byun, S.J., and Kim, Y.C. Immunopotentiating activity of water extracts of some crude drugs. *Korean Journal of Physiology and Pharmacology*, 19(3): 193–200, 1988.

Konowalchuk, J., and Speirs, J.I. Antiviral activity of fruit extracts. *Food Science*, 41: 1013, 1976.

Kurzepa, S., and Samojlik, E. Studies on the effects of extracts from plants of the family rosaceae on gonadotropin and thyrotropin in the rat. *Endokrinol Pol.*, 14: 143, 1963.

May, G., and Willuhn, G. Antiviral activity of aqueous extracts from medicinal plants in tissue cultures. *Arzneim-Forsch*, 28(1): 1–7, 1978.

Ribeiro, R.A., et al. Acute diuretic effects in conscious rats produced by some medicinal plants used in the state of Sao Paulo, Brazil. *Journal of Ethnopharmacology*, 24(1): 19–29, 1988.

Yang, L.L., Sheu, F.M., Yen, K.Y., and Tung, T.C. Study of interferon inducer in Taiwan fold medicines. *Asian J. Pharm. Suppl.*, 6(8): 121, 1986.

REISHI MUSHROOM

Cheng, H.H., et al. The antitumor effect of cultivated *Ganoderma lucidum* extract. *Journal of the Chinese Oncology Society*, 1(3): 12–16, 1982.

Gong, Z., and Un, Z.B. The pharmacological study of lingzhi (*Ganoderma lucidum*) and the research of therapeutical principle of "fuzheng guben" in traditional Chinese medicine. *Pei-Ching I Hsueh Yuan Hsueh Pao*, 13: 6–10, 1981.

Kubo, M., Matsuda, H., Nogami, M., Arichi, S., and Takahashi, T. Studies on *Ganoderma lucidum*. IV.

Effects on the disseminated intravascular coagulation. *Yakugaku Zasshi*, 103(8): 871–877, 1983.

Lee, S.Y., and Rhee, H.M. Cardiovascular effects of mycelium extract of *Ganoderma luddum*: inhibition of sympathetic outflow as a mechanism of its hypotensive action. *Chemical and Pharmaceutical Bulletin*, 38(5): 1359–1364, 1990.

Nogami, M., Tsuji, Y., Kubo, M., Takahashi, M., Kimura, H., and Matsulke, Y. Studies on *Ganoderma lucidum*. VI. Anti-allergic effect. (1). *Yakugaku Zasshi*, 106(7): 594–599, 1986.

Nogami, M., Kubo, M., Kimura, H., and Takahashi, M. Studies on *Ganoderma lucidum*. V. Inhibitory activity on the release of histamine from the isolated mast cells. *Shoyakugaku Zasshi*, 40(2): 241–243., 1986.

Nogami, M., Ito, M., Kubo, M., Takahashi, M., Kimura, H., and Matsuike, Y. Studies on *Ganoderma lucidum*. VII. Anti-allergic effects. (2). *Yakugaku Zasshi*, 106(7): 600–604, 1986.

Shimizu, A., Yano, T., Saito, Y., and Inada, Y. Isolation of an inhibitor of platelet aggregation from a fungus, *Ganoderma lucidum*. *Chem Pharm Bull*, 33(7): 3012–3015, 1965.

Shin, H.W., Kim, H.W., Choi, E.C., Toh, S.H., and Kim, K.B. Studies on inorganic composition and immunopotentiating activity of *Ganoderma lucidum* in Korea. *Korean Journal of Physiology and Pharmacology*, 16(4): 181–190, 1985.

Sone, Y., Okuda, R., Wada, N., Kishida, E., and Misaki, A. Structures and antitumor activities of the polysaccharides isolated from fruiting body and the growing culture of mycelium of *Ganoderma lucidum*. *Agr Biol Chem*, 49(9): 2641–2653, 1985.

Tao, J., and Feng, K.V. Experimental and clinical studies on inhibitory effect of *Ganoderma lucidum* on platelet aggregation. *Journal of Tongji Medical University*, 10(4): 1990.

Wilson, J.W., and Plunkett, O.A. The fungus diseases of man. Berkeley, University of California, 1965.

ROSEMARY

Singletary, K.W., and Nelshopen, J.M. Inhibition of 7,12-dimethylbenz[a]anthracene (DMBA)-induced mammary tumorigensis and of in vivo formation of mammary DMBADNA adducts by rosemary extract. *Cancer Letters*, 60(2): 169–175, 1991.

Zhao, B.L., U, X.J., He, R.G., Cheng, S.J., and Xin, W.J. Scavenging effect of extracts of green tea and natural antioxidants on active oxygen radicals. *Cell Biophysics*, 14(2): 175–185, 1989.

SAFFLOWER

Adelstein, R., Ferguson, L.D., and Rogers, K.A. Effects of dietary N-3 fatty acid supplementation on lipoproteins and intimal foam cell accumulation in the casein-fed rabbit. *Clinical and Investigative Medicine*, 15(1): 71–81, 1992.

Huang, Y.S., et al. Effect of maternal dietary fats with variable n-3/n-6 ratios on tissue fatty acid composition in suckling mice. *Lipids*, 27(2): 104–110, 1992.

Li, D., and Randerath, K. Modulation of DNA modifcation (I-compound) levels in rat liver and kidney by dietary carbohydrate, protein, fat, vitamin, and mineral content. *Mutation Research*, 275(1): 47–56, 1992.

Mills, D.E., et al. Attenuation of cyclosporine-induced hypertension by dietary fatty acids in the borderline hypertensive rat. *Transplantation*, S3(3): 649–654, 1992.

Okuyama, H. Minimum requirements of n-3 and n-6 essential fatty acids for the function of the central nervous system and for the prevention of chronic diseases. *Proceedings of the Society for Experimental Biology and Medicine*, 200(2): 174–176, 1992.

Vajreswari, A., and Narayanareddy, K. Effect of dietary fats on erythrocyte membrane lipid composition and membrane-bound enzyme activities. *Metabolism: Clinical and Experimental*, 41(4): 352–358, 1992.

Venkatraman, J.T., Toohey, T., and Clandinin, M.T. Does a threshold for the effect of dietary omega-3 fatty acids on the fatty acid composition of nuclear envelope phospholipids exist? *Upias*, 27(2): 94–97, 1992.

SAGE

Lee, C., et al. Miltirone, a central benzodiazepine receptor partial agonist from a Chinese medicinal herb *Salvia Miltiorrhiza*. *Neuroscience Letters*, 127: 237–241, 1991.

ST. JOHN'S WORT

Aizenman, B.E. Antibiotic preparations from *Hypericum perforatum*. *Mikrobiol Zh*, 31: 128–133, 1969.

Derbentseva, N.A., and Rabinovich, A.S. Isolation, purification, and study of some physiochemical properties of novoimanin. In Solov'eva, A.I. (ed.), *Novoimanin Ego Lech Svoistva*, Kiev, 1988.

Gurevich, A.I., et al. Hyperiforin, an antibiotic from *Hypericum perforatum*. *Antibiotiki*, 16: 51–52, 1971.

Hobbs, C. St John's Wort, *Hypericum perforatum* L: a review. *HerbalGram*, 18/19: 24–33, 1989.

Meruelo, D., et al. Therapeutic agents with dramatic antiretroviral activity and little toxicity at effective doses: aromatic polycyclic diones hypericin and pseudohypericin. *Proceedings of the National Academy of Sciences*, 85: 5230–5234, 1988.

Muldner, Von H., and Zoller, M. Antidepressive wirkung eines auf den wirkstoffkomplex hypericin standardisierten hypericum-extraktes. *Arzneim-Forsch*, 34: 918, 1984.

Negrash, A.K., and Pochinok, P.Y. Comparative studies of chemotherapeutic and pharmacological properties of antimicrobial preparations from common St. John's Wort. *Fitonotsidy Mater Soveshch*: 198–200, 1969.

Okpanyl, S., Lidzba, H., Scholl, B.C., and Miltenburger, H.G. Genotoxicity of a standardized Hypericum extract. *Arzheimittel-Forschung*, 40(8): 851–855, 1990.

Sajic, J. Ointment for the treatment of burns. *Ger. Offen* 2: 406, 452 (CL. A61K), August 21, 1975.

Suzuki, O., et al. Inhibition of monoamine oxidase by hypericin. *Planta Medica*, 50: 272–274, 1874.

SAW PALMETTO

Champault, G., et al. Actualite therapeutique: traitement medical de l'adenome prostatique. *Annals Urological*, 6: 407–410, 1984.

Griffiths, D.J., and Abrams, H. The assessment of prostatic obstruction from urodynamic measurement and from residual urine. *British Journal of Urology*, 51: 129–134, 1979.

Hinman, F., and Cox, C.E. Residual urine volume in normal male subjects. *Journal of Urology*, 97: 641–645, 1967.

Murray, M.T. Herbal treatment for liposterolic extract of *Serenoa repens* in the treatment of benign prostatic hyperplasmia (BPH). *Phyto-Pharmica Review*, 1(5): 1988.

Tasca, A., et al. Trattamanto della sintomatologia ostruttive d'adenoma prostatico con estratto di serenoa repents. *Minerva Urologica e Nefrologica*, 37: 87–91, 1985.

SCHISANDRA

Ahumada, F., et al. Studies on the effect of *Schisandra chinensis* extract on horses submitted to exercise and maximum effort. *Phytotherapy Research*, 3(5):175–179, 1989.

Chang, I. H., Kim, J. H., and Han, D.S. Toxicological evaluation of medicinal plants used for herbal drugs (4). Acute toxicity and antitumor activities. *Korean Journal of Physiology and Pharmacology*, 13(2): 62–69, 1983.

Chen, Y.Y., Shu, Z., and U, L.N. Studies of *Fructus shizanorae*. IV. Isolation and determination of the active compounds (in lowering high SGPT levels) of *Schisandra chinensis*. *ChungKuo K. O. Hsueh*, 19: 276, 1976.

Haneke, J. L., Wikman, G., and Hernandez, D.E. Antidepressant activity of selected natural products. *Planta Medica*, 1986(6): 542–543, 1986.

Hendrich, S., and Bjeldanes, L.F. Effects of dietary cabbage, brussels sprouts, illictum verum, *Schisandra chinensis* and alfalfa on the benzopyrene metabolic system in mouse liver. *Chem. Toxicol.*, 21(4): 479–486, 1983.

Hendrich, S., and Bjeldanes, L.F. Effects of dietary *Schisandra chinensis*, brussels sprouts and illicium verum extracts on carcinogen metabolism systems in mouse liver. *Food Chem. Toxiol.*, 24(9): 903–912, 1989.

Hernandez, O. E., Haneke, J. L., and Wikman, G. Evaluation of the anti-ulcer and antisecretory activity of extracts of aralla elata root and *Schisandra chinensis* fruit in the rat. *Journal of Ethnopharmacology*, 23(1): 109–114, 1988.

Hikino, H., Kiso, Y., Taguchi, H., and Ikeya, Y. Antihepatotoxic actions of lignoids from *Schisandra chinensis* fruits. *Planta Medica*, 50(3): 213–218, 1984.

Kim, M.S., Lee, M.G., Lee, J.H., Byun, S.J., and Kim, Y.C. Immunopotentiating activity of water extracts of some crude drugs. *Korean Journal of Physiology and Pharmacology*, 19(3): 193–200, 1988.

Koda, A., Nishiyori, T., Nagai, H., Matsuura, N., and Tsuchiya, H. Anti-allergic actions of crude drugs and blended Chinese traditional medicines. Effects on Type I and Type IV allergic reactions. *Nippon Yakurigaku Zasshi*, 80: 31–41, 1982.

Liu, G.T., Wang, G.F., Wei, H.L., Bao, T.T., and Song, Z.Y. A comparison of the protective actions of biphenyl dimethyldicarboxylate trans-stilbene, alcoholic extracts of fructus schizanorae and ganoderma against experimental liver injury in mice. *Yag Hsueh Hsueh Pao*, 14: 598–604, 1979.

Liu, G.T., and Wei, H.L. Protection by fructus schizanorae against acetaminophen hepatotoxicity in mice. *Yao Hsueh Hsueh Pao*, 22(9): 650–654, 1987.

Nishiyori, T., Matsuura, N., Nagai, H., and Koda, A. Anti-allergic action of Chinese drugs. *Jap. J. Pharmacol. Suppl.*, 31: 115, 1981.

Pao, T.T., Liu, K.I., Hsu, K.F., and Sung, C.Y. Studies on schisandra fruit. I. Its effect on increased SGPT levels in animals caused by hepatotoxic chemical agents. *National Medical Journal of China*, S4: 275, 1974.

Shin, K.H., and Woo, W.S. A survey of the response of medicinal plants on drug metabolism. *Korean Journal of Physiology and Pharmacology*, 11: 109–122, 1980.

Shipochliev, T., and Ilieva, S. Pharmacologic study of Bulgarian *Schisandra chinensis*. *Farmatseyacsofia*, 17(3): 56, 1967.

Volicer, L., Sramka, M., Janku, I., Capek, R., Smetana, R., and Ditteova, V. Some pharmacological effects of *Schisandra chinensis*. *Arch. Int Pharmacodyn Ther.*, 163: 249, 1966.

Wahlstrom, M. *Adaptogens.* Utgivare, Goteborg, 1987.

Woo, W.S., Shin, K.H., Kih, I.C., and Lee, C.K. A survey of the response of Korean medicinal plants on drug metabolism. *Arch. Pharm. Res.*, 1: 13–19, 1978.

Yin, H.Z. A report of 200 cases of neurosis treated by "shen wei he ji" (decoction of ginseng, schisandra fruit and others). *Zhejiang-Zhongyi Zazhi*, 17(9): 411, 1982.

Yu, J., and Chen, K.J. Clinical observations of AIDS treated with herbal formulas. *International Journal of Oriental Medicine*, 14(4): 189–193, 1989.

SCULLCAP

Lu, Z. Clinical comparative study of intravenous piperacillin sodium or injection of scutellaria compound in patients with pulmonary infection. *Journal of Modern Developments in Traditional Medicine*, 10(7): 413–415, 1990.

SEAWEEDS

Barchi, J.J., et al. Identification of a cytoxin from *Tolypothrix byssoidea* as tubercidin. *Phytochemistry*, 22: 2851–2852, 1983.

Chang, J., and Lewis, A.J. Prostaglandins and cyclooxygenase inhibitors, in immunomodulation agents and their mechanisms, E.L. Fenischel and M.A. Chirigos (eds.). New York, NY: Marcel Dekker, 1984.

Chida, K., and Yamamoto, I. Antitumor activity of a crude fucoidan fraction prepared from the roots of kelp (*laminaria* species). *Kitasato Archives of Experimental Medicine*, 60(1-2): 33–39, 1987.

Fukuyama, K., Wakabayashi, S., Matsubara, H., and Rogers, L.J. Tertiary structure of oxidized flavodoxin from a eukaryotic red alga *Chondrus crispus* at 2.35-A resolution. Localization of charged residues and implication for interaction with electron transfer partners. *Journal of Biological Chemistry*, 265(26): 15804–15812, 1990.

Gustafson, K.R., et al. AIDS-antiviral sulfolipids from cyanobacteria (blue-green algae). *Journal of the National Cancer Institute*, 81 (16): 1989.

Hoppe, H.A., Levring, T., and Tanaka, Y. (eds.). *Marine algae in pharmaceutical science*. Berlin, New York: Walter de Gruyter, 1979.

Maruyama, H., Nakajima, J., and Yamamoto, I. A study on the anticoagulant and fibrinolytic activities of a crude fucoidan from the edible brown seaweed *Laminaria religiosa,* with special reference to its inhibitory effect on the growth of sarcoma-180 ascites cells subcutaneously implanted into mice. *Kitasato Archives of Experimental Medicine*, 60(3), 105–121, 1987.

Miyazawa, Y., Murayama, T., Ooya, N., Wang, L.F., Tung, Y.C., and Yamaguchi, N. Immunomodulation by a unicellular green algae (*chlorella pyrenoidosa*) in tumor-bearing mice. *Journal of Ethnopharmacology*, 24(2-3): 135–146, 1988.

Teas, J. The dietary intake of *laminaria,* a brown seaweed and breast cancer prevention. *Nutrition and Cancer*, 4: 217–22, 1983.

Vane, J.R. *Nature*, 231: 232, 1971.

Watanabe, S., and Fujita, T. Immune adjuvants as antitumor agents from marine algae. Patent-Japan Kokai Tokkyo Koho, 61 197,525: 1986.

Yamamoto, I., Takahashi, M., Tamura, E., and Maruyama, H. Antitumor activity of crude extracts from edible marine algae against L-1210 leukemia. *Botanica Marina, XXV*: 455–457, 1982.

Yamamoto, I., Tukahashi, M., Tumura, E., Maruyama, H., and Mori, H. Antitumor activity of edible marine algae: effect of crude fucoidan fractions prepared from edible brown seaweeds against L-1210 leukemia. *Hydrobiologia*, 116/117: 145–148, 1984.

Zhukova, G.E., Novokhatskii, A.S., and Telltchenko, M.M. Inactivation of some RNA-contained viruses with green and blue-green algae. *Vestn Mosk Univ Biol Pochvoved*, 27(4): 108, 19n.

SENNA

Elujoba, A.A., Ajulo, O.O., and Iweibo, G.O. Chemical and biological analyses of Nigerian Cassia species for laxative activity. *Journal Pharm Biomed Anal*, 7(12): 1453–1457, 1989.

SHIITAKE MUSHROOM

Iizuka, C. Antiviral substance. Patent-Fr Demande Fr-2, 485,373: 30 pp, 1980.

Imaki, M., et al. Study on digestibility and energy availability of daily food intake (Part 1 Shiitake mushroom). *Japanese Journal of Hygiene*, 16(1): 905–912, 1991.

Kabir, Y., Yamaguchi, M., and Kimura, S. Effect of shiitake (*Lentinus edodes*) and maitake (*Grigola frondosa*) mushrooms on blood pressure and plasma lipids of spontaneously hypertensive rats. *Journal of Nutritional Science and Vitaminology*, 33(5): 341–346, 1987.

Kamm, Y.J., Folgering, H.T., van den Bogart, H.G., and Cox, A. Provocation tests in extrinsic allergic alveolitis in mushroom workers. *Netherlands Journal of Medicine*, 38(1-2): 59–61, 1991.

Maeda, Y.Y., and Chihara, G. The effects of neonatal thymectomy on the antitumor activity of lentinan. *International Journal of Cancer*, 11: 153–161, 1973.

Mizoguchi,Y., et al. Protection of liver cells against experimental damage by extract of cultured *Lentinus edodes mycelia* (LEM). *Gastroenterologia Japonica*, 22(4): 459–464, 1987.

Mizoguchi, Y., et al. Effects of extract of cultured *Lentinus edodes mycelia* (LEM) on polyclonal antibody response induced by pokeweed mitogen. *Gastroenterologia Japonica*, 22(5): 627–632, 1987.

Nanba, H., and Kuroda, H. Antitumor mechanisms of orally administered shiitake fruit bodies. *Chemical and Pharmaceutical Bulletin*, 35(6): 2459–2464, 1987.

Nanba, H., Mori, K., Toyornasu, T., and Kuroda, H. Antitumor action of shiitake (*Lentinus edodes*) fruit bodies orally administered to mice. *Chemical and Pharmaceutical Bulletin*, 35(6): 2453–2458, 1987.

Sugano, N., Choji, Y., Hibino, Y., Yasumura, S., and Maeda, H. Anticarcinogenic action of an alcohol-insoluble fraction (lap1) from culture medium of lentinus edodes mycelia. *Cancer Letters,* 27(1): 1–6, 1985.

Sugano, N., Hibino, Y., Chojl, Y., and Maeda, H. Anticarcinogenic action of water-soluble and alcohol-insoluble fractions from culture medium of lentinus edodes mycelia. *Cancer Letters*, 17(2): 109–114, 1982.

Suzuki, F., Koide, T., Tsunoda, A., and Ishida, N. Mushroom extract as an interferon inducer. I. Biological and physiochemical properties of spore extracts of *Lentinus edodes.*

Takatsu, M., Tabuchi, M., Sofue, S., and Minami, J. Anticancer substances produced by basidiomycetes. Patent-Japan Kokal, 75 12(293): 1975.

Tarvainen, K., et al. Allergy and toxicodermia from shiitake mushrooms. *Journal of the American Academy of Dermatology*, 24(1): 61–66, 1991.

Tochikura, T.S., Nakashima, H., Ohashi, Y., and Yamamoto, N. Inhibition (in vitro) of replication and of the cytopathic effect of the human immunodeficiency virus by an extract of culture medium of *Lentinus edodes mycelia. Medical Microbiology and Immunology*, 177(5): 235–244, 1988.

SOAPWORT

Cazzola, M., et al. Cytotoxic activity of an anti-transferrin receptor immunotoxin on normal and leukemic human hematopoietic progenitors. *Cancer Research*, 51 (2): 536–541, 1991.

Gasperi-Campani, A., et al. Inhibition of growth of breast cancer cells in vitro by the ribosome-inactivating protein saporin 6. *Anticancer Research*, 11(2): 1007–1111, 1991.

Teece, R., et al. Production and characterization of two immunotoxins specific for M5b ANLL leukaemia. *International Journal of Cancer*, 49(2): 310–316, 1991.

Tochikura, T.S., Nakashima, H., Ohashi, Y., and Yamamoto, N. Inhibition (in vitro) of replication and of the cytopathic effect of human immunodeficiency virus by an extract of the culture medium of *Lentinus edodes mycelia. Medical Microbiology and Immunology*, 177(5): 235–244, 1988.

SQUIRTING CUCUMBER

Yesilada, E., Tanaka, S., Sezik, E., and Tabata, M. Isolation of an anti-inflammatory principle from the fruit juice of *Ecballium elaterium. Journal of Natural Products*, 51(3): 504–508, 1988.

SWEET FERN

Mannan, A., Khan, R.A., and Asif, M. Pharmacodynamic studies on *Polypodium vulgare* (Linn.). *Indian Journal of Experimental Biology*, 27(6): 556–560, 1989.

TURMERIC

Ammon, H.P., and Wahl, M.A. Pharmacology of *Curcuma longa. Planta Medica*, 57(1): 1–7, 1991.

Chandra, D., and Gupta, S.S. Anti-inflammatory and anti-arthritic activity of volatile oil of *Curcuma longa* (haldi). *Indian Journal of Medical Research*, 60: 1972.

Donatus, I.A., Sardjoko, S., and Vermeulen, N.P. Cytotoxic and cytoprotective activities of curcumin. Effects on paracetamol-induced cytotoxicity, lipid peroxidation and glutathione. *Biochemical Pharmacology*, 39 (12): 1869–1875.

Kulkarni, R.R., et al. Treatment of osteoarthritis with a herbomineral formulation: a double-blind, placebo-controlled, cross-over study. *Journal of Ethnopharmacology*, 33(1-2): 91–95, 1991.

Nagabhushan, M., and Bhide, S.V. Anti-mutagenicity and anti-carcinogenicity of turmeric (*Curcuma longa*). *Journal of Nutrition, Growth and Cancer*, 4: 83–89, 1987.

Polassa, K., Seslkaran, B., Krishna, T.P., and Krishnasawan, K. Turmeric (*Curcuma* longa)-induced reduction in urinary mutagens. *Food and Chemical Toxicology*, 29(10): 699–706, 1991.

Rafatullah, S., et al. Evaluation of turmeric (*Curcuma longa*) for gastric and duodenal antiulcer activity in rats. *Journal of Ethnopharmacology*, 29(1): 25–34, 1990.

Shalini, V.K., and Srinivas, L. Fuel smoke condensate induced DNA damage in human lymphocytes and protection by turmeric (*Curcuma longa*). *Molecular and Cellular Biology*, 95(1): 21–30, 1990.

Tonnesen, H.H. Studies on curcumin and curcuminoids. XIII. Catalytic effect of curcumin on the peroxidation of linoleic acid by 15-lipoxygenase. *International Journal of Pharmaceutics*, 50: 67–69, 1989.

VALERIAN

Fehri, B. *Valeriana officinalis* and *Cratasgus oxyacantha*: toxicity from repeated administration and pharmacologic investigations. *Journal de Pharmade de Belgique*, 16(3): 165–176, 1991.

Houghton, P.J. The biological activity of Valerian and related plants. *Journal of Ethnopharmacology*, 22(2): 121–142, 1989.

Kohnen, R., and Oswald, W.D. The effects of valerian, propranolol, and their combination on activation, performance, and mood of healthy volunteers under social stress conditions. *Pharmacopsychiatry*, 21(6): 117–118, 1989.

Lindahl, D., and Landwall, L. Double blind study of a valerian preparation. *Pharmacology, Biochemistry and Behavior*, 32(1): 1065–1066, 1989.

Molodoshnikova, L.M. Medicinal valerian. *Feldsher i Akusherka*, 53(1): 11–16, 1989.

Narimanov, A.A., and Gavriliuk, B.K. The synergism of the action of gamma radiation and cardiovascular preparations on lymphoid cells in culture. *Radiobiolgiia*, 29(2): 189–191, 1969.

WALL GERMANDER

Tariq, M., et al. Anti-inflammatory activity of *Teucrium polium*. *International Journal of Tissue Reactions*, 11 (1): 185–189, 1989.

WALNUT (BLACK)

Galay, F.D., et al. Black walnut *(Juglans nigra)* toxicosis: a model for equine laminitis. *Journal of Comparative Pathology*, 104(3): 313–326, 1991.

Galay, F.D., et al. Gamma scintigraphic analysis of the distribution of perfusion of blood in the equine root during black walnut *(Juglans nigra)*-induced laminitis. *American Journal of Veterinary Research*, 51(4): 688–695, 1990.

Galay, F.D., Beasley, V.R., Schaeffer, D., and Davis, L.E. Effect of an aqueous extract of black walnut *(Juglans nigra)* on isolated equine digital vessels.

American Journal of Veterinary Research, 51(1): 83–88, 1990.

Minnick, P.D., Brown, C.M., Braselton, W.E., Meerdink, G.L., and Slanker, M.R. The induction of equine laminitis with an aqueous extract of the heartwood of black walnut *(Juglans nigra)*. *Veterinary and Human Toxicology*, 29(3): 230–233, 1987.

Uhlinger, C. Black walnut toxicosis in ten horses. *Journal of the American Veterinary Medical Association*, 195(3): 343–344, 1989.

WATER LILY

Emboden, W. The sacred journey in dynastic Egypt shamanistic trance in the context of the narcotic water lily and the mandrake. *Journal of Psychoactive Drugs*, 21(1): 61–75, 1969.

Gomorti, J.M., Cohen, D., Eyd, A., and Pomerans, S. Water lily sign in CT of cerebral hydatid disease: a case report. *Neuroradiology*, 30(1): 358, 1989.

Lee, D.H., Garvin, D.K., and Wimpee, C.F. Molecular evolutionary history of ancient aquatic angiosperms. *Proceedings of the National Academy of Sciences of the United States of America*, 88(2): 10119–10123, 1991.

Swanston-Flatt, S.K., Day, C., Bailey, C.J., and Flatt, P.R. Traditional plant treatments for diabetes. Studies in normal and streptozotopin diabetic mice. *Diabetaolgoia*, 33(8): 162–164, 1990.

WINTERGREEN

Boakes, R.A., Rossi-Arnaud, C., and Garcia-Hoz, V. Early experience and reinforcer quality in delayed flavour—food learning in the rat. *Appetite*, 9(3): 191–206, 1987.

Cauthen, W.L., and Hester, W.H. Accidental ingestion of oil of wintergreen. *Journal of Family Practice*, 29(5): 880–881, 1989.

WORMWOOD

Chawira, A.N., Warhurst, D.C., Robinson, B.L., and Peters, W. The effect of combination of qinghaosu (artemisinin) with standard antimalarial drugs in the suppressive treatment of malaria in mice. *Transactions of the Royal Society of Tropical Medicine and Hygiene*, 81(1): 551–558, 1987.

Elford, B.C., Roberts, M.F., Phillipson, J.D., and Wilson, R.J. Potentiation of the antimalarial activity of qinghaosu by methoxylated flavones.

Transactions of the Royal Society of Tropical Medicine and Hygiene, 81(3): 131-136, 1987.

elSohly, H.N., Croom, E.M., and elSohly, M.A. Analysis of the antimalarial sesquiterpene artemisinin in *Artemisia annua* by high-performance liquid chromatography (HPLC) with post-column derivatization and ultraviolet detection. *Pharmaceutical Research*, 1(3): 258–260, 1987.

Lang, X., and Ye, S.T. An investigation on in vivo allergenicity of *Artemisia annua* leaves and stems. *Asian Pacific Journal of Allergy and Immunology*, 5(2): 125–128, 1987.

Lwin, M., Maun, C., and Aye, K.H. Trial of antimalarial potential of extracts of *Artemisia annua* grown in Myanmar. *Transactions of the Royal Society of Tropical Medicine and Hygiene*, 85(1): 119, 1991.

Phillipson, J.D., and Wright, C.W. Can ethnopharmacology contribute to the development of antimalarial agents? *Journal of Ethnopharmacology*, 32(1-3): 155–165, 1991.

Ramay, B. Botany of Artemisia. *Allergie at Immunoligia*, 19(6): 250, 252, 1987.

Tawfik, A.F., Bishop, S.J., Ayalp, A., and el-Feraly, F.S. Effects of artemisinin, dihydroanemisinin and arteether on immune responses of normal mice. *International Journal of Immunopharmacology*, 12(1): 385–389, 1990.

Woerdenbag, H.J., Lugt, C.B., and Pras, N. *Artemisia annua* L.: a source of novel antimalarial drugs. *Pharmaceutisch Weekblead*, 12(5): 169–181, 1990.

Zhao, K.C., and Song, Z.Y. The pharmacokinetics of dihydroqinghasu given orally to rabbits and dogs. *Pharmaceutica Sinica*, 25(2): 17–119, 1990.

YAM (WILD)

Huai, Z.P., Ding, Z.Z., He, S.A., and Sheng, C.G. Research on correlation between climatic factors and diosgenin content in *Dioscorea zingiberensis* Wright. *Pharmaceutical Sinica*, 21(9): 702–706, 1989.

Liu, Y.T., and Liu, S.O. Factors influencing the production of Chinese yam (*Dioscorea batatas Decne*), *Bulletin of Chinese Materia Medica*, 12(10): 15–17, 51, 53, 1987.

Sagara, K., Ojima, M., Suto, K., and Yoshida, T. Quantitative determination of allantoin in Dioscorea rhizome and an Oriental pharmaceutical preparation, hachimi-gan, by high-performance liquid chromatography [letter]. *Planta Medica*, 5S(l): 93, 1989.

YARROW

De Pasquale, R., et al. Effect of cadmium on germination, growth and active principle contents of *Achillea millefolium L. Pharmacological Research Communications*, Suppl 5: 115–119, 1988.

Hausen, B.M., Brauer, J., Weglewski, J., and Rucker, S. AlphaPeroxyachifolid and other new sensitizing sesquiterpene lactones from yarrow (*Achillea millefolium L.,* compositae). *Contact Dermatitis*, 21(1): 271–280, 1991.

Krivenko, V.V., Potebnia, G.P., and Loiko, V.V. Experience in treating digestive organ diseases with medicinal plants. *Vrachebnoe Delo*, (3): 76–79, 1989.

Lamaisoin, J.L., and Camat, A.P. Study of azulen in 3 subspecies of *Achillea millefolium L. Annales Pharmaceutiques Francaises*, 16(2): 139–143, 1988.

Schultz, H., and Albroscheit, G. High-performance liquid chromatographic characterization of some medical plant extracts used in cosmetic formulas. *Journal of Chromatography*, 112: 353–361, 1988.

YERBA SANTA

Liu, Y.L., Ho, D.K., and Cassady, J.M. Isolation of potential cancer chemopreventive agents from *Eriodictyon californicum. Journal of Natural Products*, 55(3): 357–363, 1992.

IMAGE CREDITS

Page ii: rawpixel.com. **vi**: *Nouveau Larousse Illustré* (1898), by Pierre Larousse and Claude Augé. rawpixel.com. **viii**: rawpixel.com. **5**: Fructuts Mandragorae, *Tacuinum Sanitatis*, by Ibn Butlan 1390. Wikipedia.org. **9**: rawpixel.com. **10**: Metamorphosis insectorum surinamensium, Library of Congress, http://hdl.loc.gov/loc.rbc/General.00300. **14**: *Köhler's Medizinal-Pflanzen in Naturgetreuen Abbildungen*, Vol 1–3, 1863. archive.org. **18**: *Medical Botany* by John Stephenson and James Morss Churchill, 1836. archive.org. **21**: Rare Book Division, The New York Public Library Digital Collections. "Anemone tenuifolia flore semipleno vivido cinnabaris rubore splenoens." https://digitalcollections.nypl.org/items/510d47dd-d4d3-a3d9-e040-e00a18064a99. **23, 25**: *Medical Botany* by John Stephenson and James Morss Churchill, 1836. archive.org. **26**: *Köhler's Medizinal-Pflanzen in Naturgetreuen Abbildungen*, Vol 1–3, 1863. archive.org. **31**: Flora Graeca, John Sibthorp, 1813. archive.org. **36**: *Billeder af Nordens Flora*, by August Mentz, 1917. Archive.org. **39**: *Flora von Deutschland, Österreich und der Schweiz*, by Prof. Dr. Otto Wilhelm Thomé, 1885. **41**: *Köhler's Medizinal-Pflanzen in Naturgetreuen Abbildungen*, Vol 1–3, 1863. archive.org. **44**: *Animal Coloration: An Account of the Principal Facts and Theories Relating to the Colours and Markings of Animals*, plate IV, Frank Evers Beddard, M.A., 1892. **47**: *Atlas des Plantes de France*, A. Masglef, 1891. archive.org. **51**: *Medical Botany* by John Stephenson and James Morss Churchill, 1836. archive.org. **52**: *Medicinal Plants*, by Robert Bentley and Henry Trimen, Vol. 1–4, 1880. archive.org. **53**: *American Medicinal Plants*, by Charles Millspaugh, MD, 1887. archive.org. **55**: *Medical Botany* by John Stephenson and James Morss Churchill, 1836. archive.org. **59**: *Köhler's Medizinal-Pflanzen in Naturgetreuen Abbildungen*, Vol 1–3, 1863. archive.org. **61**: *Arbres, Arbrisseaux, Plantes, Fleurs et Fruits* by Laurent de Chazelles, 1796. **64**: *English Botany or, Coloured Figures of British Plants*, James Sowerby, 1877. archive.org. **66**: *Medical Botany* by John Stephenson and James Morss Churchill, 1836. archive.org. **68**: Rare Book Division, The New York Public Library Digital Collections. "Ruscus Myrtifolius aculeatus [Butcher's Broom]." https://digitalcollections.nypl.org/items/510d47dd-c18e-a3d9-e040-e00a18064a99. **71**: *Medical Botany* by John Stephenson and James Morss Churchill, 1836. archive.org. **73**: *Köhler's Medizinal-Pflanzen in Naturgetreuen Abbildungen*, Vol 1–3, 1863. archive.org. **77**: *Medical Botany* by John Stephenson and James Morss Churchill, 1836. archive.org. **80**: Rare Book Division, The New York Public Library Digital Collections. "Vitex Agnus-castus = Gatilier commun. [Chaste tree; Hemp tree; Sage tree; Wild pepper]." https://digitalcollections.nypl.org/items/510d47dc-92a1-a3d9-e040-e00a18064a99. **82**: *Natural History of Carolina, Florida, and the Bahama Islands*, by Mark Catesby, 1754. archive.org. **83**: Castanea sativa, USDA Pomological Watercolor Collection, 1917. archive.org. **87, 91**: *Medical Botany* by John Stephenson and James Morss Churchill, 1836. archive.org. **92**: *Dictionnaire Universel D'histoire Naturelle*, illustrated by Charles Dessalines D' Orbigny, 1892. **94**: *Officinellen Pflanzen der Pharmacopoea Germanica*, by F.G. Kohl, 1895. archive.org. **97**: *American Medicinal Plants*, by Charles Millspaugh, MD, 1887. archive.org. **100**: *Flora Londinensis, or, Plates and descriptions of such plants as grow wild in the environs of London*, William Curtis, 1777. Smithsonian Libraries. **102**: *English Botany or, Coloured Figures of British Plants*, James Sowerby, 1877. archive.org. **103**: *Atlas des Plantes de France*, A. Masglef, 1891. archive.org. **105**: *The Botanical Magazine*, William Curtis, 1794. archive.org. **106**: *Medical Botany* by John Stephenson and James Morss Churchill, 1836. archive.org. **109**: *Annales des Sciences Naturelles*, Vol. 3, 1865. archive.org. **111, 112**: *The Botanical Magazine*, William Curtis, 1787. archive.org. **116**: *Medical Botany* by John Stephenson and James Morss Churchill, 1836. archive.org. **119**: *Köhler's Medizinal-Pflanzen in Naturgetreuen Abbildungen*, Vol 1–3, 1863. archive.org. **120**: *The Flora Homoeopathica*, by Edward Hamilton, 1852. archive.org. **122, 126**: *Köhler's Medizinal-Pflanzen in Naturgetreuen Abbildungen*, Vol 1–3, 1863. archive.org. **129, 131**: *Medical Botany* by John Stephenson and James Morss Churchill, 1836. archive.org. **133, 137**: *Medical Botany*, by William Woodville, MD, 1810. archive.org. **141**: *Ueber den Ginkgo*, by Prof. Freyherrn v. Jacquin, 1819. Wellcome Collection. **143**: *Natural History of Carolina, Florida, and the Bahama Islands*, by Mark Catesby. archive.org. **145**: *Vegetable Materia Medica of the United States, or Medical Botany*, by William Barton, 1825. archive.org.

151: *Köhler's Medizinal-Pflanzen in Naturgetreuen Abbildungen*, Vol 1–3, 1863. archive.org. **154**: *Medicinal Plants*, by Robert Bentley and Henry Trimen, Vol. 1–4, 1880. archive.org. **157**: *The Natural History of the Tea-Tree*, by John Coakley Lettsom, MD, 1772. archive.org. **160**: *Flore des Serres et des Jardins de l'Europe*, by Louis Van Houtte, 1845. archive.org. **161**: *Köhler's Medizinal-Pflanzen in Naturgetreuen Abbildungen*, Vol 1–3, 1863. archive.org. **163**: *Medicinal Plants*, by Robert Bentley and Henry Trimen, Vol. 1–4, 1880. archive.org. **166**: *Köhler's Medizinal-Pflanzen in Naturgetreuen Abbildungen*, Vol 1–3, 1863. archive.org. **169**: *The Spirit of the Woods: Illustrated by Coloured Engravings*, by Rebecca Hey, 1837. archive.org. **170**: *Illustrations of Indian Botany*, by Robert Wight, 1840. archive.org. **172**: Rare Book Division, The New York Public Library Digital Collections. "Ilex Aquifolium = Houx Commun. [Holly trees]." https://digitalcollections.nypl.org/items/510d47dc-8bd8-a3d9-e040-e00a18064a99. **174, 176**: *Köhler's Medizinal-Pflanzen in Naturgetreuen Abbildungen*, Vol 1–3, 1863. archive.org. **178, 180, 183, 184, 185, 186**: *Medical Botany*, by John Stephenson and James Morss Churchill, 1836. archive.org. **189**: Plants of the Coast of Coromandel, by William Roxburgh, MD, 1795. archive.org. **190**: *Flore des Serres et des Jardins de l'Europe*, by Louis Van Houtte, 1845. archive.org. **191**: *Medical Botany*, by John Stephenson and James Morss Churchill, 1836. archive.org. **194**: *Flora Regni Borussici: Flora des Königreichs Preussen*, 1842. archive.org. **196**: *Medical Botany*, by John Stephenson and James Morss Churchill, 1836. archive.org. **198**: *Köhler's Medizinal-Pflanzen in Naturgetreuen Abbildungen*, Vol 1–3, 1863. archive.org. **201**: *Atlas der Officinellen Pflanzen*, Otto Carl Berg, 1891. archive.org. **202**: Rare Book Division, The New York Public Library Digital Collections. "Magnolia glauca = Magnolia glauque." https://digitalcollections.nypl.org/items/510d47dc-8d28-a3d9-e040-e00a18064a99. **206**: *Atlas der Officinellen Pflanzen*, Otto Carl Berg, 1891. archive.org. **208**: *Medical Botany*, by John Stephenson and James Morss Churchill, 1836. archive.org. **210**: *Köhler's Medizinal-Pflanzen in Naturgetreuen Abbildungen*, Vol 1–3, 1863. archive.org. **213**: *Medical Botany*, by John Stephenson and James Morss Churchill, 1836. archive.org. **214, 217**: *Flora von Deutschland, Österreich und der Schweiz*, by Prof. Dr. Otto Wilhelm Thomé, 1885. archive.org. **218**: *Köhler's Medizinal-Pflanzen in Naturgetreuen Abbildungen*, Vol 1–3, 1863. archive.org. **220**: *The Flora Homoeopathica*, by Edward Hamilton, 1852. archive.org. **222**: *Medical Botany*, by John Stephenson and James Morss Churchill, 1836. archive.org. **223**: *Medicinal Plants*, by Robert Bentley and Henry Trimen, Vol. 1–4, 1880. archive.org. **225**: *Flora von Deutschland, Österreich und der Schweiz*, by Prof. Dr. Otto Wilhelm Thomé, 1885. archive.org. **226**: *Medicinal Plants*, by Robert Bentley and Henry Trimen, Vol. 1–4, 1880. archive.org. **228**: Papaver, c. 1815 – c. 1830, Rjik Museum. **230**: *The Model Book of Calligraphy* (1561–1596) by Georg Bocskay and Joris Hoefnagel. Original from The Getty. rawpixel.com. **231**: *Billeder af Nordens Flora*, by August Mentz, 1917. archive.org. **233**: Iris germanica (Bearded Iris), 1812, After Pierre-Joseph Redouté; Engraver: de Gouy. Rawpixel.com. **234**: *Annales de la Société Royale d'Agriculture et de Botanique de Gand*, 1845. archive.org. **235**: Papaw or papaya (Carica papaya). Coloured etching by J. Pass, c. 1800. Rawpixel.com. **237**: *Edwards's Botanical Register*, by Sydenham Edwards, John Lindley, and James Ridgway, 1838. **239**: Dr. Willibald Artus' *Hand-Atlas Sämtlicher Medizinisch-Pharmaceutischer Gewächse*, Jena, 1848. **241, 242**: *Medical Botany*, by John Stephenson and James Morss Churchill, 1836. archive.org. **244**: *Choix des Plus Belles Fleurs*, 1833. Archive.org **245**: Rare Book Division, New York Public Library Digital Collections. "Bromella ananas." https://digitalcollections.nypl.org/items/510d47dd-f14c-a3d9-e040-e00a18064a99. **246**: *Natural History of Carolina, Florida, and the Bahama Islands*, by Mark Catesby, 1754. archive.org. **248**: *Flora Regni Borussici: Flora des Königreichs Preussen*, 1836. archive.org. **249**: *Flora Batava*, vol. 4, J. Kops, 1822. plantillustrations.org. **250**: *Paxton's Magazine of Botany and Register of Flowering Plants*, Vol. 2, 1836. archive.org. **252**: *Medical Botany*, by John Stephenson and James Morss Churchill, 1836. archive.org. **254**: *Afbeeldingen der Fraaiste, Meest Uitheemsche Boomen en Heesters*, by Johan Carl Krauss, 1802. **256**: *Medicinal Plants*, by Robert Bentley and Henry Trimen, Vol. 1–4, 1880. archive.org. **258**: *Icones Plantarum*, by Ignatz Albrecht, 1800. archive.org. **259**: *Horticulture: Jardin Potager et Jardin Fruitier*, by François Hénrincq, 1870. archive.org. **260**: USDA Pomological Watercolor Collection, 1917. Rawpixel.com. **262**: *Herbier de la France*, Vol. 1–3, 178–1783. archive.org.

265: *The Botanical Register*, by Sydenham Edwards, Vol. 2, 1815. archive.org. **266**: Rare Book Division, New York Public Library Digital Collections. "Salvia officinalis = Sauge officinale. [Garden sage]." https://digitalcollections .nypl.org/items/510d47dc-9269-a3d9-e040-e00a1 8064a99. **268**: *English Botany or, Coloured Figures of British Plants*, Vol. 2, James Sowerby, 1873. archive.org. **270**: *Medical Botany*, by John Stephenson and James Morss Churchill, 1836. archive.org. **271**: plantillustrations .org. **273**: *Flore des Serres et des Jardins de l'Europe*, by Louis Van Houtte, 1845. archive.org. **275**: *Medicinal Plants*, by Charles F. Millspaugh, 1892. archive.org. **277**: *Nouveau Larousse Illustré: Dictionnaire Universel Encycloedique*, Pierre Larousse, 1906. archive.org. **278**: *El Mundo Ilustrado*, 1879. archive.org. **280**: *Medical Botany*, by John Stephenson and James Morss Churchill, 1836. archive.org. **281**: *Die officinellen Pflanzen der Pharmacopoea Germanica*, by Dr. F.G. Kohl,1895. archive .org. **282**: *La Botanique de J.J. Rousseau*, by Pierre-Joseph Redouté. Library of Congress, Rare Book and Special Collections Division. **284**: *Herbier de la France*, Vol. 1–3, 178–1783. archive.org. **285**: *The Native Flowers and Ferns of the United States in their Botanical, Horticultural and Popular Aspects*, Vol. 1, by Thomas Meehan, 1879. archive.org. **286**: *Flora von Deutschland, Österreich und der Schweiz*, by Prof. Dr. Otto Wilhelm Thomé, 1885. **287**: *Köhler's Medizinal-Pflanzen in Naturgetreuen Abbildungen*, Vol 1–3, 1863. archive.org. **288**: *Billeder af Nordens Flora*, by August Mentz, 1917. archive.org. **289**: *Medical Botany*, by John Stephenson and James Morss Churchill, 1836. archive.org. **290**: *American Medicinal Plants*, Vol. 1, by Charles Millspaugh, MD, 1892. archive.org. **291**: Partridgeberry (*Mitchella repens*), by Mary Vaux Walcott, Smithsonian American Art Museum, Gift of the artist. **292**: *Medical Botany*, by John Stephenson and James Morss Churchill, 1836. archive.org. **294**: *Herbier de la France*, Vol. 1–3, 178–1783. archive.org. **295**: *Flora Medico-Farmaceutica*, Vol. 1, by Felice Cassone, 1847. archive.org. **296**: *Medical Botany*, by John Stephenson and James Morss Churchill, 1836. archive.org. **297**: *Nederlandsche Flora en Pomona*, Vol. 2, 1879. archive.org. **298**: *Medical Botany*, by William Woodville, MD, 1810. archive.org. **300**, **301**: *Medical Botany*, by John Stephenson and James Morss Churchill, 1836. archive.org. **302**: *The Botanical Magazine*, William Curtis, 1794. archive.org. **303**: *Köhler's Medizinal-*

Pflanzen in Naturgetreuen Abbildungen, Vol 1–3, 1863. archive.org. **305**: *Flore d'Amérique*, by Etienne Denisse, 1843. archive.org. **308**, **309**: *Medical Botany*, by John Stephenson and James Morss Churchill, 1836. archive.org. **311**: *English Botany or, Coloured Figures of British Plants*, James Sowerby, 1877. archive.org. **312**: Rare Book Division, New York Public Library Digital Collections. "Juglans nigra = Noyer à fruits noirs. [Black walnut]." https://digitalcollections.nypl.org/items/510d47dc-8f93 -a3d9-e040-e00a18064a99. **314**: *Köhler's Medizinal-Pflanzen in Naturgetreuen Abbildungen*, Vol 1–3, 1863. archive.org. **315**: *Medical Botany*, by John Stephenson and James Morss Churchill, 1836. archive.org. **317**: *Medicinal Plants*, by Robert Bentley and Henry Trimen, Vol. 1–4, 1880. archive.org. **319**: *The Botanical Magazine*, William Curtis, 1818. archive.org. **320**: Rare Book Division, New York Public Library Digital Collections. "Hamamelis Virginica = Hamamélide de Virginie. [Witch-hazel]." https://digitalcollections.nypl.org/items/510d47dc-946a -a3d9-e040-e00a18064a99. **322**: *Phytographie Médicale*, Vol. 2, Joseph Roques, 1825. archive.org. **323**: *The Botanical Magazine*, William Curtis, 1820. archive.org. **324**: *Medical Botany*, by John Stephenson and James Morss Churchill, 1836. archive.org. **326**: *American Medicinal Plants*, by Charles Millspaugh, MD, 1892. archive.org. **329**: Illustration by Lizzie Harper, lizzieharper. co.uk. **331**, **332**, **335**, **338**, **342**, **345**, **346**, **348**, **349**: rawpixel.com. **350**: *Medical Botany*, by John Stephenson and James Morss Churchill, 1836. archive.org. **352**: rawpixel.com. **355**: *Histoire des Plantes Grasses* by Pierre-Joseph Redouté, 1799. **356**: rawpixel.com. **359**: *Edwards's Botanical Register*, by Sydenham Edwards, John Lindley, and James Ridgway, 1838. **360**: *Medical Botany*, by John Stephenson and James Morss Churchill, 1836. archive.org. **362**: Rare Book Division, New York Public Library Digital Collections.USDA "Olea Europæa = Olivier d'Europe.A et B. Olivier d'Entrecasteaux. C. Caillet-roux." https://digitalcollections.nypl.org/items /510d47dc-902e-a3d9-e040-e00a18064a99. **365**: rawpixel.com. **366**: *Passion Flower* (1799), by Sydenham Teak Edwards. Edward Pearce Casey Fund, 2009. rawpixel.com. **368**: Library of Congress, ppmsca 44344, https://hdl.loc.gov/loc.pnp/ppmsca.44344. **374**: *Sketches Towards a Hortus Botanicus Americanus*, by William Jowit Titford, 1811. Wellcome Collection. **422**: rawpixel.com.

HERB INDEX
English/Latin   Latin/English

No plant is complete by common name alone. Common names often vary according to country, sometimes by region. The correct name for every plant is, by convention, based on a Latin binomial. The first name is the genus to which the plant belongs, the second name the precise species.

In the following lists you will find common English names and their universal Latin equivalents. While Latin names may sometimes vary according to new discoveries by taxonomists or plant hunters, I have chosen those names most frequently found in modern guides to herbs.

ENGLISH / LATIN

LATIN / ENGLISH

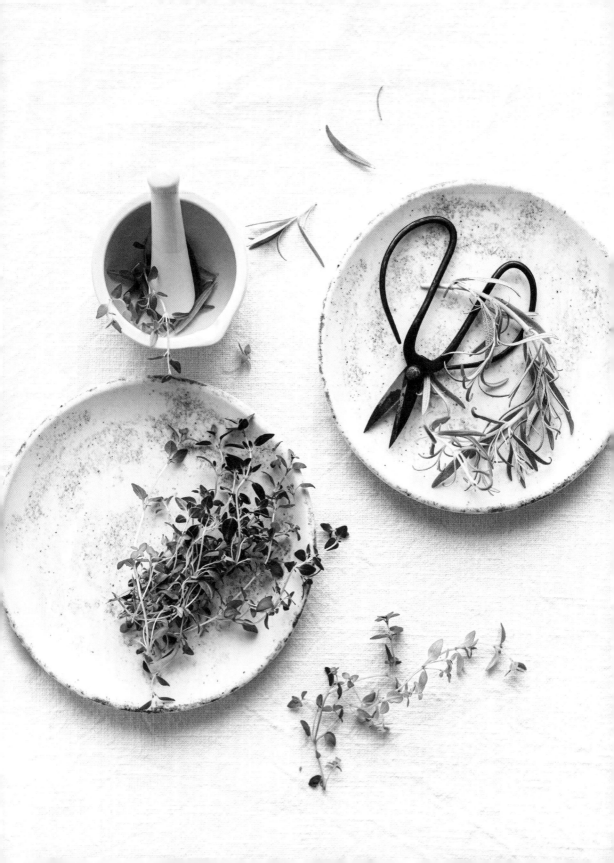

INTEGRATED INDEX